WITHDRAWN
University of
Illinois Library
at Urbana-Champaign

Vaccinia Viruses as Vectors
for Vaccine Antigens

Vaccinia Viruses as Vectors for Vaccine Antigens

Proceedings of the Workshop on Vaccinia Viruses as Vectors for Vaccine Antigens, held November 13–14, 1984, in Chevy Chase, Maryland, U.S.A.

Editor:

Gerald V. Quinnan, Jr., M.D.
Director, Division of Virology
Center for Drugs and Biologics
Food and Drug Administration
Bethesda, Maryland

Elsevier
New York · Amsterdam · Oxford

©1985 by Elsevier Science Publishing Co., Inc.
All rights reserved.

This book has been registered with the Copyright Clearance Center, Inc. For further information, please contact the Copyright Clearance Center, Salem, Massachusetts.

Published by:
Elsevier Science Publishing Co., Inc.
52 Vanderbilt Avenue, New York, New York 10017

Sole distributors outside the United States and Canada:
Elsevier Science Publishers B.V.
P.O. Box 211, 1000 AE Amsterdam, the Netherlands

Library of Congress Cataloging in Publication Data

Workshop in Vaccinia Viruses as Vectors for
    Vaccine Antigens (1984: Chevy Chase, Md.)
    Vaccinia viruses as vectors for vaccine antigens.

    Includes index.
    1. Vaccines—Congresses. 2. Vaccinia—Congresses. 3. Viral antigens—Congresses. 4. Smallpox—Congresses. I. Quinnan, Gerald V. II. Title.
    [DNLM: 1. Antigens, Viral—immunology—Congresses. 2. Vaccinia Virus—genetics—congresses. 3. Vaccinia Virus—immunology—congresses. 4. Viral Vaccines—immunology—congresses. QW 165.5.P6 W926v 1984]
QR189.W674   1984   615'.372   85-12960
ISBN 0-444-00984-1

Manufactured in the United States of America

CONTENTS

Preface ix

Participants xi

Part I: BIOLOGY OF VACCINIA AND OTHER ORTHOPOX VIRUSES   1
         Chairpersons: G. Schild and J. Nakano

   Vaccinia Virus   3
      D. Baxby

   Aspects of the Biology of Orthopox Viruses Relevant to the
   Use of Recombinant Vaccines as Field Vaccines   9
      K.R. Dumbell

   Molecular Biology of Vaccinia Virus:
   Structure of Pox Virus DNA   15
      W.K. Joklik

   Molecular Biology of Vaccinia Virus: Strategies for
   Cloning and Expression of Foreign Genes   27
      B. Moss

   Genetic Basis for Vaccinia Virus Virulence   37
      R.M.L. Buller and B. Moss

Part II: SMALLPOX VACCINES   47
         Chairperson: G.V. Quinnan, Jr.

   Complications of Smallpox Vaccination   49
      I. Arita and F. Fenner

   Utilization of Vaccine in the Global Eradication of
   Smallpox   61
      D.A. Henderson and I. Arita

   Vaccinia Virus Vaccines: Virulence and Attenuation of
   Vaccinia Strain Variation   69
      J.M. Neff

   A Comparative Study of Four Smallpox Vaccines in
   Children   77
      K. McIntosh

   Low Neurovirulent Variant of Lister Strain of
   Vaccinia Virus   85
      S. Kato

   Properties of Attenuated Mutant of Vaccinia Virus,
   LC16m8, Derived from Lister Strain   87
      S. Hashizume, H. Yoshizawa, M. Morita and K. Suzuki

   Immunogenicity of Vaccinia Viruses:
   Responses to Vaccination   101
      J.D. Millar

   Smallpox Vaccine In Vivo Production and Testing   109
      D.P. Metzgar

Tissue Culture Smallpox Vaccine 113
A.C. Hekker

Capability of Developing Countries to Produce Vaccinia
Vector Vaccine 117
I. Arita

Part III: EXPERIMENTAL RECOMBINANT VACCINIA VIRUS VACCINES 127
Chairpersons: R. Chanock and W. Dowdle

Vaccinia Virus Recombinants as Live Vaccines Against
Hepatitis B Virus and Malaria 129
G.L. Smith and B. Moss

Vaccinia Vectored Vaccines 137
E. Paoletti, M.E. Perkus, A. Piccini, S. Wos, and
B.R. Lipinskas

Infectious Vaccinia Virus Recombinants Express Herpes
Simplex Virus Glycoprotein D and Protect Against
Lethal and Latent Infections of HSV 153
K. Cremer, C. Wohlenberg, M. Mackett, B. Moss,
and A.L. Notkins

Induction of Virus Neutralizing Antibodies and
Protection Against Rabies Using a Vaccinia Rabies
Glycoprotein Recombinant 163
B. Dietzschold, T.J. Wiktor, and H. Koprowski

Influenza Virus Specific Cell-Mediated Immunity to
Vaccinia Virus Recombinants 169
J.R. Bennink, J.W. Yewdell, G.L. Smith, and B. Moss

Intranasal Vaccination with Recombinant Vaccinia
Containing Influenza Hemagglutinin Prevents Both
Influenza Virus Pneumonia and Nasal Infection:
Intradermal Vaccination Prevents only Viral
Pneumonia 175
P.A. Small, Jr., G.L. Smith, and B. Moss

Infectious Vaccinia Virus Recombinants that Express
the Epstein-Barr Virus Membrane Antigen gp340 179
M. Mackett and J.R. Arrand

Vaccinia Virus Recombinants Expressing Vesicular
Stomatitis Genes Immunize Mice and Cattle 187
T. Yilma, M. Mackett, J.K. Rose, and B. Moss

Infectious Vaccinia Virus Recombinant that Expresses
the Surface Antigen of Porcine Transmissible
Gastroenteritis Virus (TGEV) 201
S. Hu, J. Bruszewski, and R. Smalling

Part IV: OTHER VIRUSES AS VECTORS FOR VACCINE ANTIGENS 209
Chairpersons: R. Chanock and W. Dowdle

Genetic Engineering of Herpes Simplex Virus Genomes
for Attenuation and Expression of Foreign Genes 211
B. Roizman and M. Arsenakis

Part V: CONSIDERATIONS OF THE SAFETY, EFFICACY AND POTENTIAL
          APPLICATIONS OF RECOMBINANT VACCINIA VIRUSES   225
             Chairperson: G. Noble

          Potential Applications of Vaccinia Virus Vectors for
          Immunoprophylaxis   227
             F. Brown

          Considerations of Safety, Efficacy and Potential
          Applications of Vaccinia Vectors for Immunoprophylaxis:
          An Alternative Approach for Control of Human Diseases
          For Which Vaccines are Available   231
             D.T. Karzon

          Considerations of Safety, Efficacy, and Potential
          Application of Vaccinia Vectored Vaccines for
          Immunoprophylaxis Against Animal Diseases   237
             F.A. Murphy

          Panel Discussion: Needs for Further Laboratory and
          Clinical Research, Safety and Ethical Considerations. .   241
             F. Dienhardt, K. Warren, W. Jordan, and
             G.V. Quinnan, Jr.

          Index   253

PREFACE

The use of viruses as vectors for expression of heterologous antigens in mammalian cells _in vivo_ exemplifies an exciting recent advance in the application of recombinant DNA technology for vaccine production. In many respects vaccinia virus is highly suited for this purpose. Vaccinia virus vaccines were used extensively world-wide during the smallpox eradication campaign, and were generally very well tolerated, highly immunogenic, easily manufactured and readily applied in mass vaccination efforts. Even with its outstanding performance record, however, the possibility of reintroducing the use of this virus on a wide scale in man or animals raises many public health and ethical concerns. Although very rarely, serious or fatal complications of vaccinia virus infections did occur, and they occurred in contacts of vaccinees as well as in vaccinees themselves. The potential occurrence and significance of similar complications must be evaluated in considering approaches to development of recombinant vaccinia virus vaccines. Even if there were no known risks, the reintroduction of the virus into populations that are not exposed currently should be done only after careful consideration of the benefits to be achieved. Other major questions that must be addressed at the outset include: What strain(s) of vaccinia virus should be used? How should vaccines be manufactured? What tests should be done to assure acceptability of vaccines for use in field trials? What biologic properties of vaccine strains should be evaluated? In whom should vaccine trials be performed?

This book represents the proceedings of a Workshop on Vaccinia Viruses as Vectors for Vaccine Antigens, cosponsored by the United States Public Health Service, the World Health Organization, and the National Institute for Biologic Standards and Control, London, held November 13 and 14, 1984, in Chevy Chase, Maryland. The purpose of the Workshop was to begin developing answers to the questions indicated above. The data presented and relevant to these questions emanate both from studies performed during the smallpox eradication campaign and from exciting recent laboratory work on molecular biology, expression of foreign genes, determinants of virulence, and immunology of vaccinia virus infections. It is evident from these data that there are unlikely to be any insurmountable objections to the use of recombinant vaccinia virus vaccines, and that they offer great promise for use as safe and effective immunogens. Work on developing candidate strains for human administration will hopefully progress rapidly. The use of vectors other than vaccinia virus may also prove feasible.

This Workshop was followed by a meeting of consultants to the World Health Organization with the purpose of advising on evidence relevant to the public health, ethical and scientific concerns about these recombinant vaccines, and formulating draft requirements for the use of recombinant vaccinia virus vaccines. These draft requirements will be under continued development for many months. However, the intent of the World Health Organization to publish them should be viewed as an indication of the enthusiasm with which this approach has been greeted. The list of human and veterinary diseases against which vaccines of this type might be used is long and the death and suffering that might be prevented are great. The process of developing any vaccine is an arduous one, and it is never certain at the outset that any specific approach will result in a safe and effective product. It is clear that the long history of vaccinia virus is far from over and there are many opportunities ahead.

The program for this meeting was developed with the assistance of Drs. G.C. Schild, B. Moss, R. Chanock, D.A. Henderson, G. Tourigiani and F. Assaad. We gratefully acknowledge the contributions of Hilda Kopit for meeting coordination, Cathy Hobbs for editorial assistance, and Lois Baker for typing.

                                          Gerald V. Quinnan, Jr., M.D.

PARTICIPANTS

Dr. Gordon Ada
Department of Microbiology
Australian National University
P.O. Box 4
Canberra ACT
Australia 2601

Dr. Isao Arita
Chief, Smallpox Eradication Unit
World Health Organization
1211 Geneva 27
Switzerland

Dr. Fakry Assaad
Chief, Communicable Diseases
World Health Organization
1211 Geneva 27
Switzerland

Dr. Derrick Baxby
Department of Medical Microbiology
University of Liverpool
Duncan Building
Royal Liverpool Hospital
Liverpool L7 8XW, U.K.

Dr. Jack R. Bennink
The Wistar Institute
36th at Spruce Streets
Philadelphia, PA 19104

Dr. D.J. Boyle
John Curtin School of Medical
  Research
The Australian National University
Microbiology Department
Canberra City A.C.T. 2601
Australia

Dr. Fred Brown
Welcome Biotechnology Ltd.
Ash Road Pirbright
Woking Surry
GU24 ONQ
England

Dr. Don Burke
Walter Reed Army Institute of
  Research
6825 16th Street, N.W.
Washington, DC 20307

Dr. Robert Chanock
Chief, Laboratory of Infectious
  Diseases
National Institute of Allergy and
  Infectious Diseases
Building 7, Room 301
8800 Rockville Pike
Bethesda, MD 20205

Dr. Friedrich Deinhardt
Max v Pettenkofer Institute
Pettenkoferstrasse 9a
D 8000 Munich
Germany

Dr. Bernhard Dietzschold
The Wistar Institute
36th at Spruce Street
Philadelphia, PA 19104

Dr. Walter Dowdle
Center for Infectious Diseases
Centers for Disease Control
Atlanta, GA 30333

Dr. Keith Dumbell
Department of Medical Microbiology
Medical School
University of Capetown
Observatory, Cape
7925 South Africa

Dr. Sydney Ellis
Food & Drug Administration
HFN-171, Division of Drug Biology
200 C Street, S.W.
Washington, DC 20204

Dr. Joseph Esposito
Center for Infectious Diseases
Centers for Disease Control
Atlanta, GA 30333

Dr. John Furesz
Director, Bureau of Biologics
Drugs Directorate
Health Protection Branch
Tunneys Pasture
Ottawa K1A-OL2
Canada

Dr. Scott Halstead
Associate Director for Health
  Sciences
Rockefeller Foundation
1133 Avenue of the Americas
New York, NY 10036

Dr. Anton Hekker
Director, WHO Collaborative
  Centre for Vaccinia
Rijks Institute
Bilthoven
Netherlands

Dr. Donald A. Henderson
Dean
The Johns Hopkins University
School of Hygiene and Public Health
615 North Wolf Street
Baltimore, MD 21205

Dr. Ralph Henderson
World Health Organization
1211 Geneva 27
Switzerland

Dr. Shawfen Sylvia Hu
1900 Oak Terrace Lane
Thousand Oaks, CA 91320-1789

Dr. Wolfgang K. Joklik
Department of Microbiology and
  Immunology
Duke University Medical Center
Durham Medical Center
Durham, NC 27710

Dr. William Jordan
National Institute of Allergy
  and Infectious Diseases
NIH, Bldg. 31, Room 7A52
8800 Rockville Pike
Bethesda, MD 20205

Dr. David Karzon
Department of Pediatrics
School of Medicine
Vanderbilt University
Nashville, TN 37232

Prof. Shiro Kato
Research Institute for
  Microbial Diseases
University of Osaka
3-1 Yamada oka
Suita City, Osaka
Japan

Dr. Hilary Koprowski
The Wistar Institute
36th at Spruce Streets
Philadelphia, PA 19104

Dr. Michael Mackett
Patterson Laboratories
Christie Hospital
Wilmslow Road
Withington, Manchester
B209 BX
England

Dr. James Maynard
Center for Infectious Diseases
Centers for Disease Control
Atlanta, GA 30333

Dr. Kenneth J. McIntosh
Chief, Division of Infectious
  Diseases
Children's Hospital Medical Center
300 Longwood Avenue, Rm. 616
Boston, MA 02115

Dr. Donald Metzgar
Connaught Laboratories
Swiftwater, PA 18370

Dr. J. Donald Millar
Director, National Institute for
  Occupational Safety and Health
Centers for Disease Control
Atlanta, GA 30333

Dr. Carl H. Mordhorst
Orinithosis Department
Stratens Seruminstitut
DK 2300 Copenhagen 5
Denmark

Dr. Bernard Moss
Laboratory of Viral Diseases
National Institute of Allergy and
  Infectious Diseases
Building 5, Room 318
8800 Rockville Pike
Bethesda, MD 20205

Dr. Frederick Murphy
Virology Division
Centers for Disease Control
Atlanta, GA 30333

Dr. James Nakano
Center for Infectious Diseases
Centers for Disease Control
Atlanta, GA 30333

Dr. John Neff
Childrens Orthopedic Hospital
 and Medical Center
4800 Sandpoint Way
P.O. Box C5371
Seattle, WA 98105

Dr. Gary Noble
Centers for Disease Control
Atlanta, GA 30333

Dr. Dennis Panicali
NY State Department of Health
Center for Laboratories and Research
Empire State Plaza
Albany, NY 12201

Dr. Enzo Paoletti
Center for Laboratories in Research
New York State Department of Health
L2C400
Albany, NY 12201

Dr. Lendon Payne
Karolinska Institute
Department of Virology
Stockholm, Sweden

Dr. Gerald V. Quinnan, Jr.
Director, Division of Virology
Office of Biologics Research and
 Review
Center for Drugs and Biologics
8800 Rockville Pike
Bethesda, MD 20205

Dr. William Robinson
Stanford University Medical School
Palo Alto, CA 94305

Dr. Bernard Roizman
Committee of Virology
University of Chicago
939 East 57th Street
Chicago, IL 60637

Dr. Geoffrey Schild
Division of Viral Products
NIBSC
Holly Hill, Hampstead
London NW 3 6RB
England

Dr. Parker A. Small, Jr.
Department of Immunology and
 Medical Microbiology
J. Hillis Miller Health Center
University of Florida
Box J-266, JHMC
Gainesville, FL 32610

Dr. S. Suehiro
Institute of Bio Active Science
Nippon, Zoki Pharmaceutical Co.
HYOGO, Japan

Dr. Geoffrey Smith
Department of Pathology
University of Cambridge
Cambridge, England

Ms. Jill Taylor
Center for Laboratories in Research
New York State Department of Health
L2C400
Albany, NY 10019

Dr. Patricia E. Taylor
200 Central Park South
Apt. 18A
New York, NY 12201

Dr. Giorgio Tourigiani
Chief, Immunology
World Health Organization
1211 Geneva 27
Switzerland

Dr. Dennis Trent
Centers for Disease Control
P.O. Box 2087
Fort Collins, CO 80522

Dr. Gordon Wallace
National Institute of Allergy and
 Infectious Diseases
Building 7, Room 305
8800 Rockville Pike
Bethesda, MD 20205

Dr. Ken Warren
Rockefeller Foundation
1133 Avenue of the Americas
New York, NY 10036

Dr. Richard Whitley
Department of Pediatrics
University of Alabama
Birmingham, AL 35294

Dr. Roy Widdus
Institute of Medicine
National Academy of Sciences JH751
2101 Constitution Ave., N.W.
Washington, DC 20418

Dr. Tilahun Yilma
Department of Veterinary
 Microbiology and Pathology
Washington State University
Pullman, Washington 99164

PART I

BIOLOGY OF VACCINIA AND OTHER ORTHOPOX VIRUSES

Chairpersons: G. Schild and J. Nakano

VACCINIA VIRUS

DERRICK BAXBY*

*Department of Medical Microbiology, University of Liverpool, Liverpool, United Kingdom

Vaccinia is a member of the genus Orthopoxvirus. Table I lists the other members, and indicates which are human pathogens. In some cases reliable information is lacking, and ectromelia virus is the only Orthopoxvirus species known not to be a human pathogen. Genetic and serological relationships within the genus are very close and recombinants and hybrids may occur [1].

TABLE I. Orthopoxviruses.

Species	Reservoir	Other hosts	Human infection
Variola	(Man)	None	(Yes), eradicated
Vaccinia	None	See Table III	Yes
Cowpox	Rodent?	Cattle, Cats	Yes
Monkeypox	?	Monkeys	Yes
Camelpox	Camel	None	No?
Raccoonpox	Raccoon	?	?
Taterapox	Gerbil	?	?
Ectromelia	Lab. mouse	?	No

Definition of Vaccinia

When compared to e.g. polio or rubella vaccines, any definition of smallpox vaccine is inadequate. This is because the vaccine strains used this century were introduced in the 19th century before licensing procedures were necessary.

The usual working definition of vaccinia virus is that it is a virus of unknown origin, not found naturally, which is maintained in vaccine institutes and research laboratories.

Origins of Vaccinia

Possible origins of vaccinia virus are listed in Table II and have been discussed at length elsewhere [2]. Derivation has usually been proposed from smallpox and/or cowpox viruses. Some vaccines were probably derived from cowpox in the early 19th century, but there are fundamental reasons for believing that no surviving vaccine was derived

TABLE II. Origins of vaccinia.

1. From smallpox, by arm-to-arm passage.
2. From smallpox, by adaptation to animals.
3. From cowpox.
4. From smallpox and cowpox, by hybridization.
5. From horsepox.

© 1985 Elsevier Science Publishing Co., Inc.
VACCINIA VIRUSES AS VECTORS FOR VACCINE ANTIGENS, Quinnan, Editor

from smallpox or cowpox viruses. Polio or measles vaccine strains are attenuated variants of the virulent parents, and are very closely related to the parents. In fact, it is sometimes difficult to distinguish between vaccine and wild-type.

The situation with vaccinia is quite different. For vaccinia to have been derived from smallpox or cowpox would require considerable changes in the genome; in fact, the transformation of one virus into another. This is most unlikely. The genomes of vaccinia virus strains are very similar to each other but different from those of smallpox and cowpox viruses [3], and the suggestion that one Orthopoxvirus species may be transformed easily and quickly into another has been discounted [4].

Smallpox vaccines were developed from horsepox virus in the 19th century but horsepox is now extinct. However, it is possible that the clinical suitability of horsepox vaccines led to their retention, and to the rejection of cowpox vaccines. This would explain the survival of a closely related collection of vaccine strains, not found naturally, which were not obviously derived from cowpox or smallpox.

The problem of the origin of vaccinia is not purely academic at a time when we are considering not just reintroducing human vaccination but also considering extending its use to animals. As recently as 1980 it was claimed that vaccinia virus was attenuated smallpox virus, and the death of a fetus, in fact from generalized vaccinia, was cited as evidence that reversion to virulence can and does take place [5]. This suggestion was correctly criticized as absurd [6]. However, at a time when pressure groups are becoming increasingly vocal, we should take every opportunity to establish that, whatever its origins, vaccinia now represents an independent stable species with no tendency to "revert" to a more virulent form.

Vaccinia as a Typical Poxvirus

Vaccinia virus is easily grown and has been widely used as a typical poxvirus [7]. The assumption that the structure and replication of all Orthopoxviruses is essentially the same is justified, and so data obtained on vaccinia virus could be transferred to smallpox virus.

The complex structure and large size of the virion facilitates analysis by electron microscopy of uncoating, replication and assembly, and the inhibition of cellular protein synthesis in infected cells facilitates the biochemical analysis of these events.

One of the features that attracted molecular biologists to vaccinia virus is the fact that it is a DNA virus which replicates in the cytoplasm. This led to an appreciation of the importance of virion-associated enzymes in poxvirus replication. These factors, and an appreciation of the role played by smallpox vaccination in the control and eradication of smallpox, are more or less responsible for the holding of this Workshop.

Pathogenesis of Vaccinia

Vaccinia is a dermotropic virus which usually requires inoculation into the superficial layers of the skin in order to infect. Infection is usually localized. However, there are virus strains, originally called rabbitpox but now more properly considered as variants of vaccinia, which produce generalized infection in rabbits, and which may infect by the respiratory route [8].

Infection produces a lesion caused by epidermal hyperplasia and proliferation, and inflammatory infiltration which progresses from a papule through a vesicle and pustule to a crust. A transient viremia probably occurs. Generalized lesions are rare in the immunocompetent person but serious complications can occur in the immunodeficient and eczematous individual [9]. Vaccination induces an adequate humoral and cellular immune response. Studies during the early 1970s showed that an antigen on the envelope of virions released naturally from infected cells was the important inducer of humoral immunity [10].

Host Range of Vaccinia Virus

Vaccinia has a wide host range (Table III) but we may need to distinguish between hosts which become infected naturally, and those which are susceptible only to experimental infection.

TABLE III. Host range of vaccinia virus.

Man[a]	Cow[a]	Buffalo[a]
Pig[a]	Camel[a]	Rabbit[a,b]
Elephant	Monkey	Sheep
Rodents	?	?

a. Naturally-acquired infections occur.
b. Only reported in laboratory animals.

There is no good evidence that vaccinia virus becomes established in animal populations. Smallpox vaccination has been conducted on a massive scale in both developed and developing countries. In addition, particular attention has been paid to possible animal reservoirs of smallpox virus. If vaccinia had any tendency to become established in an animal population it would have certainly been recognized.

Human Vaccinia. By historical precedent and common consent, man is the principal, if artificial, host of vaccinia virus. Other contributors to this Symposium will discuss the morbidity and mortality associated with smallpox vaccine. However, it is important to note that the problem is not confined to complications in vaccinees but also extends to infection in contacts. Avoidable incidents still occur. As recently as April 1983 a young girl in Nevada was vaccinated mistakenly and transmitted infection to seven friends at a slumber party [11].

Smallpox vaccine was intended to prevent smallpox, and there is doubt about its ability to provide long-term protection against revaccination. On revaccination the lesion is usually more superficial and transient than a primary vaccination, and complications are virtually non-existent. Nevertheless, an infection does occur on revaccination and may be transferred to eyes, genitals, etc., or to contacts.

Now that smallpox has been eradicated it might be reasonable to regard any transfer of vaccinia to a contact as a complication of the original vaccination.

Bovine Vaccinia. Cowpox is the Orthopoxvirus usually associated with bovine infection. However, although bovine cowpox does occur, it is rare and the virus is probably not enzootic in cattle [12]. Vaccinia virus infects cattle producing lesions indistinguishable from those caused by cowpox virus, and laboratory studies are needed to identify the infecting virus. Bovine vaccinia is introduced into cattle by contact with a recently-vaccinated individual.

In Holland Dekking investigated a number of outbreaks of teat infection in cattle, and isolated vaccinia virus from eight of them [13]. Bovine vaccinia mammillitis has also been reported in Russia [14] and Egypt [15] and doubtless other incidents have occurred, both reported and unreported.

Once animals are infected with vaccinia there is a risk that infection may spread from them to farmworkers. This was illustrated by a large outbreak in El Salvador. There, an outbreak involved about 450 cows and also 22 farmworkers.

Other Hosts. Occasional outbreaks of vaccinia have been reported in camels [16], buffaloes [17], and pigs [18]. However, no information is available about the incidence of vaccinia infection in animals. Smallpox vaccine was produced in sheep in some countries but no evidence has been found of natural infection occurring.

A wide range of animals can be infected experimentally with vaccinia virus and it is possible that the range of animals susceptible to natural infection is also wide.

DISCUSSION

In considering the possible use of smallpox vaccine as a vector for other genes, certain general points should be considered:

1) Because vaccinia does not occur in nature, its distribution is what health authorities choose to make it.

2) The risks of smallpox vaccination were accepted when smallpox was a problem [9]. However, the eradication of smallpox meant that smallpox vaccination complications should no longer occur. Their risk will now need to be reconsidered, and compared to the risk presented by each infection it is hoped to control.

3) In the context of this Workshop the wide host range of vaccinia virus is both an advantage and a disadvantage.

   An advantage because its infectivity for the major livestock species such as cattle, sheep, pigs, camels, and buffaloes offers the prospect of using recombinant vaccines to control important veterinary infections.

   A disadvantage because, although vaccinia does not establish in animals, widespread use in a particular species may cause spread to other species.

   Widespread use in animals may also lead to appreciable levels of human infection. Such infections, even in previously vaccinated individuals at inconvenient sites, or transmitted to contacts, may prompt objection to the use of recombinant vaccines.

4) The above comments are based on the behaviour of established vaccine strains, and it may be possible that the use of suitably attenuated strains may overcome these objections.

REFERENCES

1. D. Baxby in: Topley and Wilson's Principles of Bacteriology, Virology and Immunity, Vol. 4. G.S. Wilson and F. Brown, eds. (London, Edward Arnold 1984).
2. D. Baxby in: Jenner's Smallpox Vaccine. (London, Heinemann Educational Books 1981).
3. M. Mackett and L.G. Archard, J. Gen. Virol. 45, 683-701 (1979).
4. F. Fenner, K.R. Dumbell, S.S. Marennikova, and J.H. Nakano, WHO Smallpox Eradication Document WHO/SE/80.154 (1980).
5. P.E. Razzell in: Edward Jenner's Cowpox Vaccine, 2nd ed. (Firle, Sussex, Caliban Books 1980).
6. D.A. Henderson, Book Review, J. Hist. Med. 37, 236-258 (1982).
7. S. Dales and B.E.T. Pogo, Virology Monographs 18, 1-109 (1981).
8. H.S. Bedson and M.J. Duckworth, J. Path. Bact. 85, 1-20 (1963).
9. Symposium. Am. J. Epid. 93, 222-252 (1971).
10. E.A. Boulter and G. Appleyard, Prog. Med. Virol. 16, 86-108 (1973).
11. Report. M.M.W.R. 32, 403-404 (1983).
12. D. Baxby, Brit. Med. J. 1, 1376-1381 (1977).
13. F. Dekking in: Zoonoses, J. van der Hoeden, ed. (Amsterdam, Elsevier 1964).
14. N.N. Maltseva, E.M. Shelukhina, M.A. Yumasheva, and S.S. Marennikova, J. Hyg. Epid. Microb. Imm. 10, 202-209 (1966).
15. H. el Dahaby, A. el Sabbagh, M. Nassar, M. Kammell, and M. Iskander, J. Arab. Vet. Med. Assoc. 26, 11-24 (1966).
16. S.E. Krupenko, Veterinariya No. 8, 61-62 (1972).
17. D. Baxby and B.J. Hill, Arch. ges. Virusforsch. 35, 70-79 (1971).
18. L.H. Schwarte in: Diseases of Swine. H.W. Dunne, ed. (Ames, Iowa. Iowa State Univ. Press 1964).

DISCUSSION

Dr. Nakano: But there is a disease called Uasin Gishu in Kenya, Africa. It is a skin disease in horses, and it is a pox virus, and the consensus is that it is probably not one of the orthopox viruses that we are familiar with. Would you comment on whether this is an orthopox virus?

Dr. Baxby: All the information I know is in the literature. It was compared in terms of histology in the infected horse and some traditional biological characteristics to vaccinia and cowpox. It does seem to be orthopox virus, but in many respects differs from the other orthopox viruses which are in existence.

Dr. Moss: I do not think you meant at the very end, Dr. Baxby, that a vaccination does not protect against infection with vaccinia virus. We all know that it does protect, that there is a local infection which occurs at the site of inoculation, but there is very little evidence for complications or spread with the secondary vaccination.

Dr. Baxby: Well, I think the point you make is valid, but in fact it is possible to revaccinate on an annual basis or even more often. We do need to be concerned that if in the future we vaccinate animal populations and the animal handlers have had the traditional smallpox vaccine, then if they get infected on their fingers with vaccinia, they are going to get an infection, a mild one, yes, but there is a possibility that they were going to transmit it to eyes, genitals, or elsewhere.

Dr. Dumbell: It is sure when you revaccinate you can produce a visible, local lesion, but if you were to do a growth curve on a primary vaccination and a revaccination, you would get vastly different results.

ASPECTS OF THE BIOLOGY OF ORTHOPOXVIRUSES RELEVANT TO THE USE OF
RECOMBINANT VACCINIAS AS FIELD VACCINES

KEITH R. DUMBELL*

*Department of Medical Microbiology, Medical School, University of
Capetown, Observatory, Cape, 7925 South Africa

　　　Vaccinia virus is a minor human pathogen. It was a successful and
acceptable vaccine for the prevention of the much more serious disease,
smallpox, for as long as smallpox remained endemic. The eradication of
smallpox removed the need for, and was a strong contraindication to any
further immunizations with vaccinia virus.

　　　A new situation has arisen with the development of a growing range
of genetically engineered, recombinant vaccinias that are potential
immunogens against serious infections not only of humans but also of
animals.　Closed laboratory studies may demonstrate the efficacy of
these new recombinants as immunogens; consideration of the prevalence
and morbidity of the corresponding diseases may justify the use of
minor pathogens to combat them.　When however, the minor pathogens are
engineered recombinants it is also necessary to consider the distribution
and life histories of those natural agents with which the recombinants
might interact.

　　　The background information on the Orthopoxoviruses may be obtained
from any major textbook of Virology and will be reviewed briefly and
incompletely.　Two aspects seem to warrant closer attention; these are
the stability of the genome which is being manipulated as a vector of
new immunogens and the assessment of pathogenicity.

　　　The orthopoxviruses are grouped as one genus within the subfamily
of poxviruses of vertebrates.　The principal members, each represented
by many isolates are:　vaccinia, variola, cowpox, monkeypox, camelpox
and ectromelia.　Three other members of the genus are each represented
by only one or a few isolates; they are raccoon pox, taterapox and a
poxvirus isolated from the Uasin gishu disease of horses.　The natural
distributions of these viruses are shown in Table I, which indicates the
separate transmission cycles of the main species.　Little can be said
about the distribution and consistency of species represented by single
isolates.

　　　The origins of vaccinia are obscure, but in recent times it has
been produced in large quantities as smallpox vaccine and liberally
distributed in this way.　Limited circulation of vaccinia virus has
been detected in some outbreaks of "cowpox" in Holland, and in "buffalo
pox" in India, though one isolate of buffalo pox was a minor variant of
vaccinia [1].

　　　The important antigens of the orthopoxviruses are unrelated to
those of other genera of poxviruses; within the genus there is little
antigenic diversity and the members are differentiated primarily by the
characters of the pathological effects they produce in a variety of
laboratory animals and cell culture systems.　Although the principal
orthopoxviruses have been given species status, the antigenic overlap
is almost complete:　there are no species-specific neutralizing antibodies such as are found in most virus groups.　Profiles of the size
distribution of intracellular virus polypeptides are characteristic for
four of the main species, vaccinia, variola, cowpox and monkeypox [2].

Cross absorption of antisera has revealed a few single reactions that are specific enough to identify certain species [3,4].

The genome of orthopoxviruses is a linear, double-stranded DNA molecule, some 180-220 kilobases long and closed with a hairpin loop at either end. Digestion of the DNA with restriction endonucleases gives profiles of DNA fragment sizes which are characteristic of the different species [5]. Linear maps have been constructed, showing the relative locations of the cleavage sites for three endonucleases on representative

TABLE I. Distribution and host-range of orthopoxvirus species.

Species	Geographical source	Maintenance host(s)	Experimental host range	Comments
Cowpox	Europe	Unknown	Broad	Detected in sporadic infections of man, cows, cats, also outbreaks in zoos.
Monkeypox	West and Central Africa	Unknown	Broad	Detected in sporadic human infection in rain-forest belt of Africa & by imported outbreaks in zoos & primate colonies in Europe and USA.
Camelpox	Middle East, East Africa	Camel	Narrow	Apparently confined to camel. Human infection probably does not occur.
Variola	Formerly worldwide	Man	Narrow	Now eradicated.
Vaccinia	Laboratories & vaccine institutes	-	Broad	Some natural maintenance as e.g., buffalopox in India. Sproadic isolates occur but may well derive from wide use of vaccine.
Ectromelia	Laboratory mice	Laboratory mice	Narrow	
Raccoonpox	Eastern USA	? Raccoon	?	The only new-world orthopoxvirus
Taterpox	West Africa	-	-	A single isolate from a gerbil (tatera kempi)
Uasin gishu	East Africa	-	Narrow	A few isolates from horses in Kenya. This is not the extinct 'horsepox' of Europe.

strains of cowpox, vaccinia, monkeypox, variola and ectromelia viruses
[6]. These maps can be aligned to show remarkable conservation of
restriction sites between the species in the central half of the genome.
The outer quarters cannot be so aligned but there is extensive cross-
hybridization between DNA fragments from these outer regions of the
various species. DNA sequences, unique to a particular species have
not been demonstrated (except for cowpox, which has a substantially
longer genome than the others), but any such sequences must be fairly
short, in view of the hybridization results. It would seem that the
total gene pool of the orthopoxvirus genus is largely represented in
each of the species, that there is a fairly consistent arrangement of
functional genes in the central part of the genome and that rearrangements
of sequences in the outer quarters of the genome characterize the
different species. The functions of this, as of any viral gene pool,
can be divided into two main classes. There are firstly, the functions
associated with self replication of the genes and secondly, functions
associated with their dissemination, encapsulted in virions, through
the body of the current host and between one host and the next. The
conditions imposed on successful dissemination must be subject to
continual variation, whereas the necessities for replication in vertebrate
cytoplasm would be relatively constant. It might be expected that the
central conserved region of the genome would harbour the functions
concerned with replication and the outer regions those functions more
concerned with dissemination. In support of this general division may
be cited the genome structure of the deletion mutants. Substantial
deletions of 20-30 kilobases have been found near either terminus of
the genome of viable mutants [7-9], showing that the unique sequences
in these regions are not essential to replication.

Variola, camelpox and ectromelia viruses each have a very narrow
host range in nature; cowpox and monkeypox, on the other hand can infect
spontaneously a wide range of host animals. Vaccinia will infect a
variety of experimental hosts and it is probably not a coincidence that
it is in vaccinia, cowpox and monkeypox that major genetic mutations
have been detected as frequent occurrences.

The striking white-pock mutants of cowpox result from a major
deletion of DNA sequences which maps near the right terminus of the
genome map [10]. The white-pock mutants of rabbitpox (a vaccinia virus)
may have major deletions at either the right hand end (the u mutants)
or the left hand end (the p mutants) of the genome map [7]. The full
genomic structure of these cloned and stable mutants was later elucidated
by Moyer et al. [11], for the rabbitpox p mutants and by Archard et al.
[9], for the cowpox mutants. In each case the mutant contained an
inverted terminal repeat, much larger than that of the parent. This
restored, approximately, the original length of the genome and the
terminal hairpin loop and involved duplication of additional sequences
mapping at the opposite end of the parental genome. As Moyer et al.
[11] pointed out, this structure could be derived by a single recombination event between two wild-type genomes aligned in opposite polarity.
The true situation is likely to be more complex. Williamson and Mackett
[12] made a partial analysis of DNA taken at the earliest possible
stage after the generation of white-pock mutants of cowpox. All their
mutants showed the expected deletions of wild-type DNA, but the endonuclease digests showed a more complex set of fragments than that found
in fully established whitepock mutants. The mixture was not therefore
simply due to failure to separate the mutant from wild-type virions but
to an unresolved complex of mutant DNA. Further, a stable population
with a constant genome structure could be derived by further subcloning.
Now "cloning" is not a natural phenomenon in the transmission of

poxviruses. As far as we know they are contact diseases and it is likely that normally infection will be transmitted by a cluster of virions. Cowpox, monkeypox and vaccinia may thus infect each new host with some immediate availability of genetic diversity, and may thus enable these viruses to establish infection in an abnormal species of host. This hypothesis is open to test by analysing the DNA of poxviruses adapted to different hosts, but so far this has not been done.

The relevance to the present objectives is that the ideal poxvirus vector for foreign immunogens should be one in which the capacity for spontaneous variability has been greatly reduced or eliminated.

It is almost invariably true that virulence is a multifactorial phenomenon. The virulence of orthopoxviruses has a strong component related to the host species. Ectromelia and smallpox, for example, are highly virulent to mouse and man respectively. But these viruses have a limited host range as judged by infectivity alone. The wider infective spectrum of vaccinia, cowpox and monkeypox enables these viruses to express virulence characteristics in different species of host. Rabbitpox, a vaccinia virus, is virulent for mice and rabbits; variola virus is virulent for neither. Yet when recombinants were prepared from rabbitpox and variola minor, it was found [13] that some were virulent for mice and others for rabbits. If virulence for two different species of rodents can so easily segregate, it would seem unwise to draw conclusions about human virulence from observations on experimental animals.

Primary vaccination normally produces a local skin lesion, some inflammation of regional lymph nodes and a transient fever. Yet, as Dr. Arita will detail, there are rare and serious complications in a few individuals of every million vaccinated. The cutaneous complications appear to depend on natural or induced defects in cell-mediated response; these complications could, to an extent, be reduced by excluding from vaccination those people with appropriate contraindications. The etiology of postvaccinial encephalitis and encephalopathy is not understood though the incidence was shown to be affected by the particular strain of vaccinia used [14].

In planning what vaccinia to use as a vector for immunizing people, there would seem to be no adequate experimental substitute for the extensive experience gained with those strains which have been widely used. The vaccinia strains that were extensively used to control smallpox may not be the ideal poxvirus vectors for foreign immunogens. Many questions need to be answered about the pathogenic mechanisms, and about host responses to them before a substantially improved vector could be designed and constructed. In the meantime, clinical application might proceed cautiously on the basis of present information. The strains of vaccinia which have given the most favourable field experience against smallpox could be used as vectors. The expected number of complications could be reasonably well predicted, and there are areas where the present morbidity from hepatitis, for example, would considerably outweigh the morbidity to be expected from the appropriate recombinant vaccinia given as an immunizing agent. Justification for the use of vaccinia also presupposes that no safer alternative immunogen should be available which is both equally efficient and is affordable by the health authority concerned.

REFERENCES

1. D. Baxby and B.J. Hill, Archiv. fur die ges. Virusforsch 35, 70-79 (1971).
2. L. Harper, H.S. Bedson and A. Buchan, Virology 93, 435-444 (1979).
3. R. Gispen and B. Brand-Saathof, J. Infect. Dis. 129, 289-295 (1974).
4. J.J. Esposito, J.F. Obijeski and J.H. Nakano, J. Med. Virol. 1, 35-47 (1977).
5. J.J. Esposito, J.R. Obijeski and J.H. Nakano, Virology 89, 53-66 (1978).
6. M. Mackett and L.C. Archard, J. Gen. Virol. 45, 683-701 (1979).
7. J.R. Lake and P.D. Cooper, J. Gen. Virol. 48, 135-147 (1980).
8. R. Drillien, F. Koehren and A. Kirn, Virology 111, 488-499 (1981).
9. L.C. Archard, M. Mackett, D.E. Barnes and K.R. Dumbell, J. Gen. Virol. 65, 875-886 (1984).
10. L.C. Archard and M. Mackett, J. Gen. Virol. 45, 51-63 (1979).
11. R.W. Moyer, R.L. Graves and C.T. Rothe, Cell 22, 545-553 (1980).
12. J.D. Williamson ad M. Mackett, J. Hyg. Camb. 89, 373-381 (1982).
13. H.S. Bedson and K.R. Dumbell, J. Hyg. Camb. 62, 141-146 (1964).
14. K. Berger and U. Heinrich in: International Symposium on Smallpox Vaccine. (Bilthoven, The Netherlands 1972) Symp-Series Immunobiol. Standard, Vol. 19.

MOLECULAR BIOLOGY OF VACCINIA VIRUS: STRUCTURE OF POXVIRUS DNA

WOLFGANG K. JOKLIK*

*Department of Microbiology and Immunology, Duke University Medical Center, Durham, North Carolina 27710

The genus Orthopoxvirus of the family Poxviridae comprises a group of rather closely related viruses, the best known of which are variola virus, monkeypox virus (MPV), vaccinia virus, cowpox virus (CPV), rabbitpox virus (RPV) and ectromelia (mousepox virus). These viruses possess a similar morphology, they share a variety of antigenic determinants, their protein components resemble each other in relative amount and size, and they possess ds DNA-containing genomes that are about 200 kbp long (about 125 million daltons) and exhibit 70-90 percent homology, depending on which viruses are being compared [1].

The basis of the relatedness of orthopoxvirus genomes became apparent when their restriction endonuclease sites were mapped. Figure 1 illustrates this point. It represents the cleavage maps for two enzymes, HindIII and SmaI. It is clear that the genomes of all six principal members of the genus Orthopoxvirus resemble each other closely in their central portions, where almost all restriction sites have been conserved; but that they vary both in size and cleavage site distribution (and therefore in sequence) in their terminal regions. A great deal of additional and more extensive work has led to the following model for Orthopoxvirus genomes as exemplified by the CPV genome (Figure 2). Orthopoxvirus genomes consist of a central region about 120 kbp long which is flanked by two regions, region 1 and region 2, each about 40 kbp long. Presumably the central region of the orthopoxvirus genome encodes functions related to virus multiplication, while the two flanking regions contain information related to type-specificity and to the interaction of orthopoxviruses with their host cells, particularly as it relates to host range, the effect of infection on host functions, and the extent of the ability of each virus to multiply.

The molecular structure of the orthopoxvirus genome exhibits several interesting features. For example, none of the orthopoxvirus mRNAs examined so far are spliced. This may be yet another reflection of a possibly fundamentally different origin of herpesviruses, adenoviruses and papovaviruses on the one hand, the genomes of which probably originated from the genetic material of eukaryotic cells, and poxviruses on the other, which by this criterion may have originated from a prokaryotic genome. Further, like other large DNA-containing viral genomes, the orthopoxvirus genome encodes numerous genes, the expression of which is regulated according to a very complex temporal pattern, the simplest and best known manifestation of which are the early and late multiplication cycle periods [2]. Clearly a large portion of the orthopoxvirus genome has regulatory functions. It is also clear that the orthopoxvirus genome contains genes that are not necessary for ability to multiply in all cell types. An example is the thymidine kinase (TK) gene, expression of which is not necessary in cells that express this enzyme themselves; as a result, foreign genes can be cloned into the TK gene, as Moss and Paoletti and their colleagues have demonstrated. It is the practical application of this circumstance to the production of vaccines for both humans and animals that provides the raison d'etre for the present workshop. However, this is clearly not the only region of the orthopoxvirus genome into which foreign genes may be cloned. It is known that the genomes of many white pock variants of CPV, RPV and MPV are rearranged, with long stretches of DNA being

© 1985 Elsevier Science Publishing Co., Inc.
VACCINIA VIRUSES AS VECTORS FOR VACCINE ANTIGENS, Quinnan, Editor

deleted and others duplicated, yet these variants are capable of multiplying in a variety of cultured cells, as well as in the cells of the chorioallantoic membrane (CAM) of the developing chick embryo [3-6]. No doubt foreign genes could be inserted there also.

In fact, considerable attention has been focused in recent years on the nature of the terminal regions of orthopoxvirus genomes. Three aspects of their molecular structure are particularly interesting. First, it has been found that the two strands of the orthopoxvirus genome are covalently crosslinked at their ends [7] and that it possesses at its extreme ends a 104 nucleotide long sequence that is not perfectly base paired and that exists in two forms, the so-called flip-flop loops [8]. Second, very close to these loops, or, more precisely, within 90 bp

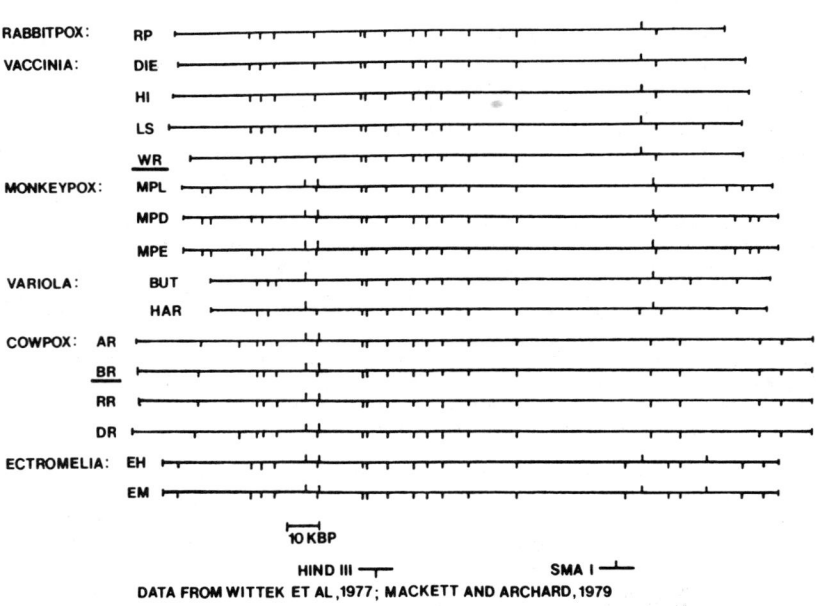

FIG. 1. Physical map locations of the HindIII and SmaI restriction endonuclease cleavage sites in the genomes of various strains of RPV, vaccinia virus, MPV, variola virus, CPV and ectromelia virus. The strains are: RPV strain Utrecht; vaccinia virus strains DIE, HI (Hall Institute), LS (Lister) and WR; MPV strains Congo, Denmark and Espana; variola virus strains Butler and Harvey; CPV red strains Austria, Brighton, Ruthin and Daisy; and ectromelia virus strains Hampstead and Moscow.

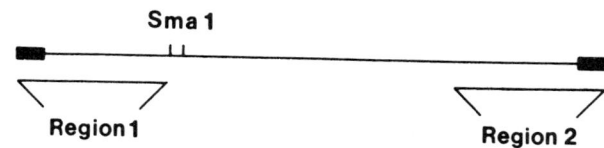

FIG. 2. The genome of CPV-BR. The locations of the SmaI cleavage sites are indicated, and the two flanking regions are designated region 1 and region 2 depending on their location relative to them. The black rectangles represent the ITRs. The size of each flanking region is about 40 kbp [13].

from them in the case of vaccinia virus and CPV DNA, there exist two sets of sequences that are composed of tandemly repeated short (about 50 bp long) "repeat units." These repeated sequence sets are 500-1500 bp long and are separated by a unique sequence about 300 bp long [9,10]. Third, orthopoxvirus genomes possess inverted terminal repeats [11,12] that may differ enormously in length; the ITRs of some viruses, such as those of variola virus, are no more than 1-2 kbp long, while those of others, like those of some of the white pock variants of CPV-BR, are 50 kbp long [13]. Typically, the two ends of the orthopoxvirus genome are about 10 kbp long, identical, and inverted relative to each other; their terminal 2 kbp contains the repeaated sequence sets described above; and at the very ends of the ITRs there are the two identical crosslinked flip-flop loops.

Our present purpose is to discuss, in turn, the nature, genesis and significance of these three sequence elements of orthopoxvirus genomes. Most of the information that will be discussed relates to vaccinia virus and CPV, and to a certain extent also to RPV and MPV. It is likely, however, that all orthopoxvirus genomes possess sequence elements similar to those to be discussed, though no doubt there will be many individual variations.

The Flip-flop Terminal Loops

A very unusual feature of the orthopoxvirus genome is that its two DNA strands are covalently joined at their ends; thus, if orthopoxvirus genomes are melted, single-stranded circles result, the circumference of which is twice their length [7]. The nature of the terminal cross links and of the sequences near each end was investigated by Baroudy et al. [8] who isolated the restriction endonuclease fragment containing the ends of vaccinia DNA and sequenced it. The vaccinia virus genome is a continuous single DNA strand collapsed into a linear configuration in which the two opposing single strand sequences are perfectly basepaired

throughout their length except for 104 nucleotides at each end. This
104 nucleotide region exists in two forms which are inverted complementary
versions of each other (Figure 3). These so-called "flip-flop" loop forms

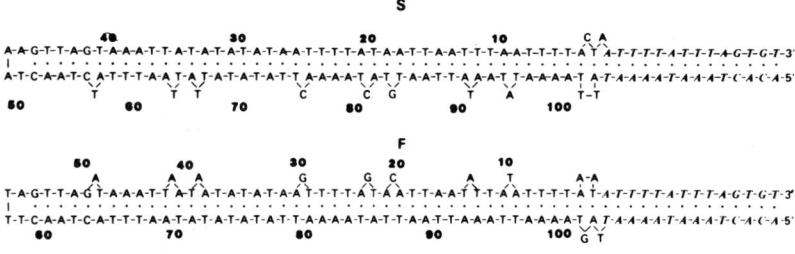

FIG. 3. The two forms of the flip-flop terminal loop structures at the
ends of vaccinia virus DNA. Both forms, which are the inverted comple-
ments of each other, are shown with maximum base-pairing. The nucleotides
of the divergent 104 nucleotides are numbered. The sequence in italics
on the right is that of the body of the vaccinia virus genome [14].

are not perfectly basepaired since even in their optimum configuration 10
of the 104 residues cannot form basepairs. They exist in the vaccinia
virus genome in approximately equal amounts. The manner in which they
are generated is not known, but would be expected to involve a site-
specific nuclease that cleaves where the flip-flop sequences are joined
to the bulk of the vaccinia virus genome. There is no reason to doubt
that flip-flop loops are present at the ends of the genomes of all
orthopoxvirus genomes.

The Repeated Sequence Sets

The regions adjacent to the flip-flop loops have been cloned and sequenced for vaccinia virus [14] and for CPV-BR [10]. The arrangement of these sequences is shown in Figure 4. Next to the flip-flop sequences

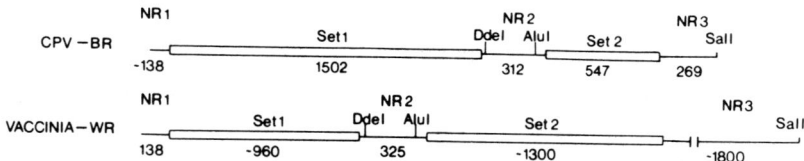

FIG. 4. Comparison of the regions adjacent to the flip-flop loops in CPV and vaccinia virus WR DNA. The numbers represent base pairs [10,14,13].

there is a unique region of 86 nucleotides (NRI) in which CPV-BR and vaccinia virus differ in only 2 residues. This is followed by (i) a region (Set 1) that is composed of tandemly repeated sequence elements that are about 50 residues long (see below); (ii) a unique region, NR2, about 300 residues long that is very similar for the two viruses, being 97% homologous and containing identically situated DdeI and AluI restriction endonuclease cleavage sites; (iii) a further set of tandemly repeated sequence elements (Set 2); and (iv) unique sequences specific for each virus (NR3). There is a SalI restriction endonuclease cleavage site 269 residues downstream from the end of Set 2 in the case of CPV-BR and about 1800 residues in the case of vaccinia virus. These regions are also very similar for the two viruses, at least the first 100 residues or so, which are 98% homologous [10,15].

The tandemly repeated sequence elements of CPV-BR and vaccinia virus DNA, that is, their repeat subunits, are related, but their arrangement is different. In the case of vaccinia virus there are only two repeated sequence elements, A and B (Figure 5), which are repeated as AB units 13 times in repeat set 1 and 18 times in repeat set 2 [9,8]. In the case of CPV-BR there are four repeated sequence elements [10] (Figure 6). There are two noteworthy features concerning them. First,

```
COWPOX TYPE A UNIT     CCATCAGAAAGAGGTTTAATATTTTTGTGAGA
VACCINIA REPEAT UNIT   CCATCAGAAAGAGGTTTAATATTTTTGTGAGACCATCGAAGAGAGAAAGAGA-TAAAACTTTTTTACGACT
COWPOX TYPE B* UNIT                                     CCATTGAAGAGAGAAAGAGAATAAAATATTTTTACGACT
```

FIG. 5. Relation between the 70 bp repeat unit of vaccinia virus WR DNA (which can be thought of as being composed of two subunits, A and B) and repeat subunits A and B* of CPV DNA [10].

```
A    CCATC------AGAAAGAG-----GTTT---AATATTTTTGTGAGA
B    CCATTGAAGAGAGAAAGAGAAAGAGAATAAAAATATTTTAGTGACT
B*   CCATTGAAGAGAGAAAGAGAA------T-AAAATATTTTTACGACT
C    CCATTGAAGAGAGAAAGAGAA------TAAAAATATTTTT------GTAAAACTTTTTTATGAGA
```

FIG. 6. Sequence composition of the four repeat subunits in CPV DNA. The sequences are aligned to reveal homology. Colons indicate mismatches. The 19 residues at the righthand end of the A and C subunits share 75% homology [10].

they are very closely related and no doubt arose from each other by deletion and unequal crossover events; it is likely that the original primordial element from which the others are derived is the A element. Second, the two vaccinia virus repeat elements are very similar, in fact almost identical, to CPV-BR elements A and B*; in fact, they are 96% homologous. As for the arrangment of the four CPV repeat elements, it is clearly more complex (Figure 7) than that of the two vaccinia virus repeat elements.

Thus, very close to the ends of the orthopoxvirus genome, there are sets of repeated sequence elements that do not encode proteins, yet have been highly conserved. No doubt the function of these repeated sequence elements relates to regulation of replication and regulation of

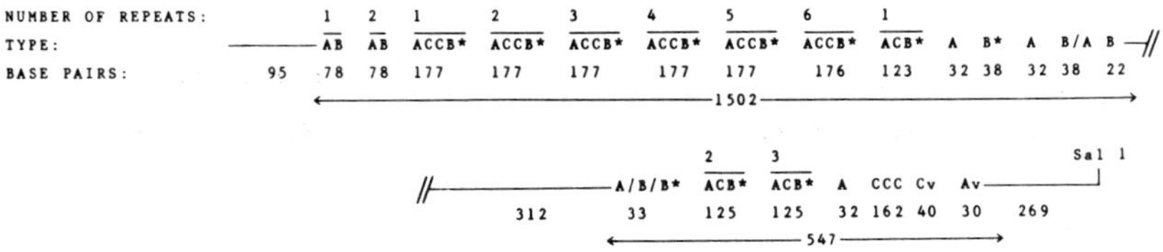

NUMBER OF REPEATS:		1	2	1	2	3	4	5	6	1					
TYPE:		AB	AB	ACCB*	ACCB*	ACCB*	ACCB*	ACCB*	ACCB*	ACB*	A	B*	A	B/A	B —//
BASE PAIRS:	95	78	78	177	177	177	177	177	176	123	32	38	32	38	22

←————————————1502————————————→

			2	3						Sal I
//————	A/B/B*	ACB*	ACB*	A	CCC	Cv	Av ————			
	312	33	125	125	32	162	40	30	269	

←————————547————————→

FIG. 7. Structure of the two repeat sets in the terminal SalI fragment of CPV-BR DNA. They are flanked by NR (nonrepeated sequence region) 1 and NR3, and are separated by NR2 [10].

transcription. Studies are currently underway in our laboratory to determine, using recombinant DNA techniques, whether these repeated sequence elements can be modified and what effect such modification has on the ability of orthopoxviruses to replicate.

The presence of repeated sequence elements at the termini of orthopoxvirus genomes explains a puzzling feature of the vaccinia virus genome. It was noticed some time ago that the length of the terminal restriction endonuclease cleavage fragment of certain orthopoxviruses, for example, those of a particular isolate of the WR strain of vaccinia virus, was highly heterogeneous. When the virus is cloned or plaque-purified, the fragment becomes homogeneous; upon passaging, it again becomes heterogeneous [16]. Clearly, there is a mechanism that renders the terminal region of the vaccinia virus genome heterogeneous. Moss et al. [17] suggested that this was due to the fact that unequal crossover occurs between two vaccinia virus genomes aligned so that repeated sequence Set 1 is lined up with repeated sequence Set 2; upon homologous crossover, one of the products would then contain three repeated sequence sets rather than two, and this process would continue until genomes are formed that contain up to twelve repeated sequence sets and are up to 12 kbp larger than the original parent strain. This tendency toward heterogeneity is genetically determined, since some vaccinia virus strains exhibit it, while others do not. This type of heterogeneity is not exhibited by cowpox virus, at least by the strain of CPV-BR studied by Pickup et al. [19]. Nor has this tendency toward length heterogeneity been noted for other orthopoxvirus genomes.

The ITRs of Orthopoxvirus Genomes

Orthopoxvirus genomes possess long inverted terminal repeats (ITRs). The length of these ITRs varies in the various orthopoxvirus prototype strains. Thus, the ITRs of vaccinia virus, CPV and MPV are about 10 kbp long, while those of RPV and ectromelia virus are about one-half this length, and those of variola virus are very short (less than 2 kbp) [18,19]. The reason why orthopoxvirus genomes possess ITRs is probably related to their mode of replication; it should be noted that adenovirus and herpesvirus genomes also possess ITRs. Models for the replication of poxvirus genomes have been discussed by Moyer and Graves [20] and Baroudy et al. [8].

The manner in which ITRs are generated has been examined in some detail for CPV-BR by Pickup et al. [13]. The ITR in this virus strain is about 9.7 kbp long. The junctions of both ITRs with the remainder of the viral genome have been identified and sequenced; the sequences are presented in Figure 8. There are no statistically significant

region 1-ITR TCGTAGCTAAAACTCAAGTAAGAGGGTTTTATTATCTCCGTCATACGTAAATGCCTTCTTAAGCTATTTG

region 2-ITR CCTTAAAGCTTCTGATGGTAACTGTGTTACATGTGCTCCGTCATACGTAAATGCCTTCTTAAGCTATTTG

FIG. 8. Nucleotide sequences at the junctions between the ITRs and unique region DNA in regions 1 and 2 of the genome of CPV-BR. Both sequences are shown in a 5' to 3' orientation, such that the 5' end would correspond to the inner end of that sequence in the genome [13].

direct or staggered homologies between the ITR sequences and the adjoining genomic sequences, nor any significant alternate purine/pyrimidine stretches indicative of ability to assume the Z configuration, nor any significant dyad symmetries. Thus the sequences around the junctions of ITRs and the remainder of the genome possess no features that would provide a clue as to why the ITR sequences should be joined at those two particular locations.

Insight into the genesis of ITRs came from an unexpected quarter, namely analysis of the genomes of a series of white pock variants of CPV-BR. CPV-BR produces red ulcerated hemorrhagic pocks on the CAM of developing chick embryos. About 1 percent of pocks, however, are white. The white pock producing variants can be isolated; many are stable genetically in that they never revert to producing red pocks. These features, namely their very high rate of generation and their total lack of reversion, together with the ease with which they can be selected and isolated, make them attractive objects for studies of the nature of their genomes. Pickup et al. [13] isolated a large number of such variants and selected ten for detailed study. Restriction endonuclease analysis of their DNAs revealed that they lack some regions of the genomes of parental wild-type red pock producing virus, that they possess two copies of other regions of which the wt strain possesses only one, and that they possess some restriction endonuclease fragments that are not present in the genome of wt virus, which is due to the presence of rearranged sequences. However, they all contain the entire wt virus ITR.

Detailed restriction endonuclease analysis revealed that the genomes of the ten variants could be represented schematically as depicted in Figure 9. All variants possess an intact region 1, but in all of them, with one exception, 32-38 kbp of the terminal region of the about 40 kbp long region 2 were deleted and replaced by a region of variable length that is identical with the terminal portion of region 1

FIG. 9. Structures of region 2 of ten white pock variants of CPV-BR. The genomes are aligned at a coordinate that maps at 40 kbp from the right terminus of CPV-BR DNA. Horizontal lines correspond to nonrepeated CPV-BR DNA; black rectangles correspond to the ITR. Open rectangles correspond to region 1 DNA sequences inverted relative to their orientation at the other end of the genome. Double vertical lines at the left-hand end of open rectangles correspond to the location of novel junctions between region 1 and 2 DNA sequences; single vertical lines represent novel junctions that were sequenced (see text). The broken line in variant W10 corresponds to the sequences deleted in this variant. W+ indicates the genome of CPV-BR [13].

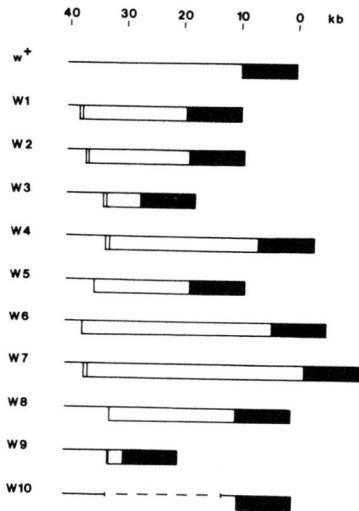

inserted in the opposite direction. Thus all these variants possess new ITRs: in all cases the new ITR is longer than that of wt virus, the shortest being that of variant W9 (12 kbp) and the longest that of variant W7 (50 kbp). In all these variants the lack of 22-28 kbp (actually 32-38 kbp, but 10 kbp correspond to the wt ITR) does not affect their ability to multiply either in the CAM or in BHK cells. This agrees with the notion discussed above that the sequences in regions 1 and 2 do not encode functions essential for orthopoxvirus multiplication, but that they encode functions concerned with the interaction of orthopoxviruses with their host cells.

The reason why in all variants the amount of material that is deleted is about the same, namely 32-38 kbp long, is probably that it cannot be shorter because the gene that causes pocks to be red is located about 30 kbp from the end of the CPV genome (Pickup et al., unpublished results), and that it cannot be longer because a gene that is essential for virus multiplication is apparently located about 40 kbp from the right end of the CPV-BR genome.

In variant 10, the length of the ITRs is exactly the same as those of the wt virus. In all others the ITRs are enlarged, in some only slightly, in others enormously. Thus, it seems clear that ITRs are generated by the same mechanism that generates deletion/duplication variants. The simplest mechanism to account for the generation of such variants is by a single crossover recombinational event such as is illustrated in Figure 10. However, this is probably not the actual mechanism by which ITRs are generated. There are several reasons for this. First, Pickup et al. [13] isolated the junction regions of

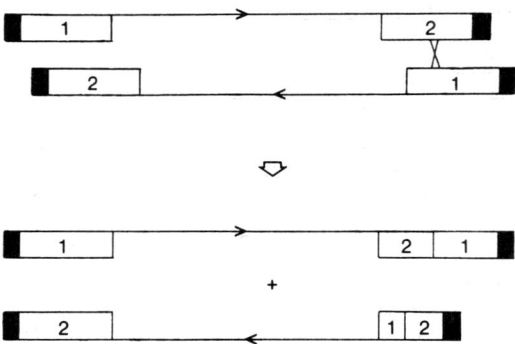

FIG. 10. A possible mechanism for generating deletion/duplication variants, and therefore ITRs, by crossover between sequences in regions 1 and 2 on two genomes aligned in opposite direction. Crossover between region 2 sequences aligned in the same direction would yield simple deletion variants like variant W10.

three of the deletion-substitution variants (W5, W6 and W8) and of the straight deletion variant W10, and sequenced them. As is the case for the ITR junction regions in wt virus depicted in Figure 8, no homology was found among the sequences that would have to recombine. Recombination would therefore have to be of the type generally referred to as nonhomologous or illegitimate. While evidence that joining of nonhomologous sequences occurs frequently is accumulating rapidly--examples being the highly efficient manner in which fragments of retrovirus proviral DNA are reconstituted [21,22] and the ends of unrelated DNAs are joined after transfection into eukaryotic cells [23]--its detailed mechanism is not known. Second, this type of recombination would be expected to yield roughly equal numbers of deletion-substitution and straight deletion variants; but analysis of the genomes of white pock variants of CPV-BR, MPV and RPV [3-6] indicates that the frequency of deletion-substitution variants is roughly ten times that of straight deletion variants. A mechanism that would generate deletion/duplication variants with those frequency ratios is the nonreciprocal transfer of genetic information between the terminal regions of different genomes or of the same genome, that is, a mechanism involving strand invasion and gene conversion. If, for example, a double-stranded break or a single-stranded nick were introduced into an ITR, the resulting free 3'-end might be able to invade the duplex at the other end of the genome and either repair or replace the gapped end with a newly synthesized copy of the intact end. The loop structure at the DNA terminus would facilitate the synthesis of a double-stranded replica of the template terminus. Intramolecular exchanges of this type would produce deletions/duplications, while intermolecular exchanges would produce both deletions/duplications and simple deletions, depending on the ends involved. This mechanism would tend to yield an excess of deletions/duplications over simple deletion variants; therefore, it may resemble more closely the actual mechanism that generates white pock variant genomes.

While details concerning the precise mechanism of formation of ITRs remain to be worked out, it is clear that genetic rearrangements in regions 1 and 2 of orthopoxvirus genomes occur with high frequency. Because of the nature of the selection involved, the system studied here, namely the formation CPV-BR white pock variants, involves only 6-10 kbp of region 2. Judging from the frequency of generation of such variants (about 1 percent per progeny virus particle), the overall frequency of such rearrangements involving the roughly 80 kbp of regions 1 and 2 may amount to about 10 percent of virus particles produced. Clearly the length of ITRs in the wt strain of CPV-BR is not fixed in a genetic sense; in fact, the length of ITRs in various red pock producing and therefore phenotypically wt$^+$ strains of CPV-BR may be quite different. It is not known at this time whether pressures exist that cause ITRs of certain lengths to be selected; in other words, whether there are pressures that tend to stabilize ITR length.

However that may be, the significance of ITRs is that they increase the genetic potential of orthopoxviruses; for the generation of new ITRs could produce new orthopoxvirus strains, that is, strains with altered virus-host cell interactions. Among the consequences of the generation of new ITRs are deletion of large segments of DNA, alteration of the relationship of control sequences to coding sequences, and the creation of novel coding sequences by changing reading frames. In fact, it seems that there must be pressures that limit the generation of new ITRs, since if the rate of generation of ITRs is as high as that suggested from this study of white pock variants of CPV-BR, namely 10 percent of progeny virus particles, new virus strains should be generated more rapidly than actually appears to be the case. On the other hand, it must be pointed out that no one has yet tested whether new orthopoxvirus strains are not actually produced at such a high rate; such studies could only be carried out by examining appropriate and as yet unspecified genetic markers. However that may be, the genetic potential for generating new orthopoxvirus strains is clearly very great, and this is a factor that must be kept in mind when considering the use of orthopoxviruses as vectors for vaccine antigens.

REFERENCES

1. H.K. Muller, R. Wittek, W. Schaffner, D. Schumperli, A. Menna and R. Wyler, J. Gen. Virol. 38, 135 (1977).
2. K.-I. Oda and W.K. Joklik, J. Mol. Biol. 27, 395 (1967).
3. R.W. Moyer, R.L. Graves and C.T. Rothe, Cell 22, 545 (1980).
4. R.W. Moyer and C.T. Rothe, Virology 102, 119 (1980).
5. J.J. Esposito, C.D. Cabradillo, J.H. Nakano and J.F. Obijeski, Virology 109, 231 (1981).
6. L.C. Archard, M. Mackett, D.E. Barnes and K.R. Dumbell, J. Gen. Virol. 65, 875 (1984).
7. P. Geshelin and K.I. Berns, J. Mol. Biol. 88, 785 (1974).
8. B.M. Baroudy and B. Moss, Nucl. Acids Res. 10, 5673 (1982).
9. R. Wittek and B. Moss, Cell 21, 277 (1980).
10. D.J. Pickup, D. Bastia, H.O. Stone and W.K. Joklik, Proc. Natl. Acad. Sci. USA 79, 7112 (1982).
11. C.F. Garon, E. Barbosa and B. Moss, Proc. Natl. Acad. Sci. USA 75, 4863 (1978).
12. R. Wittek, H.K. Muller, A. Menna and R. Wyler, FEBS Letters 90, 41 (1978).
13. D.J. Pickup, B.S. Ink, B.L. Parsons, W. Hu, and W.K. Joklik, Proc. Natl. Acad. Sci. USA 81, 6817 (1984).
14. B.M. Baroudy, S. Venkatesan and B. Moss, Cell 28, 315 (1982).
15. S. Venkatesan, B.M. Baroudy and B. Moss, Cell 125, 805 (1981).

16. R. Wittek, A. Menna, H.K. Muller, D. Schumperli, P.G. Boseley and R. Wyler, J. Virol. 28, 17 (1978b).
17. B. Moss, E. Winters and N. Cooper, Proc. Natl. Acad. Sci. USA 78, 1614 (1981).
18. M. Mackett and L.C. Archard, J. Gen. Virol. 45, 683 (1979).
19. R. Wittek, A. Menna, D. Schumperli, S. Stoffel, H.K. Muller and R. Wyler, J. Virol. 23, 669 (1977).
20. R.W. Moyer and R.L. Graves, Cell 27, 391 (1981).
21. J.J. Kopchick and D.W. Stacey, J. Biol. Chem. 258, 11528 (1983).
22. P.K. Bandypadhyay, S. Watanabe and H.M. Temin, Proc. Natl. Acad. Sci. USA 81, 3476 (1984).
23. J.H. Wilson, P.B. Berget and J.M. Pipas, Molec. Cell Biol. 2, 1258 (1982).

MOLECULAR BIOLOGY OF VACCINIA VIRUS: STRATEGIES FOR CLONING AND
EXPRESSION OF FOREIGN GENES

BERNARD MOSS*

*Laboratory of Viral Diseases, National Institute of Allergy and Infectious Diseases, National Institutes of Health, Bethesda, Maryland 20205

INTRODUCTION

The objectives of this chapter are to review aspects of the molecular biology of vaccinia virus that are most relevant to the development of vectors for expression of foreign genes, and to consider some of the strategies that have been used to create recombinant viruses. More comprehensive treatment of the biology of poxviruses may be found elsewhere [1,2]. Poxviruses, of which vaccinia virus is the prototype, are distinguished by their large size and complex morphology, high molelcular weight DNA genome, coding for enzymes needed for DNA and RNA synthesis, packaging of the latter within the infectious virus particle, and cytoplasmic site of replication.

VIRON STRUCTURE

Poxviruses are the largest and most complex of all animal viruses. Two infectious forms of vaccinia virus exist. The intracellular one, which is predominant, contains a lipoprotein envelope, a biconcave core, and lateral bodies fitted into the concavities. The extracellular form, the amount of which may vary from less than 1 percent to more than 20 percent of the total infectious virus depending on the vaccinia virus strain and cultured cell used [3], has an additional lipoprotein envelope apparently acquired from golgi membrane [4,5]. Although a minor commponent in vitro, the intracellular form is thought to be important for virus dissemination in vivo [6,7].

GENOME

The genome of vaccinia virus consists of a linear double-stranded DNA molecule of approximately 185,000 base-pairs (bp) located within the core structure [8]. The DNA has several characteristic features in addition to its large size. The sequence at the two ends of the genome are identical for about 10,000 bp [9,10]. This very long inverted terminal repetition contains sets of tandem repeats that are 54, 70 and 125 bp long [11,12] as well as several complete genes [13]. Perhaps most unusual is the covalent linkage of the two DNA strands [8] by incompletely base-paired hairpin loops at each end of the genome [14]. The 104 nucleotide hairpin structure exists in two isomeric forms that are inverted and complementary in sequence. It seems likely that the hairpins are necessary for replication of the ends of the linear DNA.

The length of the vaccinia virus genome can vary appreciably while maintaining its ability to be replicated or packaged. For example, a viable 9,000 bp deletion mutant of vaccinia virus has been isolated [15,16] and rabbitpox mutants with even larger deletions have been found [17]. The vaccinia virus genome also can be expanded by at least 25,000 bp [18]. The ability of different lengths of DNA to be packaged may be related in part to the non-icosahedral structure of the virion.

Although intact vaccinia virus DNA molecules can be isolated, the DNA is not infectious [19]. Evidently, additional virion components such as the enzymes described below are needed to start the infectious cycle.

Published 1985 by Elsevier Science Publishing Co., Inc.
VACCINIA VIRUSES AS VECTORS FOR VACCINE ANTIGENS, Quinnan, Editor

ENZYME COMPONENTS OF THE VIRION

Two-dimensional gel electrophoresis of virions disrupted with sodium dodecyl sulfate suggest that there are at least 100 polypeptides [20]. These include structural proteins as well as enzymes involved in transcription, mRNA modification and possibly other functions. The list of isolated enzymes includes a multisubunit DNA-dependent RNA polymerase [12,21], a two-subunit poly(A) polymerase [22], a two-subunit enzyme complex containing RNA triphosphatase, RNA guanylyltransferase (capping enzyme), and RNA guanine-7-methyltransferase activities [23,24], an RNA (nucleoside-2'-) methyltransferase [25], a 5'-phosphate polynucleotide kinase [26], a DNA-dependent ATPase [27], a nucleic acid dependent nucleoside triphosphatase [27], an endoribonuclease [28], two deoxyribonucleases [29,30], a DNA topoisomerase [31], a protein kinase [32], and an alkaline protease [33]. For a description of these enzymes and additional references see Moss [2].

EXPRESSION OF THE GENOME

Following adsorption and penetration of host cells, the virus core is released into the cytoplasm where transcription occurs (Figure 1)

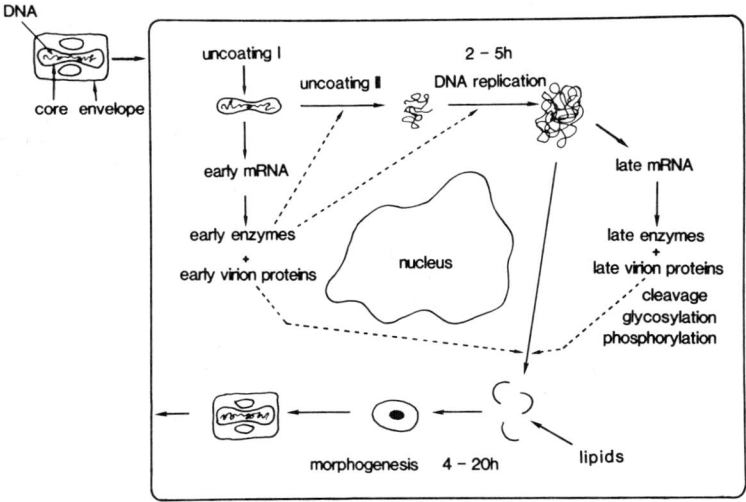

FIG. 1. Vaccinia virus growth cycle.

DNA-RNA hybridization studies indicate that about half of the genome is expressed at this early or pre-replicative stage [34,35]. There appears to be about 100 early genes distributed throughout the length of the DNA [36]. Some of these genes have been precisely mapped and several have been sequenced [37-39]. All of the genes thus far examined have continuous coding segments and no evidence of RNA splicing has been found. In addition, several RNAs were found to be initiated at the mature 5' ends [40]. Most if not all vaccinia virus mRNAs are polyadenylated [41], but it is not known whether this occurs at the site of transcriptional termination or cleavage.

Following the onset of DNA replication, the late class of genes is expressed and many of the early genes are no longer functionally active. Late genes, which include the major structural proteins, also are distributed throughout the genome, however they appear to be concentrated in the central region [36]. The nucleotide sequence of the one late gene reported thus far also contains a continuous coding segment [39]. Although late mRNAs have discrete 5' ends, their 3' ends are extremely heterogeneous and can apparently extend thousands of nucleotides past the 5' coding portion [42,43,39]. Because of this unusual feature, the late transcripts are overlapping and complementary to each other and to early mRNA [44-46]. However, the biological significance of the length heterogeneity is not known.

For most RNA polymerases that have been studied, the transcriptional signals are located upstream of the initiation site. Although the nucleotide sequences upstream of vaccinia virus genes do not correspond closely to prokaryotic or eukaryotic signals, a consensus sequence for early genes was proposed [38]. This consensus sequence was not found upstream of a late gene that was examined [39].

The promoter regions of several vaccinia virus genes have been identified by functional methods. A cell extract obtained from vaccinia virus infected cells was shown to transcribe DNA fragments that contain 200 bp or less of DNA upstream of the RNA start site of vaccinia virus genes [48]. Moreover, these extracts were unable to transcribe DNA segments containing promoter regions from other sources.

Functional promoter regions also were identified by transient expression of chimeric genes introduced into cells infected with vaccinia virus [65]. In this assay, a fragment of vaccinia virus DNA was ligated to the coding segment of the easily assayable chloramphenicol acetyltransferase (CAT) gene within a plasmid. When the recombinant plasmid was transfected into uninfected and vaccinia virus infected cells, CAT expression only occurred in the latter. In vitro deletion mutagenesis has been used to delimit the promoter region [49].

A third method used to analyze promoter regions is by the introduction of chimeric genes into the genome of vaccinia virus. This is essentially the procedure used to prepare recombinant viruses for vaccine purposes and will be described in a later section.

REPLICATION OF VACCINIA VIRUS DNA

The cytoplasmic site of DNA replication is a special feature of poxviruses. There is evidence that vaccinia virus codes for its own DNA polymerase of approximate M_r 110,000 [50,51] and presumably for a variety of other replication factors including a DNA topoisomerase [31]. Although the details of DNA replication are not understood, the available data suggest that synthesis starts near the ends of the genome, involves a strand displacement mechanism, and concatemeric forms [52-55].

VIRUS ASSEMBLY, MATURATION AND RELEASE

Vaccinia virus assembly is a complex process that occurs within specialized areas of the cytoplasm [1]. Mature particles are moved out of the assembly areas and transported to the cell periphery. Some of the particles become wrapped in modified golgi membrane and are externalized [4,5,56].

CLONING AND EXPRESSION OF FOREIGN GENES

Consideration of the biological properties of vaccinia virus is necessary for this agent to be used effectively as a cloning and expression vector. Because vaccinia virus has a unique transcriptase, the enginering of chimeric genes with vaccinia regulatory signals fused to the foreign protein coding sequence is required for efficient expression [57]. The large size of the vaccinia virus genome precludes the simple insertion of foreign DNA. In addition, the non-infectious nature of the DNA would prevent its propagation by transfection of uninfected cells. These difficulties have been overcome by allowing homologous recombination to occur in cells infected with vaccinia virus, a process originally used for marker rescue [19,58,47]. As depicted in Figure 2, this is carried out by flanking the foreign DNA with vaccinia virus DNA sequences and then transfecting this recombinant DNA into vaccinia virus-infected cells [57,59]. The site of insertion of the foreign gene is determined by the flanking vaccinia DNA. To preserve the infectivity of the virus, the insertion must not destroy an essential gene. Several non-essential regions including those in the 9,000 bp region proximal to the left inverted terminal repetition [57], the

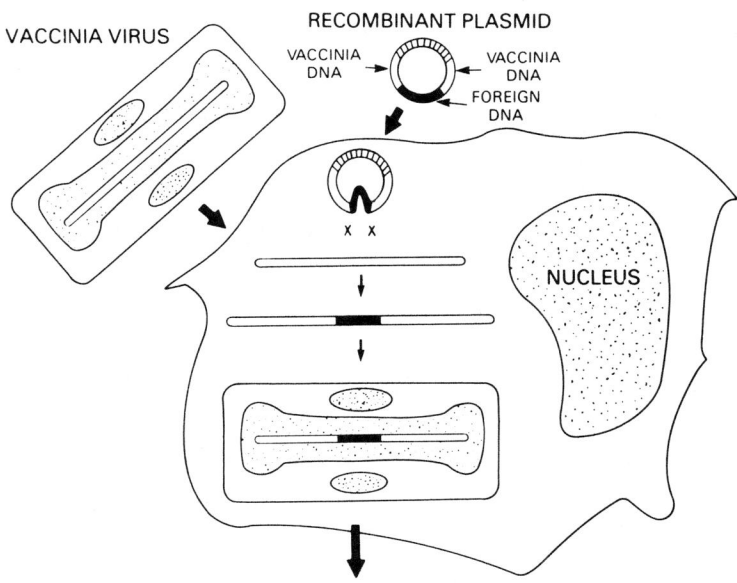

FIG. 2. Formation of vaccinia virus recombinants by homologous recombination.

thymidine kinase gene [57] and a site within the HindIII F fragment [59] have been used for this purpose. Since the recombinants comprise only a small percentage of the total progeny virus, a method of selection or screening is necessary. One general selection method has been to insert the foreign DNA into the thymidine kinase gene and, in that way, disrupt its function [57]. The TK⁻ recombinants are then selected by plaque assay in the presence of 5-bromodeoxyuridine. A similar approach was previously used to make rearrangements and deletions within the herpesvirus genome [60]. Alternatively, recombinant plaques can be screened by hybridization to the foreign DNA [59] or by expression of the foreign gene product [57,59,61].

Two approaches that use some or all of the above features for expression of foreign genes have been developed. The first consists of inserting foreign DNA into available sites within non-essential regions of the vaccinia virus genome [59,62]. Although technically simple, this procedure limits the promoters used, makes optimization of expression difficult, and can lead to the formation of fusion proteins with unpredictable properties. The second method involves the translocation of defined promoters from essential or non-essential genes and readily lends itself to optimization of expression, the synthesis of authentic or fusion products as desired, and the development of a general expression vector system [57,63]. To implement the latter procedure, a series of special plasmid vectors were constructed [63]. These plasmids contain a vaccinia virus promoter region, including the RNA start site and engineered restriction endonuclease sites for introduction of the foreign DNA, inserted into the coding region of the vaccinia thymidine kinase gene (Figure 3). The plasmids differ with regard to the vaccinia promoter and the restriction endonuclease sites. The foreign DNA segments that have been introduced typically have their natural translational initiation and termination codons so that authentic gene products will be formed.

Both the level and regulation of expression of the foreign gene are determined by the promoter used. These promoters fall into at least three classes: early, early/late, and late. In order to develop and evaluate vaccinia virus as an expression vector, a prokaryotic gene that encodes CAT was used. The assay for this enzyme is simple and quantitative and there is virtually no background since this activity is absent from eukaryotic cells [64]. Using the methods outlined in Figure 3, vaccinia virus recombinants containing the CAT gene regulated by early, early/late and late promoters were constructed [63,39]. The early promoter was excised from the TK gene, the early/late promoter from a gene that encodes a polypeptide of M_r 7,5000 (7.5K), and the late promoter from a structural polypeptide of M_r 28,000 (28K). The time courses of CAT expression in cells infected with these recombinants are shown in Figure 4. When the TK promoter was used, CAT activity was detected within 2 hr and peaked at about 6 hr. Cytosine arabinoside, an inhibitor of DNA replication, had little effect on CAT expression as expected for an early gene. With the 7.5K promoter, CAT expression occurred early but continued for a longer period than with the TK promoter. Moreover, cytosine arabinoside inhibited CAT expression by approximately 50 percent. Further analysis indicated that the 7.5K promoter contains tandemly arranged late and early transcriptional signals with separate RNA initiation sites [49]. The pattern of transcription appeared to be significantly different when the late 28K promoter was used. No CAT activity was detected until about 6 hr after infection and that was completely suppressed by cytosine arabinoside [39].

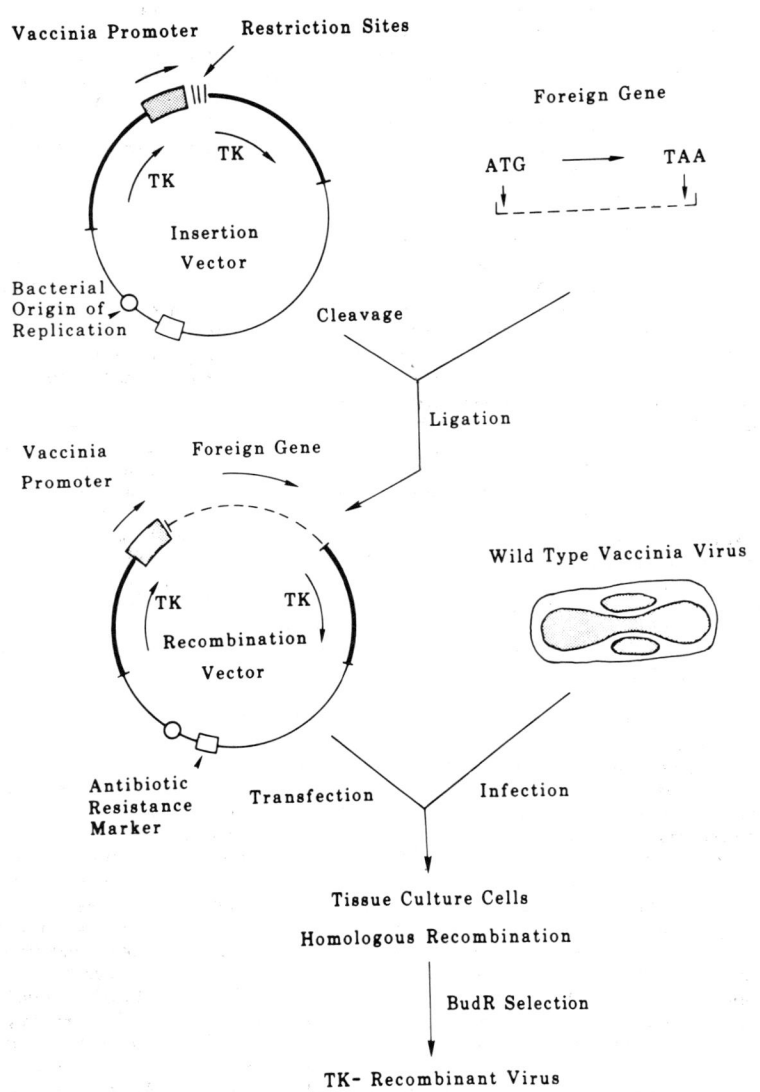

FIG. 3. System for insertion and expression of foreign genes in vaccinia virus. TK, thymidine kinase gene; ATG, translation initiation codon; TAA, translation termination codon; BudR, bromodeoxyuridine.

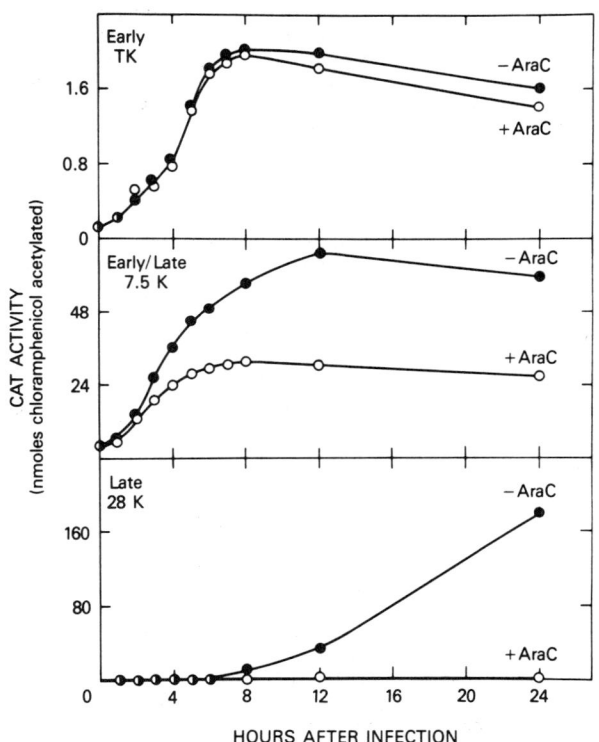

FIG. 4. Expression by vaccinia virus recombinants of chloramphenicol acetyltransferase (CAT) under control of 3 types of vaccinia virus promoters. Cells were infected with vaccinia virus recombinants in presence (+AraC) or absence of (-AraC) of cytosine arabinoside, an inhibitor of DNA replication. The promoters were isolated from the thymidine kinase (TK) gene or from genes expressing proteins of 7.5K or 28K.

CONCLUSION

With proper engineering, it appears that virtually any gene can be expressed in a vaccinia virus vector. Thus, genes from prokaryotes, e.g. CAT [63]; from DNA viruses, e.g. hepatitis B virus surface antigen [72,62]; herpes simplex virus thymidine kinase [57,59] and herpes simplex virus glycoprotein D [62,66]; from RNA viruses, e.g. influenza virus hemagglutinin [67,61]; vesicular stomatitis virus glycoprotein [68] and rabies virus glycoprotein [69,70]; and from Protozoan parasite, e.g. malaria circumsporozoite antigen [71] all have been expressed. In many cases the polypeptide products have been shown to be indistinguishable from the authentic protein, appropriately glycosylated, transported to the plasma membrane, and highly immunogenic. As our knowledge of vaccinia virus gene expression increases, the efficiency of the system will undoubtedly improve. New selection methods may make isolation of recombinant virus still easier. Since the capacity of the vaccinia virus genome for added foreign DNA is at least 25,000 bp [18], there should be no technical obstacle to the insertion and expression of multiple genes.

ACKNOWLEDGEMENTS

I am grateful for the collaborations with past and present members of my laboratory which have contributed to the development of vaccinia virus as a vector and would especially like to mention R. Wittek and J.A. Cooper for mapping the first vaccinia virus genes; S. Venkatesan and B.M. Baroudy for sequencing the genes and identifying putative promoter regions; J.P. Weir for locating and analyzing the thymidine kinase gene permitting development of a recombination and selection procedure; and M. Mackett and G.L. Smith for developing expression vector systems and demonstrating that vaccinia virus recombinants synthesize authentic foreign proteins and can be used for live immunization.

REFERENCES

1. S. Dales and B.G.T. Pogo in: Biology of Poxviruses (Virology Monographs, Vol. 18), D.W. Kingsbury and H. Zur Harusen, eds. (Springer-Verlag, New York 1981) pp. 1-109.
2. B. Moss in: Human Viral Diseases, B.N. Fields, R.M. Chanock and B. Roizman, eds. (Raven Press, New York 1985) in press.
3. L.G. Payne, J. Virol. 31, 147-155 (1979).
4. Y. Ichihashi, S. Matsumoto and S. Dales, Virology 46, 507-532 (1971).
5. C. Morgan, Virology 73, 43-58 (1976).
6. E.A. Boulter and G. Appleyard, Prob. Med. Virol. 16, 86-108 (1973).
7. L.G. Payne, J. Gen. Virol. 50, 89-100 (1980).
8. P. Geshelin and K.I. Berns, J. Mol. Biol. 88, 785-796 (1974).
9. C.F. Garon, E. Barbosa and B. Moss, Proc. Natl. Acad. Sci. USA 75, 4863-4867 (1978).
10. R. Wittek, A. Menna, K. Muller, D. Schumperli, P.G. Bosley and R. Wyler, J. Virol. 28, 171-181 (1978).
11. R. Wittek and B. Moss, Cell 21, 277-284 (1980).
12. B.M. Baroudy and B. Moss, J. Biol. Chem. 255, 4372-4380 (1980).
13. J.A. Cooper, R. Wittek and B. Moss, J. Virol. 37, 284-294 (1981a).
14. B.M. Baroudy, S. Venkatesan and B. Moss, Cell 28, 315-324 (1982).
15. D. Panicali, S.W. Davis, R.L. Weinberg and E. Paoletti, Proc. Natl. Acad. Sci. USA 80, 5364-5368 (1983).
16. B. Moss, E. Winters and J.A. Cooper, J. Virol. 40, 387-395 (1981).
17. R.W. Moyer and C.T. Rothe, Virology 102, 119-132 (1980).
18. G.L. Smith and B. Moss, Gene 25, 21-28 (1983).
19. C.K. Sam and K.R. Dumbell, Ann. Virol. 132E, 135-150 (1981).
20. K. Essani and S. Dales, Virology 95, 385-394 (1979).
21. E. Spencer, S. Shuman and J. Hurwitz, J. Biol. Chem. 255, 5388-5395 (1980).
22. B. Moss, E.N. Rosenblum and A. Gershowitz, J. Biol. Chem. 250. 4822-4729 (1975).
23. S.A. Martin, E. Paoletti and B. Moss, J. Biol. Chem. 250, 9322-9329 (1975).

24. S. Venkatesan, A. Gershowitz and B. Moss, J. Biol. Chem. 255, 903-908 (1980).
25. E. Barbosa and B. Moss, J. Biol. Chem. 253, 7692-7697 (1978).
26. E. Spencer, D. Loring, J. Hurwitz and G. Monroy, Proc. Natl. Acad. Sci. USA 75, 4793-4797 (1978).
27. E. Paoletti, H. Rosemond-Hornbeak and B. Moss, J. Biol. Chem. 249, 3273-3280 (1974).
28. E. Paoletti and B.R. Lipinskas, Virology 87, 317-325 (1978).
29. B.G.T. Pogo and M.T. O'Shea, Virology 77, 55-56 (1977).
30. H. Rosemond-Hornbeak and B. Moss, J. Biol. Chem. 249, 3292-3296 (1974).
31. W.R. Bauer, E.C. Ressner, J. Kates and J. Patzke, Proc. Natl. Acad. Sci. USA 74, 1841-1845 (1977).
32. J.H. Kleiman and B. Moss, J. Biol. Chem. 250, 2420-2429 (1975).
33. P. Arzoglou, R. Drillien and A. Kirn, Virology 95, 211-214 (1978).
34. E. Paoletti and L.J. Grady, J. Virol. 23, 608-615 (1977).
35. R.F. Boone and B. Moss,, J. Virol. 26, 554-569 (1978).
36. H. Belle Isle, S. Venkatesan and B. Moss, Virology 112, 306-317 (1981).
37. S. Venkatesan, A. Gershowitz and B. Moss, J. Virol. 44, 637-646 (1982).
38. J.P. Weir and B. Moss, J. Virol. 46, 530-537 (1983).
39. J.P. Weir and B. Moss, J. Virol. 51, 662-669 (1984).
40. S. Venkatesan, B.M. Baroudy and B. Moss, Cell 25, 805-813 (1981).
41. J.R. Nevins and W.K. Joklik, Virology 63, 1-14 (1975).
42. J.A. Cooper, R. Wittek and B. Moss, J. Virol. 39, 733-745 (1981).
43. A. Mahr and B.E. Roberts, J. Virol. 49, 510-520 (1984).
44. C. Colby, C. Jurale and J.R. Kates, J. Virol. 7, 71-76 (1971).
45. N.L. Varich, I.V. Sychova, N.V. Kaverin, T.P. Antonova and V.I. Chernos, Virology 96, 412-430 (1979).
46. R.F. Boone, R.P. Parr and B. Moss, J. Virol. 301, 365-374 (1979).
47. J.P. Weir, G. Bajszar and B. Moss, Proc. Natl. Acad. Sci. USA 79, 1210-1214 (1982).
48. C. Puckett and B. Moss, Cell 35, 441-448 (1983).
49. M.A. Cochran, C. Puckett and B. Moss, J. Virol., in press (1985).
50. M.D. Chalberg and P.T. Englund, J. Biol. Chem. 254, 7812-7819 (1979).
51. E.V. Jones and B. Moss, J. Virol. 49, 72-77 (1983).
52. M. Esteban and J.A. Holowczak, Virology 78, 57-75 (1977).
53. B.G.T. Pogo, M.T. O'Shea and P. Freimuth, Virology 108, 241-248 (1981).
54. R.W. Moyer and R.L. Graves, Cell 27, 391-401 (1981).
55. B. Moss, E. Winters and E.V. Jones in: Proceedings of the 1983 UCLA Symposium, N. Cozzarelli, ed. (A. Liss, New York, in press 1983) pp. 449-461.
56. G.V. Stokes, J. Virol. 18, 636-642 (1976).
57. M. Mackett, G.L. Smith and B. Moss, Proc. Natl. Acad. Sci. USA 79, 7415-7419 (1982).
58. E. Nakano, D. Panicali and E. Paoletti, Proc. Natl. Acad. Sci. USA 79, 1593-1596 (1982).
59. D. Panicali and E. Paoletti, Proc. Natl. Acad. Sci. USA 79, 4927-4931 (1982).
60. L.E. Post and B. Roizman, Cell 25, 227-232 (1981).
61. G.L. Smith, B.R. Murphy and B. Moss, Proc. Natl. Acad. Sci. USA 80, 7155-7159 (1983).
62. E. Paoletti, B.R. Lipinskas, C. Samsonoff, S. Mercer and D. Panicali, Proc. Natl. Acad. Sci. USA 81, 193-197 (1984).
63. M. Mackett, G.L. Smith and B. Moss, J. Virol. 49, 857-864 (1984).
64. C.M. Gorman, L.F. Moffat and B.H. Howard, Mol. Cell. Biol. 2, 1044-1051 (1982).

65. M.A. Cochran, M. Mackett and B. Moss, Proc. Natl. Acad. Sci. USA 82, 19-23 (1985).
66. K.J. Cremer, M. Mackett, C. Wohlenberg, A.L. Notkins and B. Moss, Science in press (1985).
67. D. Panicali, S.W. Davis, R.L. Weinberg and E. Paoletti, Proc. Natl. Acad. Sci. USA 80, 5364-5368 (1983).
68. M. Mackett, T. Yilma, J.K. Rose and B. Moss, Science 227, 433-435 (1985).
69. M.P. Kieny, R. Lathe, R. Drillien, D. Spehner, S. Skory, D. Schmitt, T. Wiktor, H. Koprowski and J.P. Lecocq, Nature 312, 163-166 (1984).
70. T.J. Wiktor, R.I. Macfarlan, K.J. Reagan, B. Dietzschold, P.J. Curtis, W.H. Wunner, M.P. Kieny, R. Lathe, J.P. Lecocq, M. Mackett, B. Moss and H. Koprowski, Proc. Natl. Acad. Sci. USA 81, 7194-7198 (1984).
71. G.L. Smith, G.N. Godson, V. Nussenzweig, R.S. Nussenzweig, J. Barnwell and B. Moss, Science 224, 397-399 (1984).
72. G.L. Smith, M. Mackett and B. Moss, Nature 302, 490-495 (1983).

GENETIC BASIS FOR VACCINIA VIRUS VIRULENCE

R. MARK L. BULLER* AND BERNARD MOSS*

*Laboratory of Viral Diseases, National Institute of Allergy and Infectious Diseases, National Institutes of Health, Rockville, Maryland 20205

INTRODUCTION

The orthopoxvirus genus contains a highly successful group of viruses which infect a large number of animal species (see Baxby, Dumbell this volume). Vaccinia virus, in particular, has a very broad host range in nature and has been reported to infect cows [1,2], pigs [3], buffaloes [4], and camels [5]. In the laboratory the virus replicates in a large number of tissue culture cell lines. Within the vaccinia virus specie, strains can show distinct differences in pathogenesis in the host. For example, during the smallpox eradication program a significantly higher incidence of post-vaccinial encephalitis was noted following vaccination with the Copenhagen strain of vaccinia virus as opposed to the Lister strain [6]. The basis of the enhanced virulence of the Copenhagen strain is most certainly at the level of the DNA sequence in the virus genome, and the exact region can potentially be deduced from studying DNA structure and function.

The vaccinia virus functions important to virus virulence in the host can be investigated by direct analysis of naturally occurring variants in the virus population, by the induction and isolation of conditionally lethal mutants or by insertional inactivation of specific gene functions using recombinant DNA techniques. The following article is an attempt to integrate recent studies directed towards defining important vaccinia virus virulence functions with what is known concerning orthopoxvirus virulence functions as a whole.

Orthopoxvirus Variants

Orthopoxviruses produce two types of pocks in the chick chorioallantoic membrane: an ulcerated pock with a hemorrhagic center (U^+) and a white nodular nonulcerated pock (U^-) [7,8]. The U^- pock variants arise with a frequency which varies with the parental virus strain examined but is usually about 1%, and exhibit certain characteristics which suggest they may be deletion mutants [9,10]. Subsequently, restriction endonuclease analysis of the genomic DNAs from U^- variants of cowpox [11,12], monkeypox [13,14] and rabbitpox [15-17] have characterized net DNA deletions at ends of the genome (Figure 1). In the case of rabbitpox virus, net DNA deletions of up to 10 and 20×10^6 daltons have been mapped to the left-hand and right-hand regions of the genome, respectively. If these deletions are additive, then 30×10^6 daltons of DNA are not essential for virus replication in certain cell lines [17]. This represents approximately 25% of the viral genome. Deletions at the left-hand end of the rabbitpox genome but not the right-hand end can affect the U^- variants's ability to replicate in pig kidney (Pk-15) and rabbit cornea (RC-60) cells [15,16]. Early studies by Fenner and colleagues demonstrated that certain white pox variants of rabbitpox virus showed reduced virulence for mice and rabbits following intracerebral and intradermal routes of virus inoculation, respectively [18]. This reduction in virulence was correlated with DNA deletions at the right-hand end of the genome [15]. The rabbitpox U^- phenotype can be generated by a deletion at either terminus, but with cowpox and monkeypox viruses compensated deletions have only been reported for the right-hand terminus of the genome [12,13,14].

Published 1985 by Elsevier Science Publishing Co., Inc.
VACCINIA VIRUSES AS VECTORS FOR VACCINE ANTIGENS, Quinnan, Editor

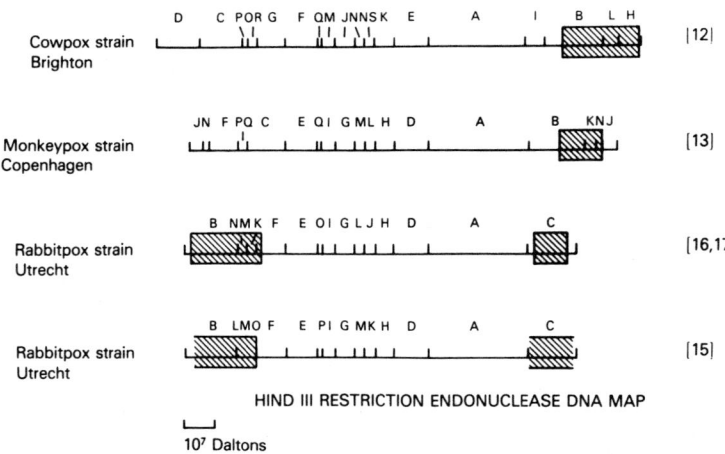

FIG. 1. The Hind III map of DNAs from U⁻ variants of cowpox strain Brighton, monkeypox strain Copenhagen, and rabbitpox strain Utrecht. The individual DNA maps were aligned with one another by choosing as a reference point the Hind III restriction enzyme site which separates fragments O and I on the original map of rabbitpox [13]. The cross-hatched box region delineates the position of the largest deletion observed in the U⁻ variants examined in the indicated references. An open-ended box indicates uncertainty with respect to the boundaries of the deletion.

Variants of vaccinia virus have been characterized by restriction endonuclease analysis to have large deletions at the left-hand end of the genome [19-21]. The WR-6/2 virus replicates normally in BS-C-1, Hela and Pk-15 cells, but has reduced virulence for mice by the intracerebral and intraperitoneal routes [22]. The Copenhagen-hr virus is unable to multiply in the human cell lines assayed. From the differences in the lengths of the deletions in WR-6/2 and Copenhagen-hr viruses and from marker rescue experiments, the function(s) required for replication in human cells are thought to lie in the Hind III N, M or K fragments (Figure 2).

One convenient model for defining orthopoxvirus virulence genes utilizes a natural virus disease of the inbred mouse: mousepox. Mousepox is caused by the ectromelia virus which shares both DNA sequence [23,24] and antigenic homology [25,26] with vaccinia virus. In the late 1940s, Fenner suggested that mousepox was analogous to generalized vaccinia and inoculation smallpox (Figure 3) [27]. Because ectromelia virus is an order of magnitude more virulent than vaccinia virus for the mouse, mousepox is a far more sensitive model system with which to analyze genes important in vaccinia virus virulence.

Ectromelia virus variants which had an altered pathogenesis in the BALB/cByJ mouse, have been isolated from T-lymphocyte-derived cell lines

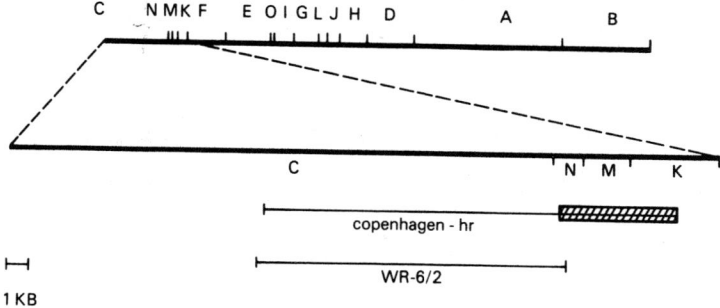

FIG. 2. The Hind III map of DNA deletion mutants of vaccinia virus. The thin horizontal line indicates the span of the deletion detected in variants Copenhagen-hr and WR-6/2. The hatched box denotes the fragment of DNA responsible for the host range phenotype in Copenhagen-hr as determined by marker rescue techniques.

which were persistently infected with ectromelia virus [28]. One such mutant, hr-1, appeared to produce less extracellular virus than wild-type virus during its replicative cycle as judged by the failure to show extensive comet formation, a term used to describe a series of secondary plaques tailing away from the primary plaque. These secondary plaques are thought to result from the natural release from infected cells of extracellular enveloped virions (EEV) which may be important in dissemination of the virus in the infected host [29,30]. BALB/cByJ mice infected with this mutant by the footpad route did not die and showed no detectable virus in spleen or liver by day 17 post-infection, whereas mice inoculated with WT virus died by day 9. Elucidating the genomic location and function of the genes(s) that are altered in hr-1 is in progress, as is the search for comparable genes in the vaccinia virus genome.

These data taken together argue that the DNA sequences near the termini of orthopoxviruses are not essential for growth in the chick chorioallantoic membrane and in certain cell lines, but are important for host range phenotypes and pathogenesis in the host. Consistent with this region of the DNA being important in virus specie specific virulence functions is the observation that the DNA sequence homology among orthopoxviruses is lower near the termini than in the central portion of the genome [23,24,31].

Conditional Lethal Mutants of Vaccinia Virus

Three separate laboratories using either vaccinia virus strain WR or strain Copenhagen have isolated over 123 virus mutants which are temperature-sensitive (ts) in functions necessary for virus replication in either primary chick embryo fibroblasts or an African green monkey kidney cell line, BSC-40 [32,34]. Using marker rescue techniques the positions of these ts mutants have been determined on the Hind III

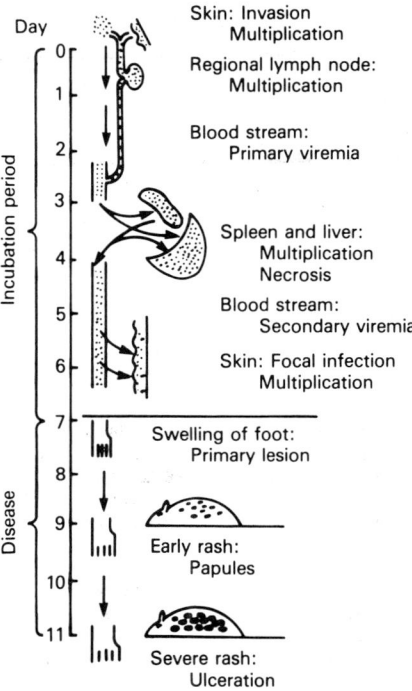

FIG. 3. Mousepox, a model for generalized vaccinia and inoculation smallpox [27].

restriction endonuclease map of vaccinia DNA (Figure 4). One striking feature of the distribution of the vaccinia virus ts mutations along the DNA restriction maps is the clustering within the central region of the genome which has been shown to be highly conserved among orthopoxvirus species [23,24]. However, it must be noted that in Figure 4B the cloned DNA fragments which were tested for marker rescue of the ts mutants comprised less than 50% of the vaccinia genome. Furthermore, the large size of Hind III fragment A used in the marker rescue experiments depicted in Figure 4C does not permit as accurate an assignment of mutant map position in this portion of the genome as does the analysis shown in Figure 4A. As seen previously (Figure 1) the DNA sequences near the left (Hind III fragments C, N, M) and the right terminus (Hind III fragment B) do not appear to be essential for replication in certain tissue culture cells, and therefore ts mutants would not be expected to be isolated from these portions of the genome.

These data can be interpreted to suggest that the highly conserved central portion of the genome contains the majority of the basic functions required for vaccinia virus replication. To date, DNA polymerase [35], thymidine kinase [36] and a number of virion structural polypeptides [37,38] have been shown to be coded by this region of the genome.

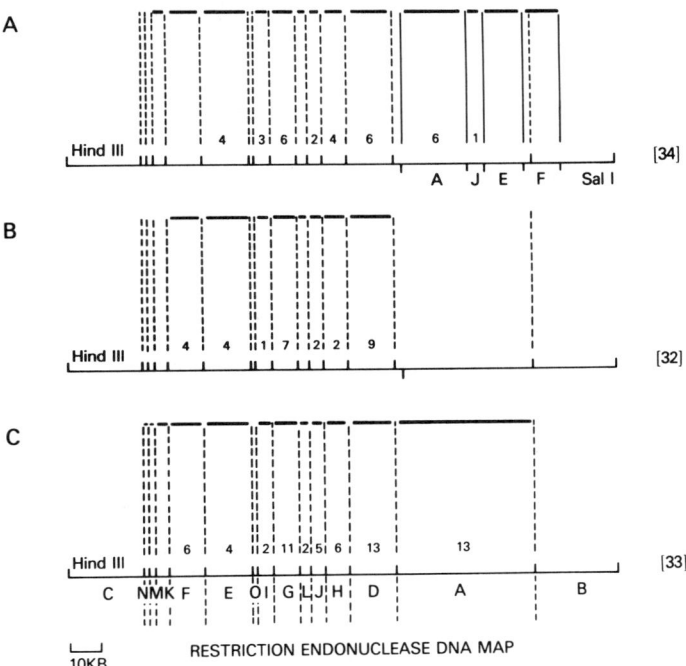

FIG. 4. The physical map of ts mutants of vaccinia virus. The vertical broken and solid lines indicate the cleavage sites on the vaccinia virus DNA genome of the restriction endonucleases Hind III and Sal I, respectively. Marker rescue experiments using Sal I were only carried out in reference 34. The horizontal broken thick lines indicate the cloned vaccinia virus DNA fragments which were used in the marker rescue experiments. The arabic numbers denote the number of mutant isolates rescued by each DNA fragment.

Insertional Inactivation of Vaccinia Virus Virulence Genes

Foreign DNA has been inserted into several regions of the vaccinia virus genome in order to create infectious vaccinia virus recombinants which have been evaluated as eucaryotic expression vectors [39,40]. One segment of the genome used for insertion of foreign DNA mapped to an Eco RI/Ava I fragment contained in the 9 kb sequence proximal to the left terminus of the genome which is defined by the 6/2 deletion (Figure 2). This region of the vaccinia virus genome is non-essential for replication in tested cell lines, but appears to be important for virus virulence in the mouse [19,22]. The site used most extensively in the construction of vaccinia virus recombinants (which have been evaluated as candidate vaccines) is located in the thymidine kinase gene (Hind III J fragment). The role of the virus-coded thymidine kinase (TK) is to

provide a sufficient pool of thymidine triphosphate for virus DNA
synthesis in host cells which are not actively dividing, and therefore
have lower endogenous levels of the precursors for DNA synthesis [41-43].
Thymidine kinase minus (TK$^-$) vaccinia virus strains, which have been
isolated either by chemical mutagenesis or by insertional inactivation
of the TK locus, showed a marked reduction in virulence for the mouse
by the intracerebral and intraperitoneal routes of inoculation [22,44].
This attenuation of the vaccinia virus recombinants can be attributed
totally to the thymidine kinase negative phenotype. Similarly, TK$^-$ HSV
type 1 and 2 and marmoset herpes viruses showed a reduced virulence in
mice compared to that of wt virus [45,46].

To further examine the effect of a TK$^-$ phenotype on vaccinia virus
virulence, two distinct strains of vaccinia virus and their respective
recombinants were used to inoculate New Zealand white rabbits. The
Wyeth strain is the New York City Board of Health (NYCBH) strain used
extensively in the U.S. and elsewhere for smallpox vaccination. The WR
strain was derived from the NYCBH strain by multiple passage in mouse
brain [47]. The virulence of TK$^-$ vaccinia virus recombinants (constructed

TABLE I. The response of rabbits to varying doses of wild-type and
thymidine kinase minus vaccinia strains.

Rabbit	Virus inoculated[a]	Virus dose	Lesion character	
			Ulcer	diameter (mm)
1	WR-wt	1.5×10^1	–	–
		1.5×10^2	+	4
		1.5×10^3	+	7
		1.5×10^4	+	8
		1.5×10^5	+	10
		1.5×10^6	+	11
	WR-vHBs4	2.1×10^1	–	–
		2.1×10^2	–	–
		2.1×10^3	–	–
		2.1×10^4	+	2
		2.1×10^5	+	2
		2.1×10^6	+	4
2	NYCBH(Wyeth)-wt	8×10^1	–	–
		8×10^2	–	–
		8×10^3	–	–
		8×10^4	+	3
		8×10^5	+	7
		8×10^6	+	8
	NYCBH(Wyeth)-v55	7×10^1	–	–
		7×10^2	–	–
		7×10^3	–	–
		7×10^4	+	1
		7×10^5	+	2
		7×10^6	+	7

[a]The backs of two New Zealand white rabbits were shaved. To rabbit
one, increasing doses of WR-wt and WR-vHBs4 virus were inoculated
subcutaneously on the left and right sides of the dorsal midline,
respectively. Similarly, rabbit two was inoculated with NYCBH(Wyeth)-wt
and NYCBH(Wyeth)-v55. At eleven days post-inoculation the site of
inoculation was scored as ulcerated or not, and a lesion diameter was
recorded.

by inserting DNA coding for the HBsAg into either the WR [48,49] or NYCBH (Wyeth) strain of vaccinia virus) was compared with parental wt virus by measuring the diameter of the lesion at the site of inoculation (Table I). The dose of virus required to ulcerate the skin was 1.5×10^2 and 2.1×10^4 pfu for WR-wt and WR-vHBs4 viruses, respectively. Furthermore, the diameter of the lesion was greater with the WR-wt than recombinant at comparable doses. The results with the NYCBH(Wyeth) strain of virus were similar, although the magnitude of the difference between TK^- recombinant and TK^+ parental virus was not as great as seen with the WR strain. In both NYCBH(Wyeth)-wt and v55 recombinant similar doses of virus were needed to detect ulceration of the skin, although the diameter of the ulcer was larger with the NYCBH(Wyeth)-wt virus at all doses tested. The NYCBH(Wyeth)-wt lesion also appeared to have more protuberant character than the comparable lesion caused by the recombinant virus. Although both the WR and Wyeth strains were derived from the NYCBH strain, the former appeared to be far more virulent for the rabbit (Table I).

Experiments carried out in chimpanzees indicated that the animal inoculated with WR-wt virus developed a larger primary lesion (diameter 37 mm) than that seen with the two animals inoculated with the recombinant WR-vHBs4 virus (diameter = 22 and 24 mm) [49]. In summary, TK^- recombinant viruses appeared less virulent than wt in the three animal species tested.

DISCUSSION

The data is consistent with a model where functions coded in the DNA from the left-hand and right-hand terminal regions of the orthopoxvirus genome are not essential for replication of the virus in certain tissue culture cell lines, but are concerned with host range and virus virulence in the animal. The TK^- recombinant viruses, which have been shown to protect animals from subsequent challenge with the appropriate infectious agents [48-54], where examined, have been shown to be less virulent for mice, rabbits and chimpanzees than the TK positive non-recombinant parental virus [22,44,49]. This may suggest that a general feature of TK^- vaccinia virus will be an attenuated virulence pattern in the host. The relative importance of the thymidine kinase gene product to virus pathogenesis will become clearer as we gain more information on the number and function of the remaining vaccinia virus virulence genes.

REFERENCES

1. El.H. Dahaby, El.A. Sabbagh, M. Nassar, M. Kamell and M. Iskander, J. Arab. Vet. Med. Ass. 26, 11-24 (1966).
2. F. Dekking in: Zoonoses, J. Van Der ed. (Amsterdam Elsevier 1964) pp. 411-418.
3. N.N. Maltseva, E.M. Akatova-Shelukhina, M.A. Yumasheva and S.S. Marennikova, J. Hyg. Epidemiol. Microbiol. Immunol. 10, 202-209 (1966).
4. D. Baxby and B.J. Hill, Arch. Ges. Virus Forsch. 35, 70-79 (1971).
5. S.S. Krupenko, Veterinariya, Moskva No. 8, 61-62 (1972).
6. M.F. Polak in: International Symposium on Smallpox Vaccine, Bilthoven, The Netherlands, 11-13 October 1972, Symposia Series in Immunobiological Standardization, Vol 19, pp. 235-242.
7. A.W. Downie and D.W. Haddock, Lancet i, 1049-1050 (1952).
8. F. Fenner and B.M. Comben, Virol. 5, 530-548 (1958).
9. C.J.M. Rondle and K.R. Dumbell, J. Hyg. 60, 41-49 (1962).
10. D. Baxby and C.J.M. Rondle, J. Hyg. 66, 191-205 (1968).

11. L.C. Archard and M. Mackett, J. Gen. Virol. 45, 51-63 (1979).
12. L.C. Archard, M. Mackett, D.E. Barnes and K.R. Dumbell, J. Gen. Virol. 65, 875-886 (1984).
13. K.R. Dumbell and L.C. Archard, Nature 286, 29-32 (1980).
14. J.J. Esposito, C.D. Cabradilla, J.H. Nakano and J.F. Obijeski, Virology 109, 231-243 (1981).
15. J.R. Lake and P.D. Cooper, J. Gen. Virol. 48, 135-147 (1980).
16. R.W. Moyer and C.T. Rothe, Virol. 102, 119-132 (1980).
17. R.W. Moyer, R.L. Graves and C.T. Rothe, Cell 22, 545-553 (1980).
18. A. Gemmell and F. Fenner, Virol. 11, 219-235 (1960).
19. B. Moss, E. Winters and J. Cooper, J. Virol. 40, 387-395 (1981).
20. D. Panicali, S.W. Davis, S.R. Mercer and E. Paoletti, J. Virol. 37, 1000-1010 (1981).
21. R. Drillien, F. Koehren and A. Kirn, Virol. 111, 488-499 (1981).
22. R.M.L. Buller, G.L. Smith, K. Cremer, A.L. Notkins and B. Moss, submitted to Nature.
23. M. Mackett and L.C. Archard, J. Gen. Virol. 45, 683-701 (1979).
24. H.K. Muller, R. Wittek, W. Schaffner, D. Schumperli, A. Menna and R. Wyler, J. Gen. Virol. 38, 135-147 (1978).
25. F.M. Burnet and W.D. Boake, J. Immunol. 53, 1-13 (1946).
26. F. Fenner, Aust. J. Exp. Biol. Med. Sci. 27, 1-18 (1949).
27. F. Fenner, Lancet ii, 915-921 (1948).
28. R.M.L. Buller in: Viral and Mycoplasma Infections of Laboratory Rodents: Effects on Biomedical Research, P. Bhatt, H. Morse, A. New and R. Jacoby, eds., in press.
29. G. Appleyard, A.J. Hapel and E.A. Boulter, J. Gen. Virol. 13, 9-17 (1971).
30. L.G. Payne and E. Norrby, J. Gen. Virol. 32, 63-72 (1976).
31. D. Schumperli, A. Menna, F. Schwendimann, R. Wittek and R. Wyler, J. Gen. Virol. 47, 385-398 (1980).
32. R.C. Condit, A. Motyczka and G. Spizz, Virol. 128, 429-443 (1983).
33. M.J. Ensinger and M. Rovinsky, J. Virol. 48, 419-428 (1983).
34. R. Drillien and D. Spehner, Virol. 131, 385-393 (1983).
35. E.V. Jones and B. Moss, J. Virol. 49, 72-77 (1984).
36. J.P. Weir, G. Bajszar and B. Moss, Proc. Natl. Acad. Sci. USA 79, 1210-1214 (1982).
37. R. Wittek, B. Richner and G. Hiller, Nucleic Acid Res. 12, 4835-4847 (1984).
38. R. Wittek, M. Hanggi and G. Hiller, J. Virol. 49, 371-378 (1984).
39. M. Mackett, G.L. Smith and B. Moss, Proc. Natl. Acad. Sci. USA 79, 7415-7419 (1982).
40. D. Panicali and E. Paoletti, Proc. Natl. Acad. Sci. USA 79, 4927-4931 (1982).
41. H.G. Klemperer, G.R. Haynes, W.I.H. Shedden and D.H. Watson, Virol. 31, 120-128 (1967).
42. M.E. Thouless and P. Wildy, J. Gen. Virol. 26, 159-170 (1975).
43. A.T. Jamieson,, G.A. Gentry and J.H. Subak-Sharpe, J. Gen. Virol. 24, 465-480 (1974).
44. R.M.L. Buller, G.L. Smith, K. Cremer, A.L. Notkins and B. Moss in: Vaccines 85: Molecular and Chemical Basis of Resistance to Viral, Bacterial and Parasitic Diseases, R. Chanock and R. Lerner, eds., in press.
45. H.J. Field and P. Wildy, J. Hyg. Camb. 81, 267-277 (1978).
46. S. Kit, H. Qavi, D.R. Dubbs and H. Otsuka, J. Med. Virol. 12, 25-36 (1983).
47. D. Stevens in: American Type Culture Collection Catalogue of Strains, Fourth edition (American Type Culture Collection, MD 1983) p. 328.
48. G.L. Smith, M. Mackett and B. Moss, Nature 302, 490-495 (1983).
49. B. Moss, G.L. Smith, J.L. Gerin and R.H. Purcell, Nature 311, 67-69 (1984).

50. G.L. Smith, B. Murphy and B. Moss, Proc. Natl. Acad. Sci. USA 80, 7155-7159 (1983).
51. K. Cremer, M. Mackett, C. Wohlenberg, A.L. Notkins and B. Moss in: Vaccines 85: Molecular and Chemical Basis of Resistance for Viral, Bacterial and Parasitic Diseases, R. Channok and R. Lerner, eds., in press.
52. M.P. Kieny, R. Lathe, R. Drillien, D. Spehner, S. Skory, D. Schmitt, T. Wiktor, H. Koprowski and J.P. Lecocq, Nature 312, 163-166 (1984).
53. T.J. Wiktor, R.I. MacFarlan, K.J. Reagan, B. Dietzschold, P.J. Curtis, W.H. Wunner, M.P. Kieny, R. Lathe, J.P. Lecocq, M. Mackett, B. Moss and H. Koprowski, Proc. Natl. Acad. Sci. USA 81, 7194-7198 (1984).
54. M. Mackett, T. Yilma, J.K. Rose and B. Moss, Science 227, 433-435 (1985).

DISCUSSION

Dr. Quinnan: Have you had an opportunity to look at all, at any other strains such as CV-1, to begin to define the genetic basis of attenuation and would you comment more on the relevance of the mouse neurotropism model to human disease?

Dr. Esposito: I just did a limited analysis of CV-1. It looks like it has a deletion at the left-hand end compared to the New York Board of Health and Lister strains.

Dr. Buller: With regard to the question concerning the relevance of mouse neurovirulence, the biology of these viruses is such that each animal model is of limited use. One might point out in this case, however, that the TK gene function may be important for neurovirulence in all species, since neural cells are resting cells.

Dr. Ada: Dr. Blandon has studied the susceptibility of different inbred strains of mice to ectromelia virus. There are two effects, one linked to H2, the other not. Susceptibility linked to H2 genes varied over 1,000-fold range. The genes that were not H2-linked were associated with variations in susceptibility over a 100,000-fold range. He correlated susceptibility with ease or the rapidity of spread of the virus from the skin to internal organs. That is, the slower the virus penetrated into the animal, the more resistant the animals were to the virus.

Dr. Buller: That's right. It seems to be a race between the virus reaching the target organ and replicating to a high enough titer to destroy it, the liver in this case, and the immune system responding. The initial observations were made by Schnell. He studied crosses of different mouse strains and found that the C57Bl mouse had an autosomal dominant resistance locus when crossed with outbred mice. Blandon followed that by crossing the C57Bl/10 mouse with the A mouse and found essentially the same thing, in that cross resistance was mainly dependent on the non-H2-linked genes.

Dr. Dumbell: Dr. Mackett and I have mapped the DIS mutant of the Japanese vaccinia strain. That has a left end deletion which starts in the K fragment, includes the M and the N fragments, and extends out to the terminal repetition. We did marker rescue experiments with a fragment which stops at the left-hand end of M and N, and found that its ability to grow in human and rabbit cells had been restored. Even though the host range of the virus was restored, however, the rescued virus continued to produce small pocks in the egg membrane, like the DIS mutant.

Dr. Boyle: Would you mention again the markers you use for measuring or quantitating the amount of extracellular virus in your ectromelia system?

Dr. Buller: There were three measures. One was comet formation, the tail extending away from the primary plaque. It is a very clear and dramatic effect. If extracellular virus is not produced, you just get a round lytic center only. The second was titration of virus in the extracellular fluid of an infected culture. The third was to separate intracellular and extracellular virus particles by gradient centrifugation.

Dr. Boyle: Have you looked at the rates of growth of TK plus and TK minus vaccinia in serum starved cells? In the case of herpes simplex virus there is a difference in the ability of the plus and minus viruses to grow in the serum-starved cells.

Dr. Buller: We haven't examined growth in serum-starved cells.

Dr. Boyle: Are viruses with inserts in other regions, for example the F region, attenuated?

Dr. Paoletti: In trying to understand attenuation in terms of reduced capacity to cause central nervous system disease, I think a more critical issue may be the blood-brain barrier. Dr. Kato described a variant strain that was attenuataed in ability to cross that barrier. I am curious to know whether that particular strain is TK plus or TK minus.

Dr. Kato: As far as I know, it is TK plus.

Dr. Buller: I think it is important to understand the pathogenesis of central nervous system disease, and it is not clear in my mind whether it is caused by virus replication in the central nervous system or an autoimmune reaction.

PART II

SMALLPOX VACCINES

Chairperson: G.V. Quinnan, Jr.

COMPLICATIONS OF SMALLPOX VACCINATION

ISAO ARITA* AND FRANK FENNER**

*Smallpox Eradication, World Health Organization, Geneva, Switzerland;
**The John Curtin School of Medical Research, The Australian National University, Canberra, Australia.

INTRODUCTION

One of the important benefits that flowed from the success of the global smallpox eradication programme was that routine smallpox vaccination could be dispensed with in all countries. Of 162 WHO member states, all except Albania had ceased smallpox vaccination of the general public by November 1984. The resulting savings, including the costs of vaccinations, port health inspections and the medical treatment required for complications of smallpox vaccination, is estimated to be US$1000 million annually.

While national health authorities and the world scientific community are gratified with this situation, a new scientific development, namely the use of vaccinia vector vaccines for the control of communicable diseases other than smallpox, necessitates a reappraisal of the situation. If the efficacy of new vaccines based on genetically engineered vaccinia virus is proved, is it justifiable to use them in national immunization programmes? Such vaccines would have four advantages: (1) production is easy, (2) production costs are low, (3) freeze-dried vaccine is very heat stable, and (4) it is easily administered. If suitable genes can be inserted and are adequately expressed, such genetically engineered vaccines have great potential to control severe and widespread diseases such as malaria or hepatitis B, especially in Third World countries. The major disadvantage could be the return of postvaccinal complications. In order to make rational decisions, the advantages of such vaccines must be weighed against the disadvantage of complications. Recently we reviewed the literature on the complications of vaccination, and to facilitate your appraisal of this matter, we would like to try to present here as clear a picure as possible of the complications of vaccination with vaccinia virus. In making this analysis we have ignored the use of attenuated vaccines. The few that were tested on a large enough scale multiplied so poorly in man that they were not sufficiently immunogenic for use as a protection against smallpox. Others that were more recently developed are G9 strain in China and LC16m8 strain in Japan. More information is required to evaluate their efficacy and their liability to produce complications.

Types of Complications

Three types of complications occurred among vaccinated subjects: (1) abnormal skin eruptions, (2) disorders affecting the central nervous system, and (3) a variety of other less severe complications.

Abnormal skin eruptions. This group included four syndromes with different predisposing factors and different prognoses (Figure 1):

Progressive vaccinia (Figure 1A) was the most severe complication of vaccination. The local lesion at the vaccination site failed to heal, secondary lesions appeared elsewhere on the body and all lesions spread progressively until the patient usually died two to five months later. It occurred only among persons with a deficient cell-mediated

Published 1985 by Elsevier Science Publishing Co., Inc.
VACCINIA VIRUSES AS VECTORS FOR VACCINE ANTIGENS, Quinnan, Editor

immune mechanism, either because of a congenital deficiency or a lymphoproliferative disorder, or from immunosuppressive treatment. The case-fatality rate was extremely high, treatment by vaccinia-immune globulin rarely being effective.

Eczema vaccinatum (Figure 1B) was much more common, and occurred among persons with eczema who were vaccinated (although eczema was a contraindication to vaccination in many countries) and also among eczematous contacts of newly-vaccinated persons. Either coincident with or shortly after the development of the local vaccinial lesion (or after an incubation period of about five days in unvaccinated eczematous contacts) a vaccinial eruption occurred on areas of skin that were eczematous at the time or had previously been so. These areas became intensely inflamed and sometimes the eruption spread to healthy skin. Constitutional symptoms were usually severe. The reported case-fatality rates varied greatly in different series of cases, but according to Kempe, 30% to 40% died. Treatment with vaccinia-immune globulin reduced the case-fatality rate to 7% [2].

Generalized vaccinia (Figure 1C) followed hematogenous spread of vaccinia virus, with the production of pustular lesions on many parts of the body. The course of the individual skin lesions resembled that at the vaccination site, but if the rash was profuse the lesions sometimes varied greatly in size. It did not seem to be associated with immunological deficiencies, and had a good prognosis. Vaccinia-immune globulin was effective in hastening resolution of the lesions.

Accidental infections (Figure 1D) could occur both in vaccinees and contacts, the most serious being those affecting the eyes or the perineum. Vaccinia-immune globulin was helpful in treatment.

Treatment

Several drugs were tried for the treatment of these complications, including cytosine arabinoside, rifampicin, urea derivative of diphenyl sulphone and methisazone. None was as effective as vaccinia-immune globulin, which was useful for all skin complications except progressive vaccinia.

Prevention

In countries with well-developed medical services, progressive vaccinia could be reduced by strictly observing the rule that congenital or acquired immunodeficiencies, and immunosuppressive treatment, were absolute contraindications to vaccination. Active eczema or a history of eczema were regarded as contraindications to vaccination in most industrialized countries. Administration of vaccinia-immune globulin at the time of vaccination reduced the frequency of eczema vaccinatum in persons with eczema in whom vaccination was essential [5]. However, if vaccinia vector vaccines are introduced, these measures are unlikely to be effective in developing countries, where vaccinia-immune globulin is not readily available and in general contraindications are not applied to immunization programmes. On the other hand, children with congenital immunodeficiencies are unlikely to survive other childhood infections.

Accidental or contact vaccinial infections will be a problem if immunization with a vaccinia vector vaccine is applied only to certain risk groups while the rest of the population remains susceptible to vaccinia. Vaccinial infections among contacts of newly vaccinated military recruits have been reported recently in the USA and Canada.

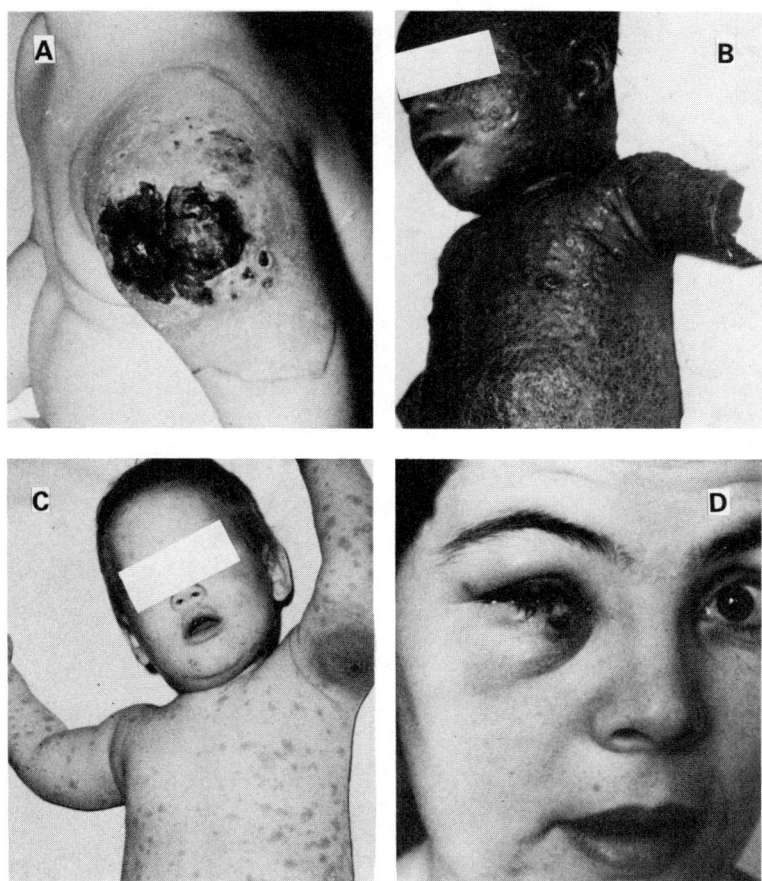

FIG. 1. Cutaneous complication of vaccinia virus infection: A. progressive vaccinia which was fatal, in a child with immunodeficiency; B. eczema vaccinatum in the unvaccinated contact of a vaccinated sibling; C. generalized vaccinia 10 days after vaccination, benign course, no residual scarring; D. accidental infection with vaccinia virus. (Photos courtesy of the late Dr. Henry Kempe.)

Disease Affecting the Central Nervous System (CNS)

CNS disease was the most serious vaccinial complication, in that it was associated with a 30% case-fatality rate and, unlike progressive vaccinia and eczema vaccinatum, its occurrence was unpredictable. In fact, many industrialized countries contributed to the global smallpox eradication programme in the hope that with the eradication of smallpox, the termination of smallpox vaccination programmes would eliminate the occurrence of postvaccinial encephalitis and encephalopathy.

For diagnosis of post vaccinial complications of the central nervous system, however, it should be borne in mind that vaccinia virus was rarely recovered from central nervous systems of fatal cases and that the diagnosis was principally based on the temporal relation of central nervous system disturbance to vaccination. The recorded cases may well have included illness from other causes, the timing of the encephalitis being purely coincidental to recent vaccination. Nevertheless, serious neurological complications were sometimes caused by smallpox vaccination.

Weber and Lange [6] studied autopsy records of 265 cases of postvaccinial CNS disease and demonstrated that the disease in children less than 2 years of age was usually an encephalopathy, with histological findings of brain edema and hyperemia. On the other hand, in older children and adults encephalomyelitis was found, with demyelinisation similar to that seen in other post-infection encephalitides, such as is seen after measles. This differentiation of encephalopathy and encephalitis was consistent with earlier observations made by de Vries (1960). The distribution of these two types of CNS disease by age and incubation period is shown in Figure 2.

Encephalopathy started with convulsions, commonly accompanied by hemiplegia and aphasia. Recovery was incomplete, the patient being left with cerebral impairment and hemiplegia. On the other hand, encephalomyelitis was marked by vomiting, malaise, disorientation, delirium, convulsions and coma. In non-fatal cases, recovery was usually complete and often rapid. Wilson [7] suggested that the overall case-fatality rate was about 30%, but encephalopathy appeared to cause more deaths than encephalomyelitis.

There were no effective treatment and no effective preventive measures for either type of CNS disease.

Other Complications of Vaccination

Fetal vaccinia occurred as a very rare complication of pregnancy; multiple sclerosis or malignant skin tumors were said to be related but their links with vaccination were probably purely coincidental. These complications were not a public health problem and hence will not be discussed further.

Frequency

We start by focussing on the first group of complications—progressive vaccinia, eczema vaccinatum, generalized vaccinia and accidental infections with vaccinia virus. A great deal has been published regarding these complications, but it is difficult to draw definite conclusions since the frequencies reported at different times and in different countries varied greatly, for various reasons. Wilson [7] reviewed ten different reports from 1931 to 1963 in the United Kingdom, Federal

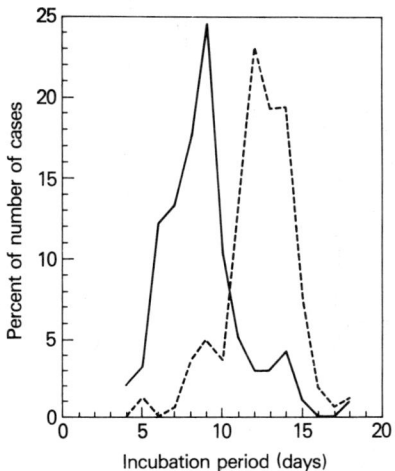

FIG. 2. Distribution of incubation period of 259 cases of post-vaccinial cerebral damage following primary vaccination. Solid line indicates encephalopathy in children <2 years of age. Dash line indicates post-vaccinial encephalomyelitis in children >2 years of age. Reproduced from Weber and Lange [6].

Republic of Germany and USA (1964) and found that the frequency of eczema vaccinatum per million primary vaccinations varied from 2.9 in Bavaria (1945-1953) to 185 in England and Wales in 1962, when mass vaccination was carried out because of outbreaks of smallpox. This great variation reflects the care with which eczematous subjects were excluded from vaccination; in earlier surveys (1951-1960) in the United Kingdom the frequency was 3.2 per million.

Two surveys conducted in the USA in 1968 are worth examining here, as they provide much the most comprehensive surveys of vaccination complications of all kinds in a large country over a period of one year. One was a national survey of smallpox vaccination complications [3] and the other a ten-state survey conducted in the same year [4] to assess the validity of the national survey. The national survey utilized essentially passive methods for collecting data, finding complications through miscellaneous routes such as the distribution of vaccinia-immune globulin and methisazone, reports of complications from state epidemiologists or Red Cross consultants or vaccine producers, and reported cases of encephalitis, etc. For the other survey physicians were approached directly. Although the sample numbers were smaller, frequencies of all complications were greater in the ten-state survey, especially for the less severe complications. The results of the ten-state survey are summarized in Table I. For comparison purposes, the results of a national survey are also cited.

TABLE I. Complications of smallpox vaccination in the USA in 1968

Status and age (years)	Number of vaccinations	Post-vaccinial encephalitis	Progressive vaccinia	Eczema vaccinatum	Generalized vaccinia	Accidental infection erythema multiforme, and others[a]
		Complication Rates (Cases per Million)				
		Results of a 10 State Survey				
Primary Vaccination[c])						
<1	71,000	42	–	14[b]	394	1,099
1-4	317,000	9.5	3.2[b]	44	233	972
>5	262,000	7.6	–	34	149	748
Revaccination[d])						
<1	–	–	–	–	–	–
1-4	55,000	–	–	–	–	200
>5	943,000	2.1	3.2	3.2	9.5	81
		Results of a National Survey				
Primary Vaccination[e])						
<1	614,000	6.5	–	8.1	70.0	27.7
1-4	2,733,000	2.2	0.4[b]	11.3	17.2	47.9
>5	2,247,000	2.7	1.8	9.3	16.9	23.6
Revaccination						
<1	0	–	–	–	–	–
1-4	478,000	–	–	2.1[b]	–	4.2
>5	8,096,000	–	0.7	0.9	1.2	1.7

a) Others include bacterial infections and severe reactions requiring medical care.
b) Computed based on 1 case.
c) Excludes 59 complications of unknown age group.
d) Excludes 4 complications of unknown age group.
e) Excludes 5 complications of unknown age group.

Based on Lane, et al. (1969 and 1970).

TABLE II. Summary of post-vaccinial complications of the central nervous system

Survey number	Country	Investigator	Year investigated	Cases per million primary vaccinations			Vaccinia strains
				Encephalopathy age <2 years	Encephalomyelitis age >2 years		
1	Austria	Berger & Puntigam (1954)	1948-53	103	1,211		–
2	Hamburg	Seelemann (1960)	1939-58	93	449		–
3	Bavaria	Herrlich (1954)	1945-53	56	121		–
4	Holland	Stuart (1947)	1930-43	50	348		–
5	Holland	van den Berg (1946)	1924-28	39	232		–
6	UK	Conybeare (1964)	1951-60	15[a]	15		Lister
7	USA (10 states)	Lane, et al (1970)	1968	42[a]	9		New York City Board of Health
8	USA (National)	Lane, et al (1969)	1968	7[a]	2		New York City Board of Health

a) Age less than one year.

Based on Wilson (1967).

Looking at the total incidence for all age groups may not be relevant, since each vaccinia vector vaccine, if used, is likely to be targeted at a certain age group in the population, which may be different from the target populations of the smallpox vaccination programme in the USA in the 1960s. In the ten-state survey, the frequency of eczema vaccinatum was 14 patients per million primary vaccinations in children under 12 months of age and 44 patients per million among those of 1 to 4 years of age. Revaccination was rarely carried out in children under 5 years of age, but the incidence of eczema vaccinatum was much lower in revaccinated subjects. Only one case of progressive vaccinia was noted after primary vaccination, in an infant with hypogammaglobulinemia. In older persons, most of whom received revaccination, the frequency of progressive vaccinia was the same as in children (although the cause was usually a lymphoproliferative disorder, rather than a congenital immunodeficiency).

Despite many studies, there is still difficulty in assessing the true incidence of postvaccinial CNS disease. Utilization of a vaccinia vector vaccine would raise the problem again, if vaccine strains similar to those used previously were employed. Using data from Wilson [7] and Lane et al. [3,4], the frequency of this disease is summarized as shown in Table II.

There is some evidence that the occurrence of CNS disease is related to the strain of vaccinia virus. For example, after the Bern strain, once used in Austria, Switzerland and West Germany, was replaced by the Lister strain in 1971, the occurrence of complications of the central nervous system declined. Surveys numbered 1 to 5 showed a high incidence of this complication, but it is believed that the vaccinia strain used at that time played a major role. If the Lister or the New York City Board of Health strains are utilized for vaccinia vector vaccine, we may expect the magnitude of CNS complications to be about that found in surveys number 6 or 7. The survey number 6 was the survey conducted by the Ministry of Health, U.K. from 1951 to 1960 during which period 39 CNS complications were recorded in 2,661,488 primary vaccinees of children under one year of age and 17 CNS complications among 1,158,881 primary vaccinees of above one year of age [1]. We assume that the survey number 7, of the ten-state survey, provides a better index of the frequency of complications in the USA than did the national survey (number 8). In summary, with children under 1 year of age, between 15 and 42 children per million receiving primary vaccination may suffer from postvaccinial encephalopathy, and primary vaccination of persons above 1 year of age, mainly children, may be accompanied by between 9 and 15 cases of postvaccinial encephalitis per million.

Just as the frequency of CNS complication varied greatly in different surveys, so did the case-fatality rates. Wilson [7] cites an average figure of 30%; the review of survey numbers 6, 7 and 8 suggests that although the numbers are small, most deaths occurred in the age group under 1 year of age (Table III).

CONCLUSION

Past knowledge and experience relating to complications of smallpox vaccination have been briefly presented to aid in evaluating whether or not the frequency of such complications would be acceptable should vaccinia virus be used as a vaccine vector.

The complications involving the CNS are important since they are severe, unpredictable and therefore cannot be avoided by withholding

TABLE III. Post-vaccinial complications of the central nervous system

		Cases (death)		
		<1 year	>1 year	Total
Survey No. 6	UK	39(16)	17(3)	56(19)
Survey No. 7	USA (10 State)	3(1)	5(0)	8(1)
Survey No. 8	USA (National)	4(3)	12(1)	16(4)
				80(24)

TABLE IV. Vaccinia vector vaccine hazards: Estimated frequency of complications using Lister or New York City Board of Health strains

Type of complication	Cases per million primary vaccinations	
	Age < one year	Age > one year
Central nervous system	10 - 40	10 - 20
Abnormal skin eruptions[a] (progressive vaccinia, eczema vaccinatum)	10	50
Accidental infection	?	?
Other (generalized vaccinia, erythema multiforme, etc.)	1,000	1,000

a) All would be eczema vaccinatum except for a few cases of progressive vaccinia.

vaccination from high-risk subjects, and there is no effective treatment. With the least pathogenic strains of vaccinia virus widely used in the smallpox eradication campaign, such as the Lister or the New York City Board of Health strains, between 10 and 40 children under 1 year of age might be expected to suffer in every 1 million primary vaccinees (Table IV).

Progressive vaccinia would be very rare, but eczema vaccinatum might be expected at a rate of 10 per million primary vaccinations of children under 1 year old, the rates of each complication being dependent on the specified contraindications to vaccination and the care with which these were excluded, or if cases of eczema, given vaccinia-immune globulin.

Accidental vaccinia infection among contacts might cause some unpleasant social problems but it is hard to estimate its frequency. All other complications including generalized vaccinia, erythema multiforme, bacterial infections, etc. are grouped together as they are mild and may not be necessary to include in an evaluation of risks and benefits. Perhaps 1000 such cases might occur among each million primary vaccinations of children under 1 year of age.

The figures for complications presented in the tables for subjects over 1 year of age also vary, but are of the same order of magnitude as in infants.

The frequency of complications in the United Kingdom and the USA occurred in well-nourished populations with good medical care services, including availability of vaccinia-immune globulin. The application of these incidence estimates of case-fatality rates, especially, to populations in developing countries should be made with caution.

These estimated hazards must be weighed against the public health importance of the target disease, taking into consideration the advantages of vaccinia vector vaccine, namely, ease of production, ease of administration, low cost and heat stability. If any further attenuation of virulence can be made, without loss of immunogenicity, so much the better. Field trials to determine the frequency of serious complications would require very large groups of subjects, since the incidence of such important complications as CNS disease may well be less than one in 100,000 primary vaccinations.

The hazards from use of vaccinia vector vaccine appear to be much smaller than those of diseases such as malaria or hepatitis B, where these are common. Benjamin Franklin wrote in his autobiography:

"In 1736, I lost one of my sons (Francis Folger), a fine boy of four years old by the smallpox. I long regretted bitterly and still regret that I had not given it to him by inoculation. This I mention for the sake of parents, who omit the operation on the supposition that they should never forgive themselves if a child died under it: my example shows that the regret may be the same either way, and that therefore the safer should be chosen."

ACKNOWLEDGEMENT

We are grateful to Dr. Keith Dumbell for his review and advice on the preparation of this paper.

REFERENCES

1. E.T. Conybeare. Monthly Bulletin of the Ministry of Health and Public Health Laboratory Service, Vol. 23, September, 150-159 (1964).
2. C.H. Kempe, J. Pediatrics 26, 170-189 (1960).
3. J.M. Lane, F.L. Ruben, J.M. Neff and J.D. Millar, N. Engl. J. Med. 281, 1201-1208 (1969).
4. J.M. Lane, F.L. Ruben, J.M. Neff and J.D. Miller, J. Infect. Dis. 122, 303-309 (1970).
5. J.C.M. Sharp and W.B. Fletcher, Lancet i, 656-659 (1973).
6. G. Weber and J. Lange, Deutsche medizinische Wochenschrift 86, 1461-1468 (1961).
7. G.S. Wilson. The Hazards of Immunization (London, Athlone 1967).

DISCUSSION

Dr. Burke: I have three related questions. First, what is the background rate of encephalitis in that same age group less than two years old? Second, what is the relative risk for an individual who has recently received a vaccination? And third, how do you define an encephalomyelitis or central nervous system disease as being due to vaccinia? What were the case definitions?

Dr. Arita: I will address the last question first. I am not expert at pathology. However, in the old literature, there is a report by Weber and Lange who studied about 250 autopsy records in Germany. They found a difference in the type of pathology observed above and below the age of two years. Below the age of two years the picture was more typical of encephalopathy, characterized predominantly by brain edema. Above the age of two years, the pathology was more typical of encephalitis with demyelinization. There is no adequate case definition to define which cases were actually due to vaccinia. Reports of isolation of vaccinia from the central nervous system have been very rare. The best indication that some of these cases may have been due to vaccinia is the apparent clustering of cases with these types of non-specific pathology within a finite period of time after vaccination.

Your first question related to the background rate of the encephalitis under two years of age. In fact, I do not know. Estimates have been made in the past by others that the rate in some European countries is 20 per million. The accuracy of these estimates is uncertain.

With regard to your second question, the relative, attributed risk of encephalitis in vaccinees compared to nonvaccinees is unknown. All we can say is that the incidence of central nervous system complications is 10 to 40 per million in primary vaccinees under two years of age.

Dr. Buller: I wanted to add that I think the background rate of central nervous system disease from vaccinations is a very important number to define. If one goes back to the literature that Dr. Arita has summarized so well, one finds that there were no isolations of virus from the central nervous system. The only indication that vaccinia virus may have been a causative was a temporal association with vaccination. There is a high probability, therefore, that the incidence of vaccinia virus encephalitis is actually much less than 10 to 40 per million.

Dr. D.A. Henderson: I think it is very hard to come up with estimates that have any reliability here. The European studies are really very uncertain. Very few of them have any denominators at all, and their methods of surveillance were poor. The only really good studies were the couple that were done here in the United States. One who conducted those is Dr. Neff whose data you have. I wondered how he reacts to estimates that were presented here.

Dr. Neff: Well, there are several points that have been made that are correct. It is extraordinarily difficult in doing these studies to make the diagnosis of post-vaccine encephalitis, because of those cases, only about one percent would be deaths. When you have a death, what you look for is perivascular infiltration and demyelinization, so that you have to use a clinical diagnosis of encephalitis and use it in a temporal pattern following vaccination. But in all these studies, there really was a very clear temporal pattern which made these illnesses very similar to the parinfectious type of encephalopathies that you would see, for example, after measles and varicella. It did seem to have a ten times higher incidence in children under the age of one than older children. There have also been a few recent, isolated case reports in the literature, predominantly from England, where the virus was isolated from the central nervous system. By and large, however, the disease mechanism was probably a post-infectious or parinfectious type of encephalitis.

It is very difficult to be able to say what the background level of encephalitis is, because that varies tremendously from season to season and area to area. About all that you can say when you look at individual cases, is that these cases of parinfectious encephalitis fit very neatly into a timeframe following vaccination and are therefore most likely related to it.

UTILIZATION OF VACCINE IN THE GLOBAL ERADICATION OF SMALLPOX

Donald A. HENDERSON* AND ISAO ARITA**

*Dean, School of Hygiene and Public Health, The Johns Hopkins University, Baltimore, Maryland 21205. **Chief, Smallpox Eradication Unit, World Health Organization, Geneva Switzerland

Immunization is potentially the most cost-effective procedure for disease control, its efficacy and practicability being governed by the characteristics of the antigen which is available. Vaccinia virus, although not ideal, is one of the best. It possesses a number of characteristics which, for the smallpox program, make it unusually suitable for developing countries--where trained personnel are few in number, where ambient temperatures are high and refrigeration is scarce and where funds, especially foreign currency, are limited.

Among the attributes of vaccinia virus, five were of particular importance. Had any one of these been lacking, the ultimate success of the program would have been seriously jeopardized. The attributes are as follows: (1) the vaccine was easy to administer; (2) it was comparatively simple to produce; (3) it was stable for long periods at ambient tropical temperatures; (4) it conferred remarkably durable immunity even after a single application; and (5) it was widely accepted, producing few recognized serious reactions.

Ease of Administration

A vaccine which can be readily administered to large numbers of persons with minimally trained staff and little equipment is especially advantageous in conducting a vaccination program in a developing country. Oral vaccine preparations are perhaps the easiest to administer but at present, few antigens can be administered successfully by this route. Most vaccines require percutaneous application but, other than for smallpox vaccine, they require the use of either needles and syringes or jet injectors.

Disposable needles and syringes would appear to be an obvious solution for large-scale vacination campaigns, but even when purchased in bulk, their cost is prohibitive. If syringes and/or needles are reused after sterilization, the costs for supplies may be reduced but the logistics and effort required to do this are formidable.

Jet injectors offer an advantage where large numbers are vaccinated during the course of a day, but the injectors now available experience mechanical problems with distressing frequency and require skilled personnel to maintain and repair them. They are not usually practicable even when a few hundred persons can be vaccinated daily. During the global smallpox eradication program jet injectors were used throughout western and central Africa and in Brazil, the first programs to be initiated. In these countries, it was possible to train or to provide sufficiently skilled personnel to repair and maintain the injectors over the three-to-five year period during which large numbers of vaccinations were performed. To continue the programs for a longer period would have been problematical given the difficulties in sustaining distribution systems for spare parts and an interest on the part of donor countries in providing necessary replacement equipment and, in many instances, foreign technicians.

In 1968, the functional and elegantly simple bifurcated needle became the instrument of choice for multiple puncture vaccination [5]. The

© 1985 Elsevier Science Publishing Co., Inc.
VACCINIA VIRUSES AS VECTORS FOR VACCINE ANTIGENS, Quinnan, Editor

needle was developed by Dr. Benjamin Rubin of Wyeth Laboratories [7], and the needle design was made available to WHO free of patent charges. We anticipated that the needles would be repeatedly sterilized and reused and so we altered their metallic content to make them more durable. They were produced by a German manufacturer at a cost of $5.00 per 1000. Field tests revealed that each needle was fully effective for 200 or more inoculations, whether sterilized by boiling or by heating over an open flame. Experience showed that village workers, with 15 to 30 minutes training, could satisfactorily reconstitute the vaccine and perform multiple puncture vaccinations. A vaccine vial containing 0.25 ml of reconstituted vaccine, the smallest quantity of vaccine which was technically feasible to freeze-dry in a container, served to vaccinate approximately 100 persons. Such a vial of vaccine cost less than $1.00 to produce.

Multiple puncture vaccination, employing the bifurcated needle, was eventually used in all countries, displacing all other techniques and instruments. It remains, by far, the most practicable method for percutaneous inoculation.

Vaccine Supply and Production

In an immunization program, personnel costs constitute the principal expenditure, the costs of vaccine usually representing only a fraction of the total. For a developing country, however, foreign currency cost rather than overall cost is the principal constraint. If vaccine cannot be produced locally, the principal foreign currency cost is for vaccine. Presently, in most immunization programs in developing countries, vaccines are donated or their costs are met largely by bilateral or multinational agencies. Provision of vaccines in this manner is not a satisfactory long-term solution, however, because it is difficult to sustain the interest of donors in continuing to make donations of substantial quantities of vaccine over long periods. Thus, local production of vaccine is preferred where the quantities of vaccine which are used warrant it.

Smallpox vaccine was able to be produced in many developing countries, but even with this effort, it was difficult to assure the continuing availability of adequate quantities for the global eradication program [8]. In most instances, donations were obtained only with difficulty and because laboratories in most industrialized countries had small capacities, contributions were proportionately small. Fortunately, during the early years of the program, two major contributors provided most of the vaccine which was needed. Approximately 140 million doses annually were provided by the Soviet Union through bilateral and multilateral contributions and 40 million doses were provided by the USA to countries in western and central Africa. The balance of perhaps 20 to 30 million doses was initially provided through contributions of other industrialized countries and through production in developing countries.

Support was provided by WHO and UNICEF to laboratories in developing countries to produce their own vaccine. In these laboratories, vaccinia virus was harvested from the skin of calves or water buffalo and, after a comparatively simple of series of steps to purify and concentrate it and to reduce the bacterial content, it was freeze-dried in vials or ampoules. Some laboratories were able to embark on large-scale production within a period of two years, although most required somewhat longer. By 1971, more than 250 million doses of vaccine were produced in the developing countries, most of which met accepted international standards as determined by independent assay in WHO collaborating laboratories (Table I) [1].

TABLE I. Estimated quantities of freeze-dried vaccine produced in developing countries--1971.

	Millions of doses
Argentina	12
Bangladesh	30
Brazil	45
Burma	15
Colombia	4
Ecuador	2
Guinea	5
India	80
Indonesia	30
Iran	15
Kenya	10
Peru	5
Thailand	15
	268
People's Republic of China	?
Mozambique	?

Experience showed that for most laboratories, a more complex production technology, such as one involving tissue cultures, would not have been possible. Indeed, not until the 1970s did any laboratory in any country succeed in producing a heat stable, freeze-dried vaccine employing vaccinia virus grown in tissue culture [4]. Nevertheless, early in the programme some concerned with biological standards proposed, as a matter of principle, to modify the international standards to require that vaccine for the jet injectors be bacteriologically sterile. The vaccine then in use had a very low bacterial count and was required to be free of pathogens but a sterile vaccine would have required production in tissue cultures. Fortunately, the application of these standards was able to be forestalled; otherwise, vaccine for the jet injectors would not have been available. No known complications are known to have occurred, however, as a result of use of the non-sterile but pathogen-free preparations.

Vaccine Stability

The logistics and problems involved in maintaining antigens at a proper temperature from the time of production until inoculation have been well documented by those concerned with the WHO Expanded Program on Immunization. The provision and maintenance of refrigerators and insulated boxes for transport are formidable problems for most developing countries. Many imaginative approaches and solutions have been devised in recent years, but despite highly commendable efforts and numerous training programs, maintenance of the "cold chain" has proved to be one of the Program's most vexing challenges. For the smallpox eradication program, however, the problem was much less difficult.

Commercially acceptable techniques for producing an exceptionally heat stable vaccine were elucidated by Collier at the Lister Institute in the 1950s [2]. One of the criteria for an acceptable vaccine was that it exhibit a potency of $10^{8.0}$ pock forming units (pfu) when assayed

on chick chorioallantoic membrane <u>after</u> incubation at 37°C for one month.
This concentration of vaccinia virus was about 50 times greater than that
required to obtain vaccine take rates of more than 95% in primary vaccines. Some laboratories, in fact, substantially exceeded these standards,
both in vaccine titer and stability. Some vaccines contained more than
10^9 pfu and retained titers of 10^8 pfu or greater for as long as 6 to 12
months at high ambient temperature.

Standard procedures in the smallpox eradication program called for
the vaccine to be stored and shipped in such a manner that it was exposed
to temperatures of greater than 4°C for no longer than one month. In
most programs, this implied storage of the vaccine in conventional refrigerators or freezers only in the capital city and provincial or state
capitals. In these cities and towns, working refrigerators as well as
electricity and/or kerosene were more readily available. From these
depots, the vaccine was distributed to health centers and field staff
once each month, a comparatively simple logistical problem. Even so,
there were a number of documented failures in the system and, unquestion-
ably, many undocumented ones. Nevertheless, repeat titrations of improp-
erly stored vaccine, when conducted, usually revealed an adequate level
of potency, the margin for permissible error in handling being so great.
No other vaccine available today approaches smallpox vaccine in its
stability.

Durability of Immunity

In 1967, conventional wisdom held that revaccination every three to
five years was essential to sustain adequate levels of vaccinal immunity.
However, this assumption was soon called into question by surveillance
data which showed that 80% to 90% or more of cases occurred among those
with no vaccination scar and no history of vaccination. The reason for
this was revealed in studies by Heiner and his colleagues [3], who found
that many who were partially protected by immunization experienced subclinical infections with a subsequent substantial increase in antibodies.
In the endemic countries, therefore, immunity was a composite of responses
to prior infection with both vaccinia and variola viruses. A single
primary vaccination provided remarkably durable protection in such areas,
sample surveys showing vaccine efficacy ratios of 80% or greater among
those vaccinated 20 years or more previously. Unfortunately, similar data
are not available from non-endemic areas.

Although successful vaccination prior to exposure was remarkably
effective in preventing naturally acquired smallpox infection, it was far
less effective in preventing vaccinia virus replication in the skin when
revaccination was performed. In fact, most individuals to whom a high
titered vaccinia virus was administered experienced a so-called "major
reaction," i.e. erythema and induration at the vaccination site at the
sixth to eighth day, even when as little as 6 to 12 months had elapsed
since their previous vaccination.

Administration of Vaccine and Acceptance of Vaccination

Vaccine was administered to all persons in the population irrespective
of age, illness or other conditions. The only stated contraindication to
vaccination was serious illness which appeared likely to result in death
of the vaccinee within a few days and whose death might be attributed to
smallpox vaccination. These policies differed from those in industrialized
countries where vaccination was not usually administered to those under
6 to 12 month of age, to pregnant women or to those with eczema. Vaccination from the time of birth was initiated on the basis of Rao's studies

in Madras, India, which showed this practice to be efficacious and safe [6]. Possible pregnancy was disregarded because of the unusually high risk of death from smallpox among pregnant women and the rarity of complications following vaccination. Eczema likewise was not considered a contraindication because of the widespread occurrence of skin infections in many developing countries and the difficulty which vaccinators, as well as trained clinicians encountered in differential diagnosis of skin conditions.

Vaccination was generally well-received. Aside from the expected reaction of a lesion on the arm and a short-lived fever, few vaccine complications were observed. Resistance to vaccination was uncommon although sometimes occurring among those who objected for religious reasons and among some rural Asian populations who feared any incapacitation during the harvest or planting season. Infrequent but serious complications such as post-vaccinal encephalitis are well-documented in industrialized countries and undoubtedly occurred in developing countries as well. However, with encephalitic symptoms due to other diseases being so widely prevalent, the frequency of those due to vaccinia virus could not be documented and were rarely noted. That vaccination was so widely accepted, indeed sought by most, became evident when government authorities endeavored to stop vaccination following eradication. Popular demand caused many governments to continue the practice for a number of years even though it was no longer needed.

SUMMARY

The availability of a protective antigen against smallpox with the characteristics of vaccinia virus was critical to the success of smallpox eradication. WHO staff and collaborating scientists in many laboratories expended considerable time and effort in assuring the adequacy of supply of smallpox vaccine and, through a variety of quality control measures, of its potency, stability and purity. To meet demand, however, required expanded production in the developing countries themselves. If international standards had required a sterile vaccine produced in tissue culture, such production would not have been possible. The vaccine itself had unique properties of stability, the best of any antigen available today, which greatly facilitated its use in the field and because vaccination left a permanent scar, assessment of vaccinal immunity in a community was comparatively easy. Finally, for a percutaneously administered antigen, the multiple puncture technique was by far the simplest and least expensive. If it were possible to utilize vaccinia virus as a carrier for other antigens, the difficulties intrinsic to providing adequate quantities of vaccine for developing countries and of conducting immunization programmes would be greatly minimized.

REFERENCES

1. I. Arita in: International Symposium on Smallpox Vaccine (Bilthoven, The Netherlands 1973). Basle, Kargar, Symposium Series in Immunobiological Standardization, pp. 79-87.
2. L.H. Collier, J. of Hygiene (London) $\underline{53}$, 76-101 (1955).
3. G.G. Heiner, N. Fatima, R.W. Daniel, J.L. Cole, R.L. Anthony, and F.R. McCrumb, Amer. J. Epidemiology $\underline{94}$, 252-268 (1971).
4. A.C. Hekker, J.M. Bos, and L. Smith, J. Biol. Standardization $\underline{1}$, 21-32 (1973).
5. D.A. Henderson, I. Arita, and E. Shafa, WHO (unpublished document, Studies of the bifurcated needle and recommendations for its use).
6. A.R. Rao in: Smallpox (The Kothari Book Depot, Bombay, 1972).

7. B.A. Rubin, WHO Chronicle 34, 180-181 (1980).
8. World Health Organization, The Global Eradication of Smallpox: Final Report of the Global Commission for the Certification of Smallpox Eradication (Geneva, 1980).

DISCUSSION

   Dr. Moss: Can you tell us something about the age of the vaccinees?

   Dr. Henderson: Originally, I think most countries believed that one should not vaccinate younger than three months or six months or nine months of age. Rao, in Madras, pioneered the work of vaccinating at birth and found this to be safe and effective, fully effective, and so progressively the principle of vaccinating at birth, or as soon thereafter as possible, was used. Good primary takes occurred as frequently as with older children, and the protection seemed to be good.

   Dr. Arita: Albania is the only one country who continues vaccination. France and Egypt stopped.

   Dr. Henderson: Dr. Arita corrects me. France and Egypt have now ceased vaccination. Only Albania continues it.

   Dr. Jordan: Do you have an estimate of what percent of the world's population you had to immunize to eradicate smallpox?

   Dr. Henderson: It's kind of an embarrassing question. We do have data from a great many countries as to what percentage of the population had received vaccinia virus at some time, as measured by vaccination scar. I think we should note, however, that the eradication could not be correlated with the percentage vaccinated, in that in some countries we were able to terminate transmission with only 40 or 50 percent vaccinated. However, I think we found that it was comparatively easy to establish programs which reached 80 percent or more of the population, as measured by having a vaccination scar, and that in well organized programs one could reach 90 percent fairly well. So that in the countries where there were really effective vaccination programs, I would say we were dealing with something in the 80 to 90 percent range when transmission was interrupted, but interruption of transmission was not directly correlated with the level of vaccination. Surveillance contributed greatly to containment.

   Dr. R. Henderson: I think some discussion of current objectives of the Expanded Program on Immunization (EPI) is relevant here. Eradication of the targeted diseases is not a realistic expectation in the near future. Our principal objective is the setting up of a delivery system that will continuously reach the youngest segment of the population. Our focus is on children less than a year of age. Those children are very difficult to reach, and even in the smallpox program where 80 or 90 percent of a total population was vaccinated, there was often a tendency to selectively miss the youngest age groups. Our emphasis in the EPI is on the delivery systems to assure that that vaccine is getting to the children before they are exposed to these diseases.

   One of the perspectives that is beginning to change in my mind is the emphasis on production of vaccines in developing countries. We are approaching a world situation where there are established permanent delivery systems. I do not see in the next 20 to 30 years many developing countries being able to pay on their own behalf the costs for those systems, and we are facing a world where either the developed countries are willing to come forward with long-term support, which has not been available in the past, or we are going to see our hopes and dreams collapse because countries are not going to pay for the gasoline to get trucks out. They are not going to pay for the training. They are not going to pay for the supervision. They are not going to pay for any of of the coaching that is needed, and I think the emphasis on the need for a vaccinia virus which can be produced in developing countries, at least for the short-term future, should be a major consideration for the people who are designing the vaccine.

VACCINIA VIRUS VACCINES: VIRULENCE AND ATTENUATION OF VACCINIA STRAIN VARIATION

JOHN M. NEFF*

*Professor of Pediatrics, University of Washington School of Medicine; Medical Director, The Children's Orthopedic Hospital and Medical Center, Seattle, Washington 98105

Origins of Vaccinia

Very little is known about the origin of smallpox vaccine. Vaccination was established long before there was any knowledge concerning the nature of the virus. Little also was known about the number of poxviruses that were circulating in the 18th and 19th century. Even during Jenner's life there was controversy over the origins of his vaccine virus. He felt that it came from a horsepox ("grease") and became more suitable for human use after passage through cows. Others felt that the virus came from cows, but the current vaccine strains are quite different from cowpox, and for that matter, other poxviruses. Also, early drawings of the pox lesions produced by vaccinia were quite different when compared to those produced by cowpox. There also is a remote possibility that the current vaccine strains may have been derived from variola or were some sort of hybrid with variola that resulted from variolation and strain mixing as the strains were propagated from human arm to arm transmission during the 19th century [1].

Variation of Pathogenicity of Different Vaccinia Strains

Regardless of the origins of vaccinia, by the 20th century there were many strains used throughout the world. During the early part of the 20th century it was quite evident that from country to country there was a great variation of the incidence of complications to smallpox vaccination, particularly post-vaccinal encephalitis [2]. The high incidence of this complication was most marked in the Netherlands where it was noted to be as high as 1 per 4000 primary vaccinees in certain groups. In contrast, the incidence of this complication in the United States has been estimated to be 2 to 6 per 1,000,000 primary vaccinees [3]. One of the explanations for differences in observed rates of this complication could be the fact that the incidence of the complication was dependent on the strain of vaccinia used. In the early 1960's there were several attempts to study and measure the pathogenicity of these strains. In the Netherlands where the complications of post-vaccinal encephalitis were high, the strain that was implicated was the Copenhagen strain. The pathogenicity of this strain was compared to the Bern strain (Germany), the Ecuador strain (South America), and the Elstree strain (Lister-Great Britain) [4].

They measured the index of pathogenicity as calculated by the number of febrile days (>38.7°C) in 100 vaccinations and demonstrated that this was considerably higher for the Copenhagen (100), and Bern strain (94), than for the Ecuador (54-58) or Elstree strain (23-28). As a result of this and other evaluations the strains that were most highly pathogenic were abandoned by vaccine producers, so that by 1972 most of the vaccines used in the WHO eradication program were derived either from the Elstree (Lister Institute) strain or the New York Board of Health strain [5]. The strain from the Moscow Institute of Virus Preparation, EM-63, was used to some degree. That strain in all probability had its origin from Ecuador and from there originally from the Massachusetts strain [6]. Thus that strain resembles to a great

degree the New York Board of Health strain which is similar to the
lassachusetts strain.

Up through the successful campaign to eradicate smallpox, the
vaccine strains were almost all produced from calf lymph. One noted
exception was Brazil, which used a chorioallantoic membrane grown (CAM)
vaccine for 90% of their vaccinations [7]. The standards established
by the WHO were that the vaccine had to produce more than 95% major
reaction takes for a primary vaccination, and 90% after revaccination
of subjects vaccinated ten or more years previously. Such a vaccine
also had to have a titer of 10^8 pock-forming units (pfu) per ml after
incubation at 37°C for one month [8].

These were the principal strains and the standards that were used
during the campaign that successfully eradicated smallpox. During the
late 1960's and 1970's, however, there was interest in developing tissue
culture vaccines which, because of their increased purity over calf
lymph, and their further attenuation, could not only be used successfully
to prevent smallpox, but also would have fewer complications. Because
smallpox was successfully eradicated by the use of the freeze-dry calf
lymph vaccine, there has been little recent work in developing the
concept of the utilization of further attenuated tissue culture vaccines.
Now, however, because of the possibility of utilizing the vaccinia
virus as a vector for vaccine antigens, there may be renewed interest
in developing tissue culture vaccines for these endeavors.

Rivers Attenuated Tissue Culture Vaccine

Some of the earlier work on the development of further attenuated
tissue culture vaccine was initiated by Thomas Rivers in 1930, who used
the New York Board of Health vaccine strain in tissue culture experiments.
The New York Board of Health vaccine strain was the strain which was
derived directly from England shortly after Jenner's work, and is now
the major strain used in the United States. The original material that
Rivers used for this vaccine was passed initially four times through
rabbit testes, and then passed on tissue culture of minced chick embryo.
After 34 passages of the chick cells the virus gradually dropped its
potency, as measured by the decreased percentage of takes in primary
vaccinees. In order to raise the titer it was passed six more times
through rabbit testicles. The virus derived from the sixth rabbit
passage was called the first revived strain, CV-I [9]. This virus was
then passed 31 times through chick embryo fibroblasts and again through
rabbit testes three times to increase potency. This was called the
second revised strain, or CV-II. This second revised strain caused a
benign pox-like lesion in humans on percutaneous vaccination [10].

CV-II Vaccinia Strain

In the Netherlands, because of the high incidence of post-vaccinal
encephalitis, in those who received the calf lymph Copenhagen strain,
there was interest in using the second revived strain of Rivers, or CV-II,
for vaccination. The original strain from Rivers was obtained and
passed 170 times on chick embryo explants, 13 times on chick embryo
fibroblasts and finally on choreoallantoic membranes with the subsequent
development of a titer of 10^8 pfu/ml. This vaccine was used in 60,000
adult military recruits, and within this group only one case of post-
vaccnal encephalitis occurred and there were no deaths. In contrast
there were 53,044 recruits who received the Copenhagen strain. They
demonstrated 13 cases of post-vaccinal encephalitis and one death.
When gamma globulin, however, was given with the calf lymph Copenhagen

strain, there was a marked reduction in the cases of post-vaccinal encephalitis. In the 53,630 primary vaccinees who received the gamma globulin modified Copenhagen strain, there were only three cases of post-vaccinal encephalitis and one death. The gamma globulin also was used with the Rivers CV-II vaccine trials. Thus, it is difficult to account for the decrease in cases of post-vaccinal encephalitis on just the use of the Rivers vaccine alone. The other aspect of this study was that there were much lower post-vaccinal neutralizing antibody titers in those who received the modified Rivers strain, CV-II, as compared to those who received the more reactive Copenhagen calf vaccine. This suggested that the CV-II strain might not be as protective against smallpox as the Copenhagen calf lymph strain [11].

There was another reason why the decrease in post-vaccinal encephalitis could not be attributed solely to the change in the strain in the Netherlands. Although there was a decreased incidence of post-vaccinal encephalitis when the Netherlands changed from the Copenhagen to the Estree strain, there was not a sharp decline in the incidence of complications but only a gradual decline suggesting other factors than just the change of the strain alone may have contributed to the decline in the incidence of post-vaccinal encephalitis [12].

Van der Noordaa also looked for a laboratory marker for CV-II as an index of pathogenicity. He compared the Copenhagen, the Elstree and the CV-II strain in human amnion (U) cells and human embryonic lung (HEL) cells. He was able to demonstrate a direct correlation between strain pathogenicity for man and between plaque size and multiplication rates in tissue culture. These measurements, especially multiplication rate, decreased in order of decreasing pathogenicity for the three vaccine strains. Copenhagen was the most pathogenetic, Elstree was in between and finally Rivers CV-II the least pathogenic [13]. He could, however, find no differences in temperature and pH sensitivity. Virus multiplication for all three strains were enhanced at 37°C as compared to 40°C and inhibited at a low pH [14].

CV I-78 Vaccinia Strain

In the United States, Henry Kempe revived an interest in the first revised strain of Rivers, or CV I. This renewed interest came about because of the number of cases of eczema vaccinatum that occurred in the United States as a result of the widespread use of vaccinia virus (New York Board of Health strain) in children. The first revived strain of Rivers (CV I) was passed an additional 39 times in chick embryo explants and 19 times in choreoallantoic membranes obtaining a titer of $10^{8.4}$ $TCID_{50}$/ml. This virus was called the CV I-78 strain. This vccine has been one of the most extensively studied attenuated vacciness [15].

A total of approximately 9,000 primary vaccinations were given, including 3,446 eczematous children. In all instances, systemic responses were milder in those who received the CV I-78 vaccine, and in the eczematous children there were no cases of eczema vaccinatum [16]. The clinical modification of this strain was also demonstrated in a small study by Neff and a multicenter NIH study that compared the pathogenicity and immunological response among three vaccine strains, Elstree, New York Board of Health, and the CV I-78 [17,18]. In both studies the individuals who received the CV I-78 vaccine had a modified clinical response as compared to the other vaccines and a lower postvaccinal neutralizing antibody response even after revaccination with the New York Board of Health vaccine. After revaccination about 65% of the CV I-78 as compared to 100% of the New York Board of Health vaccine group had positive neutralizing antibodies to vaccine after revaccination with the New York Board of Health vaccine [17].

It was evident from the studies of the CV I-78 vaccine that the vaccine was considered to be less reactive than the New York Board of Health vaccine or the Elstree strain, and it was considered to be too attenuated for protection against smallpox. Since then there have been no further clinical studies of this particular vaccine.

Now that there is a possibility of using vaccinia as a vector for vaccine antigens, we must consider once again the possibility of utilizing CV I-78 vaccine as that vector. In comparing its attenuation to that of the New York Board of Health vaccine strain, it is not certain that the use of the CV I-78 will decrease the incidence of serious complications to vaccination over the New York Board of Health strain. Although Kempe used CV I-78 as a primary vaccine in over 3,000 children with eczema, without a case of eczema vaccinatum, the true incidence of that complication in children who are vaccinated and who have eczema is not known. In a retrospective study in Maryland in 1965 Neff detected 197 children with eczema who also had received primary vaccinations with the New York Board of Health vaccine [19]. None of these children developed eczema vaccinatum. The U.S. data of the early 1970's and 1960's would indicate that the complications of eczema vaccinatum occurs at the rate of approximately 1 to 5 per 100,000 normal primary vaccinees [3]. Also, it is uncertain whether the use of CV I-78 strain will reduce the incidence of post-vaccinal encephalitis as that complication occurs in about 2 to 6 per 1,000,000 primary recipients of the New York calf lymph vaccine [3]. The number who have received CV I-78 nowhere near approaches that number.

Other Attenuated Vaccinia Strains

There have been other strains developed. There is the Yugoslavian strain (HDC), WI-38 strain which was derived from the Bern strain and grown and passed 12 times through human diploid cells [20]. This strain was used in the 1972 smallpox epidemic in Yugoslavia where 724 individuals received the vaccine as primary vaccinees. The take rate for this vaccine was 100% with clear evidence of modification. The reactivity (fever indices) to the vaccine increased with the age of the vaccinees, but in general was lower in those who received the human diploid cell vaccine.

In the Netherlands a freeze-dried vaccine was prepared by Hekker in monolayers of primary rabbit cells [21]. There have been limited field trials of this vaccine, but when compared to calf lymph vaccines in terms of take rate, antibody titers and vaccination illness, there seems to be very little difference. In Munich the MVA strain was developed from their vaccinia virus. This virus was passed 523 times through chick embryo fibroblasts. Like CV I-78, this vaccine produced a very modified local reaction, but also only sporadic humoral antibodies [22]. In Japan the Darien I (DEI) mutant strain has been developed from white mutants from the DEI strain by identifying smaller pox lesions on CAM on serial passage of vaccinia virus through 1 day eggs. The mutant has been found to grow on human embryonic cells and is highly attenuated in cynomologus monkeys [23].

CONCLUSION

In addition to the above, there are other vaccinia strains that have been developed in tissue culture and there is no question that there

are available strains of vaccinia that are more attenuated than the
standard Elstree (Lister) and New York Board of Health strains. They
do seem to produce less systemic reaction and perhaps may not have as
high a rate of serious complication as the standard vaccines. This,
however, has not really been tested since serious complications occur
very infrequently and there would have to be studies involving more
than a million primary vaccinees to determine whether or not the
complications, such as post-vaccinal encephalitis, vaccinia necrosum or
eczema vaccinatum are decreased as the result of using these new
attenuated strains. There also is some question whether or not these
strains are as protective against smallpox, as the accepted Elstree or
New York strain. This is not a relevant question now. What is more
relevant is the question of how much they protect against vaccinia
since any reduction in the multiplication of the vaccinia virus at the
time of revaccination may diminish the use of vaccinia virus as a vector
for multiple vaccinations in the same host. In conclusion, there is no
question that it is possible to develop more purified strains through
tissue culture and other techniques than through the older, time-honored
method of growing the vaccine in calf lymph. The two as yet unanswered
questions remain: (1) will any new strain provide a significantly
lower incidence of the serious complications than the Elstree or New
York strain, and (2) which strain will maximize the immunological
response to the antigens that are incorporated into vaccinia virus
either as a part of single or multiple innoculations?

REFERENCES

1. D. Baxby, J. Infect. Dis. 136, 453-455 (1977).
2. G. Stuart, Bull. World Health Organization 1, 36-53 (1947).
3. J.M. Lane, J.D. Millar and J.M. Neff, Ann. Rev. Med. 22, 251-272 (1971).
4. M.F. Polak, B.J.W. Bennders, A.R. Van Der Werff, E.W. Sanders, J.N. Van Klaveren and L.M. Brans, Bull World Health Organization 29, 311-322 (1963).
5. World Health Organization, Technical Report Series, WHO, Geneva, 493, 37 (1972).
6. S.S. Marennikova, International Symposium on Smallpox Vaccine, Bilthoven, The Netherlands, S Krager AG, Basel 19, 253-260 (1973).
7. C.F. Voegeli, International Symposium on Smallpox Vaccine, Bilthoven, The Netherlands, S Krager AG, Basel 19, 69-73 (1973).
8. World Health Organization, Technical Report Series, WHO, Geneva, 493, 36 (1972).
9. T.M. Rivers and S.M. Ward, J. Exp. Med. 58, 635-658 (1933).
10. J. Van der Noordaa. Primary vaccination of adults with an attenuated strain of vaccinia virus. The history of the second revised strain of vaccinia. Thesis, University of Leiden, 1-4 (1964).
11. J. Van der Noordaa, F. Dekking, J. Posthuma and B.J.W. Bennders, Archiv. Fur Die Gesamte Virusforschung 22, 210-214 (1967).
12. M.F. Polak, International Symposium on Smallpox Vaccine, Bilthoven, The Netherlands, S Krager AG, Basel 19, 235-242 (1973).
13. J. Van der Noordaa. Primary vaccination of adults with an attenuated strain of vaccinia virus. Comparative investigation of the vaccinia strains Copenhagen, Elstree and Rivers. Thesis, University of Leiden, 34-38 (1964).
14. J. Van der Noordaa. Primary vaccination of adults with an attenuated strain of vaccinia virus. The effect of temperature and pH on the growth of the Copenhagen, Elstree and Rivers strains of vaccinia. Thesis, University of Leiden, 39-56 (1964).
15. C.H. Kempe, V. Fulginiti, M. Minamitani and H. Shienfield, Pediatrics 42, 980-985 (1968).

16. H. Tint, International Symposia on Smallpox Vaccine, Bilthoven, The Netherlands, S Krager AG, Basel 19, 281-292 (1973).
17. J.M. Neff, International Symposium on Smallpox Vaccine, Bilthoven, The Netherlands, S Krager AG, Basel 19, 269-274 (1973).
18. G.J. Galasso, D.T. Karzon, S.L. Katz, S. Krugman, J.M. Neff and F.C. Robbins J. Infec. Dis. 135, 131-186 (1977).
19. J.M. Neff, The American Pediatric Society and the Society for Pediatric Research, Combined Program and Abstracts: 200 (1970)
20. D. Ikic, R. Weisz-Malecek, T. Manhalter and S. Serdarvic, International Symposium on Smallpox Vaccines, Bilthoven, The Netherlands, S Krager AG, Basel 19, 179-186 (1973).
21. A.C. Hekker, J. Huisman, M.F. Polak, J.Th.S. Van der Hoeven, M.H. O'Breen, J. Gertenbach and R.M. Mollema, International Symposium on Smallpox Vaccines, Bilthoven, The Netherlands, S Krager AG, Basel 19, 187-195 (1973).
22. H. Stickl, V. Hochstein-Mintzel and H. Huber, International Symposium on Smallpox Vaccines, Bilthoven, The Netherlands, S Krager AG, Basel 19, 275-278 (1973).
23. I. Tagaya, H. Amano, T. Kitamura, T. Komatsu, Y. Ueda, Y. Tanaka, N. Uchida and H. Kodama, International Symposium on Smallpox Vaccines, Bilthoven, The Netherlands, S Krager AG, Basel 19, 299-307 (1973).

DISCUSSION

Dr. Deinhardt: Dr. Neff, would you like to speculate? You said that the more attenuated vaccinia viruses do not induce such a strong immune response. Our concern is not immune responses to the vaccinia genome products, but the foreign antigens. I would be very much afraid that expression of both types of antigens would run in parallel.

Dr. Neff: I think that is a good point, and there is also the concern regarding which immune responses are important, neutralizing antibodies, the hemagglutination inhibition antibodies, or others. The revaccination response to the attenuated viruses is reduced but it is not clear what that means in terms of the protection against smallpox. Probably, in protection against smallpox, the most critical function is T cell immunity, and the evidence of the take on the arm may be the best indicator of that. But you are absolutely right. They are not as antigenic as the New York Board of Health strain.

Dr. Henderson: I would like to make two points for clarification. First, you referred to the three strains: Elstree, EM-63 and Lister. I think the only two of interest for recombinant vaccinia vaccines are the Elstree and New York Board of Health strains. The EM-63 actually stands for Ecuador-Moscow, 1963. It was thought to have come from Ecuador, and to have originally been a New York Board of Health strain. In fact, it was dropped, because it did not give a very good yield in the laboratory. The Soviet Union primarily produce their vaccine from the Elstree strain.

Second, there was an important study done by the Centers for Disease Control on complications. It was in 1965, before the St. Louis record center burned down. We looked at all illnesses coded as encephalitis and as vaccine complications among all military forces in World War II. We found there were no cases whatsoever in this group. The estimate was that there were , based on five percent of soldiers being primary vaccinees, one to two million primary vaccinees during this period, and no evidence whatsoever of post-vaccinal encephalitis. These population-based statistics give a lower estimate of frequency than the other data sources.

In trying to acquire population-based statistics in developing countries there are great difficulties. We did a study in Indonesia involving the tissue culture vaccine developed by Dr. Hekker in the Netherlands. That was really a first passage Lister strain vaccine. There were 50,000 children vaccinated. They were followed up at 30 days to assess whether there were severe complications following vaccination, and indeed there were. There were an enormous number of deaths due to just about everything one can imagine. When we went back to calculate what the normal death rate was in young children in Indonesia, it was no different than what occurred in the vaccinees. The death rate was also the same whether they received a tissue culture vaccine or the ordinary vaccine. There were cases of encephalitis, there were cases of all sorts of diseases, and it was very difficult to do any sort of study in that situation. We could not draw any conclusions. So doing a study like this in a developing country would be very difficult.

A COMPARATIVE STUDY OF FOUR SMALLPOX VACCINES IN CHILDREN

KENNETH McINTOSH*

*Children's Hospital, Boston, Massachusetts 02115

In the late 1960's, as the gradual (and eventually successful) eradication of smallpox was becoming evident, it was clear that there was a need to define the optimal vaccination technique for those parts of the world which were free of smallpox, a technique which would be essentially without morbidity but would at the same time offer partial or full protection against smallpox should the need for this arise. The National Institute of Allergy and Infectious Diseases therefore sponsored a large, multicenter** trial of smallpox vaccines which was designed to answer this need. The study compared the effect of three different vaccinia strains (one of them in two different forms), administered by two different routes, each in three different concentrations. Each child, after receiving this experimental vaccination, returned at six months for a revaccination "challenge," performed by the usual percutaneous route with the standard dose and strain of vaccine.

The three strains of vaccinia virus used were (1) the New York City Board of Health strain, administered as either a calf-lymph preparation (NYC-CL) or as a chorioallantoic membrane-grown vaccine (NYC-CAM); (2) the Lister, or Elstree, strain, prepared as sheep lymph; and (3) the CV-1 vaccine of Rivers, which had been deliberately attenuated by passage through avian cells (both in the egg and in tissue culture), and which was prepared for this trial in the chorioallantoic membrane of hens eggs. Each of the four vaccines (NYC-CL, NYC-CAM, Lister, or CV-1) was administered by either the percutaneous or the subcutaneous route, and each was prepared in three different doses. The doses used for percutaneous vaccination were 10^6, 10^7, and 10^8 pock-forming units (pfu)/ml, and those used for subcutaneous administration were 10^3, 10^4, and 10^5 pfu/ml. The vaccines were all labelled under code, and the study was performed double-blind. Many clinical parameters were measured, including daily temperatures, the size of any skin lesion (ulcer and erythema), swelling or edema, the rate of development of the skin lesion, skin rashes and systemic reactions. In addition, blood was drawn one month after primary immunization and immediately before and one month after revaccination. The serum thus obtained was examined for vaccinia hemagglutination inhibiting (HI) and neutralizing antibody. A total of 1,746 children took part in the studies, of whom 786 received primary percutaneous vaccination and are analyzed here. This study has been extensively analyzed and reported in full [1-6].

Ironically, as the study was beginning the recommendation for discontinuation of routine smallpox immunization was made by the Red Book Committee and the Advisory Committee on Immunization Practices of the U.S. Public Health Service. Nevertheless, extensive and detailed data were obtained on the comparative infectious doses, local and systemic reactivity, antibody responses, protection against percutaneous challenge, and complication rates for each of the four vaccines. Details are given in the original publications. For the purposes of this meeting,

---

**The principal investigators at the four centers participating in this trial were Abram S. Benenson, James D. Cherry, James D. Connor, and Kenneth McIntosh. Overall coordination was performed by George J. Galasso, and statistical analysis by David W. Alling. Many other individuals participated in the trials and are recognized in the original publications.

© 1985 Elsevier Science Publishing Co., Inc.
VACCINIA VIRUSES AS VECTORS FOR VACCINE ANTIGENS, Quinnan, Editor

comments will only be made about the data on primary percutaneous vaccination and the subsequent revaccination of these same children.

Infectious Dose

Figure 1 shows the rate of primary "take" after each of the percutaneous vaccinations with each vaccine dose. It is evident that the ID_{50} of the two NYC vaccines was virtually identical, very slightly over 10^6 pfu/ml administered by multiple puncture, and that the ID_{50} for the Lister strain is very similar. In contrast, the ID_{50} for the CV-1 vaccine was about 10-fold higher, somewhat more than 10^7 pfu/ml. Moreover, even at the highest concentration tested, 10^8 pfu/ml, the take rate for the CV-1 strain was only about 75%, with no evidence presented that a higher rate would be achieved by using a higher dose. From the point of view of infectivity, then, the CV-1 strain appeared to be truly attenuated.

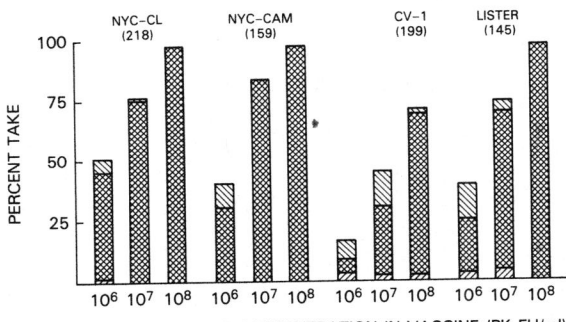

FIG. 1. Rate of major reaction and serologic response to primary percutaneous vaccination with four smallpox vaccines. Figures in parentheses indicate number of children in group. ▨ = major reaction; ▧ = neutralizing antibody and/or HI antibody present in serum taken at 28 days; pfu = pock-forming units.

Reactivity

Table I shows the fever measured during days 4-14 after primary inoculation with each of the four vaccines. Data for those with primary takes are evaluated separately from those without. While there was no placebo control group included in this study, the group without takes probably represents a fair estimation of the background rate of fever in this age group at this time.

It is clear that the two preparations of the NYC strain were, once again, virtually identical. Surprisingly, the Lister strain produced significantly more frequent fever (53% over 101°F, as opposed to 38-40%) than the two NYC strains. The CV-1 vaccine, in contrast, produced this degree of fever in only 26% of children, while the "no-take" control had fever in 20%.

TABLE I. Fever during days 4-14 after primary percutaneous vaccination
with four smallpox vaccines.

Vaccine (no. of children)	Percentage with indicated maximal temperature (F) on days 4-14			
	<100	>100	>101	>102
Takes				
NYC-CL (146)	30	70	40	18
NYC-CAM (105)	38	62	38	21
CV-1 (78)	41	59	26	13
Lister (85)	33	67	53	25
No takes (349)	46	54	20	10

This evidence for the attenuation of the CV-1 strain carried over
to the size of the cutaneous reactions seen (Figure 2). As before, the
two NYC strains were identical. The Lister strain produced slightly
smaller central lesions than these, particularly at the two lower doses,
and the CV-1 strain lesions were even smaller, at all dose levels
tested. The same data were found if surrounding erythema was measured,
rather than central lesion size.

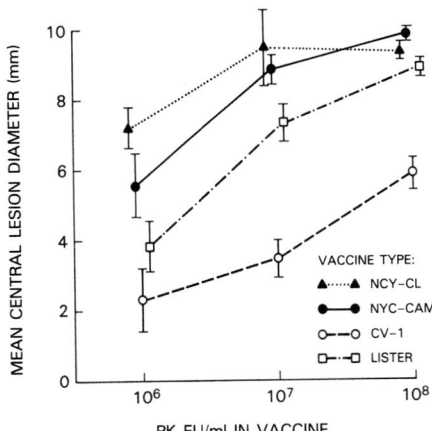

FIG. 2. Mean size ($\pm$ SE) of central lesion
10 days after primary percutaneous vaccination, as a function of the type of vaccine
used and the potency (pock-forming units,
pfu/ml) of the vaccine.

Antibody Response to Primary Vaccination

The antibody response seen 28 days after primary percutaneous
vaccination is shown in Table II. There were a number of important
differences between the vaccines, although the two NYC preparations
again behaved identically. First, in those children with primary takes
there were small but significant differences in the ability of the
three strains to induce HI antibody. The reciprocal geometric mean
titer (GMT) of HI antibody following the CV-1 vaccine was 30, as opposed
to 41 and 56 for the two NYC vaccines and 46 for the Lister. In contrast,

TABLE II. Antibody response 28 days after primary percutaneous vaccination with four smallpox vaccines (children with takes only).

Vaccine (no. of children with take)	Neutralizing antibody		HAI antibody	
	Percentage with detectable antibody[a]	Reciprocal GMT[b] (95% confidence interval)	Percentage with detectable antibody[a]	Reciprocal GMT[b] (95% confidence interval)
NYC-CL (165)	85	92 (67-128)	98	41 (36-47)
NYC-CAM (117)	84	112 (74-171)	99	56 (48-64)
CV-1 (83)	30	7 (5-10)	92	30 (24-38)
Lister (95)	82	89 (56-141)	94	46 (37-56)

[a] Titer of $\geq$ 1:10.
[b] GMT = geometric mean titer.

however, the differences in neutralizing antibody induced by the three
strains were striking. Only 30% of CV-1 vaccinees with clinical takes
developed any neutralizing antibody at all, while the rate was 82-85%
in the other three groups. Moreover, the titers achieved in those with
measurable responses to CV-1 vaccination were very much lower. The
difference seen between the CV-1 strain and the others could not be
attributed to the difference in the sizes of either the central lesion
or erythema, although there was a somewhat higher GMT neutralizing
antibody achieved in the children with the largest local reactions to
the CV-1 strain.

Response to Revaccination

Percutaneous revaccination was performed 6 months after primary
vaccination, and the highest dose (10^8 pfu/ml) of the NYC-CL vaccine
was used for this purpose in all the children. Considerable weight was
given to the rate at which a cutaneous response developed in response
to revaccination, as an index of induced immunity. A "primary-type
response" to revaccination, that is, the development of a Jennerian
central vesicle with surrounding erythema reaching a maximum on or
after the seventh day after revaccination, was judged to represent a
failure of the primary vaccination to induce immunity. As shown in
Table III, even in those children who had a major reaction after their
first vaccination, 21% of those initially receiving the CV-1 vaccine
showed such a "primary-type response," as opposed to 8-12% with the
other three vaccines. Moreover, 62% of CV-1 vaccinees who had developed
only antibody and no major reaction to their first vaccination had a
primary-type response to revaccination. This table also shows that
there was a somewhat reduced take-rate even in those children who had
shown no detectable response at all to their primary vaccination and
who should therefore have reacted exactly like primary vaccinees. In
Figure 1 it was shown that 97% of those receiving the NYC-CL vaccine at
the full 10^8 dose level reacted initially. Thus, it seems likely that
a small proportion of those with no measurable response to primary
vaccination did indeed develop some level of immunity.

Complications

The study was too small to allow for the measurement of the rate
of serious complications. Nevertheless, there were 410 children who
had primary takes with the first vaccination attempt, and these could
be analyzed. Nineteen developed satellite lesions surrounding the
primary take site, 1 developed an accidental infection, 11 had minor
rashes which were classified as either roseola vaccinatum or erythema
multiforme, and one had mild generalized vaccinia. No serious
complications were seen.

Summary

A multicenter trial of four smallpox vaccines was performed in
1,746 children in four university centers in the early 1970's. Of
these, 786 received primary percutaneous vaccination with one of the
four vaccines in one of three doses. Both the NYC Board of Health
strains and also the Lister strain were found to have ID_{50}'s of about
10^6 pfu/ml, whereas the CV-1 strain had an ID_{50} of about ten times
that. Moreover, the CV-1 strain, even when it did produce a primary-
type take, produced less fever than the other three vaccines. The
local lesions produced by the CV-1 strain were also significantly
smaller, both with regard to central lesion and also erythema. While
all four vaccines produced fairly consistent HI antibody responses

TABLE III. Development of primary-type response to revaccination after percutaneous primary vaccination against smallpox.

	No. of children with primary-type response[a] to revaccination/ no. with indicated response to primary vaccination (%)			
Primary vaccine	Major reaction[a]	Serologic response alone[b]	Take[c]	No take
NYC-CL	11/102 (11)	3/4 (67)	14/106 (13)	30/34 (88)
NYC-CAM	7/59 (12)	1/2 (67)	8/61 (13)	17/22 (78)
CV-1	8/38 (21)	3/13 (62)	16/51 (31)	60/74 (81)
Lister	4/52 (8)	1/7 (14)	5/59 (8)	27/33 (82)
Total	30/251 (12)	13/26 (50)	43/277 (16)	134/163 (82)

[a] "Major reaction" was defined as a Jennerian central vesicle with surrounding erythema reaching a maximum on or after the seventh day after vaccination; this response after revaccination was termed "primary-type response."
[b] "Serologic response" was defined as development of antibody (either HI or neutralizing, $\geq$ 1:10) one month after primary vaccination.
[c] "Take" was defined as presence of major reaction and/or serologic response; "no take" was defined as absence of both.

28 days after vaccination, the neutralizing antibody response to the CV-1 vaccine was clearly deficient. Moreover, there was less clinical immunity to revaccination at 6 months after a "take" with the CV-1 vaccine. These collaborative studies thus demonstrated that two preparations of the NYC strain, one prepared in calf lymph and one in the chorioallantoic membrane, behaved identically; that the Lister strain was very similar to the NYC strain, with minor differences in induction of fever and size of cutaneous reaction; and the CV-1 was clearly attenuated for man, producing fewer "takes" with a given dose, smaller cutaneous lesions, far lower levels of neutralizing antibody after primary vaccination, and a lower level of protection against revaccination six months later.

REFERENCES

1. A.S. Benenson, J.D. Cherry, K. McIntosh, et al., J. Infect. Dis. 135, 135-144 (1977).
2. J.D. Cherry, K. McIntosh, J.D. Connor, et al., J. Infect. Dis. 135, 145-154 (1977).
3. K. McIntosh, J.D. Cherry, A.S. Benenson, et al., J. Infect. Dis. 135, 155-166 (1977).
4. J.D. Connor, K. McIntosh, J.D. Cherry, et al., J. Infect. Dis. 135, 167-175 (1977).
5. J.D. Cherry, J.D. Connor, K. McIntosh, et al., J. Infect. Dis. 135, 176-182 (1977).
6. G.J. Galasso, M.J. Mattheis, J.D. Cherry, et al., J. Infect. Dis. 135, 183-186 (1977).

DISCUSSION

Participant: When was revaccination performed?

Dr. McIntosh: After six months, so it was obviously at a time of maximal immunity.

Participant: How was vaccine potency established?

Dr. McIntosh: The vaccines were titered in pock-forming units. The neutralization test was quantitated in plaque-forming units.

Participant: Was there a boost in neutralizing antibodies on revaccination?

Dr. McIntosh: The hemagglutination inhibiting antibody did not boost well, and that has actually been known for a long time. The neutralizing antibody does boost reasonably well, but if they are high to begin with, you do not get a boost.

Dr. Neff: There was an interesting feature of the neutralizing antibodies responses. Those that received CV-178 vaccine first and then had revaccination with the standard calf lymph vaccine, still did not develop the same frequency of neutralizing antibodies as those who had received the standard vaccine first, seeming as if there was some kind of a blocking effect. I think it was the same in the large study.

Dr. McIntosh: Yes. There is something funny about the CV-1 vaccine in its ability to induce neutralizing antibody in the first place, as shown on my slides, and also if you boost with a regular vaccine. But that may have nothing to do with effectiveness of the strain as a vector for foreign antigens.

Dr. Arita: Do you conclude that the CV-1 or CV-2 strains are good candidates for use as vectors?

Dr. McIntosh: Yes, I think they would be good choices. However, if vaccine takes are important, as I think they probably are, then you would have to use more than 10^8 pfu/ml of the CV-1 strain to get more than 75 percent takes.

LOW NEUROVIRULENT VARIANT OF LISTER STRAIN OF VACCINIA VIRUS

SHIRO KATO*

*Research Institute for Microbial Diseases, Osaka University, Suita, Yamadaoka, Japan

The eradication of smallpox in Japan was achieved in 1955. Consequently, the incidence of postvaccinal encephalitis mostly due to the primary vaccination became a very serious social problem in Japan. Responding to the social requirement, a temperature-sensitive and low neurovirulent clone named LC16m8 derived from Lister strain of vaccinia virus was isolated by Hashizume [1]. The unique characteristics of this clone having extremely low neurovirulence in monkeys made the Japanese government decide to use the clone for the primary vaccination. Before the abolition of vaccination against smallpox in 1976 in Japan, about 50,000 children were primarily vaccinated with this clone without any serious complications. Although the number of people vaccinated with this clone was not large, it may be a noteworthy fact that the original Lister strain had been used extensively in the world. The only disadvantage of this clone as well as the original Lister strain so far noticed seems to be the delayed crust formation which may cause more chances of secondary infections. This is probably because of the lack of the vaccinia virus induced-early cell surface antigen [2,3] in cells infected with Lister strain [4].

I believe that it is worthwhile to give this clone (LC16m8) careful reconsideration as a vector for recombinant vaccine because of the low neurovirulence of this clone in primates.

Since the papers of the LC16m8 have not been published in English, an English paper of the detailed characteristics of this clone was prepared by Hashizume et al. for this meeting.

REFERENCES

1. S. Hashizume, Clinical Virology 3, 229-235 (1975).
2. H. Miyamoto and S. Kato, Biken J. 11, 343-353 (1968).
3. K. Ikuta, H. Miyamoto and S. Kato, J. Gen Virol. 47, 227-232 (1980).
4. M. Ito and A.L. Barron, Proc. Soc. Exp. Biol. Med. 140, 374-377 (1972).

PROPERTIES OF ATTENUATED MUTANT OF VACCINIA VIRUS, LC16m8, DERIVED FROM LISTER STRAIN

SO HASHIZUME,* HANAKO YOSHIZAWA,* MICHIO MORITA,** AND KAZUYOSHI SUZUKI**

*Department of Pathobiology, School of Nursing, Chiba University, Inohana, Chiba 280, Japan; **Chiba Serum Institute, Ichikawa 272, Japan

SUMMARY

The further attenuated mutant, LC16m8, was established from Lister strain of vaccinia virus. The virus was obtained by passage in rabbit kidney cells at 30°C and by selecting the clone by temperature sensitivity and with small pock size on the CAM of embryonated eggs.

The mutant virus showed markedly lower neurovirulence in monkeys and rabbits than the parent virus (LO) and other vaccinia viruses of vaccine strains. The immunogenicity of the mutant exhibited, however, was almost the same as that of LO virus or Lister's calf lymph vaccine. The clinical reaction to the LC16m8 vaccine after primary vaccination was very mild; the rate of appearance of fever was only 7.7% and no other severe complications were observed in more than 10,000 children during the field trials. The LC16m8 virus has been authorized for use in Japan as a vaccine strain against smallpox for primary vaccination since 1975.

INTRODUCTION

Recently, the production and selection of infectious vaccinia virus recombinants expressing foreign genes has been achieved by two groups [1,2]. The recombinant vaccinia virus will be probably used for the production of live vaccines. However, those vaccinia viruses of vaccine strains previously used against smallpox were highly neurovirulent [3,4] and their use sometimes resulted in severe complications after vaccination, i.e. postvaccinal encephalitis or encephalopathy. The vaccinia virus for using as a vector of the recombinant vaccines should be a further attenuated vaccinia virus rather than the previously used vaccine strains.

The further attenuated vaccinia virus mutant, LC16m8, was established from a Lister strain of vaccinia virus. The virus was less neurovirulent and the vaccine of the virus showed lower side effects after vaccination than the calf lymph vaccine of the Lister strain, but the immunogenicity was almost the same as that of the Lister strain. The present paper describes properties of the mutant and some other clones derived from Lister virus.

Materials and Methods

Virus Strain. Lister strain (Elstree) which was used for preparation of vaccine against smallpox in Japan, served as the parent virus (LO) of the mutant. The virus which was prepared from infected calf lymph and purified partially by fluorocarbon, was inoculated and was passaged in primary rabbit kidney (PRK) cells at 30°C.

CV1-78 strain virus was prepared with the CAM with the approval of Dr. Kempe and was used as control virus in some experiments.

Cell Culture. PRK cells were prepared from the kidneys of infant rabbits less than 14 days old.

Virus Titration. Titrations of infectivity were mostly performed on the basis of $TCID_{50}$ with Vero cell cultures, but titrations of the LC16m8 were done by the pock count method on the CAM of embryonated eggs. For reproductive capacity of temperature (rct) marker test, the plaque count method on PRK cells was employed; appropriate dilutions were made in 199 medium and inocula were 0.2 ml for 2 oz culture bottles. Following adsorption for one hour at 37°C, the cultures were overlaid with 6 ml of agar medium (Eagle's MEM with 7% calf serum, 0.15% bicarbonate, and 1.5% agar). After the incubation period (2 days for cultures at higher temperatures, and 3 days at 37°C culture), 4 ml of second overlay medium (Eagle's MEM with 7% calf serum, 0.15% bicarbonate, 1:20,000 neutral red, and 1.5% agar) was added and cultured for an additional day.

Neutralization Test

Vero cells cultured in 24 wells plastic dishes (Limbro, FB-16-24) were used for the assay system of neutralization. L5 virus, which was LO virus passaged 5 times in PRK cells, was used as the challenge virus. The L5 virus fluid was diluted to contain 400 to 600 PFU in a volume of 0.1 ml of 199 medium containing 0.2% gelatin. To 0.1 ml of appropriate diluted serum were added 0.1 ml of 5% fresh rabbit serum solution and 0.2 ml of the challenge virus. The serum-virus mixture was incubated for 2 hours at 37°C, then overnight at 4°C. After incubation, 0.05 ml of the serum-virus mixture was inoculated into Vero cell cultures and each dilution of the samples was inoculated in 4 wells. The mixture was adsorbed for 30 minutes at 37°C, 1 ml of 199 medium containing 2% calf serum was added to each well and cultured at 37°C. Following 2 days incubation, the cells were fixed with methanol and were stained with crystalviolet solution to enable counting focuses of the virus growth to be counted. The neutralizing antibody titer was calculated by a 50% reduction of the focus.

Hemagglutination Inhibition Test

HI antibody titers were measured as described in Nakano's report [5]; chicken erythrocytes were used for the test and nonspecific hemagglutinins in sera were removed by adsorption with 50% of chicken erythrocytes.

RESULTS

Selection of the Virus Clones

LO virus was passaged in primary rabbit kidney (PRK) cells at 30°C. At the 26th passages, the growth of the virus at 40°C was somewhat poorer than that of the virus which had been passaged at 37°C. Then the low temerature culture was continued a further 10 times. The 36th passaged virus was cloned by plaque method and 50 plaques were picked off and suspended in one ml of 199 medium.

After each virus fluid was propagated one time at 30°C, 25 clones of those clone viruses were tested rct marker in Vero cells. The titer of 5 clones displayed $10^{1.5}$ or less, 9 clones more than $10^{3.5}$, and the other 11 clones between $10^{1.8}$ and $10^{2.8}$ TCID/0.2 ml in 40°C culture.

One of the clones, designated LC16, showed the lowest titer at 40°C, among the clone viruses. Compared with LO strain, the LC16 strain had rather enhanced growth in rabbit skin, but much reduced growth in the CNS of rabbit and monkey as compared with that of highly attenuated strain DIs. Following these results, a small scale (34 children) inoculation test was done. The rate of appearance of fever was 14% but crust formation was delayed notably, 2 children had not formed crust by later than 14 days after inoculation.

To prevent complication of auto-inoculation, a mutant which had lower capacity of growth in the skin was selected by using pock size marker on the CAM of embryonated eggs. Following 6 passages in PRK cells at 30°C, a single plaque which produced medium size pocks (2-3 mm) on the CAM was isolated and referred to as LC16mO. After a further 3 additional passages of LC16mO virus, the cloning was done in PRK cells, a small pock (0.5-1.0 mm) clone, LC16m8, was selected.

Susceptibility of the Virus Clones to Various Cells

As shown in Table I, when titrated on CAM, Vero, PRK, and primary chick embryo fibroblast (CEF) cells at 37°C, the LO, LC16, and LC16mO showed no difference in Vero cells and the CAM, but the titer in PRK and CEF cells was 1 to 1.5 logs lower than in Vero or the CAM. Conversely, the LC16m8 virus showed 2 logs lower in Vero cells, and 1 log lower in PRK cells, than the CAM.

TABLE I. Comparison of results with different titration systems for Lister virus and its clones.

	Titration System			
Virus	Vero $(TCID_{50})^a$	CAM $(PFU)^a$	PRK $(PFU)^a$	CEF $(PFU)^a$
Lister	8.2	8.2	7.1	6.8
LC16	7.8	8.3	6.3	nd
LC16mO	7.8	7.7	6.6	6.2
LC16m8	5.2	7.2	6.0	6.2

CAM: chorioalantoic membrane; PFU = pock forming unit.
PRK: primary rabbit kidney; PFU = plaque forming unit.
CEF: chick embryo fibroblast cells; PFU = plaque forming unit.
a: 10^n

Reproductive Capacity of the Viruses at Different Temperature

The reproductive capacities of the viruses, LO, LC16, LC16mO, LC16m8, and CV1-78 was compared by the plaque method on PRK cells at different temperatures: 37°C and 40.5°C, or 37°C and 41°C. The ceiling temperature of the LC16m8 was 40.5°C and that of the LC16 and LC16mO was 41°C, but the LO and CV1-78 grew even at 41°C (Table II).

TABLE II. Rct-marker tests with rabbit kidney cells.

Virus	Test 1			Test 2		
Strain	37.0°C	40.5°C	37°C/40.5°C	37.0°C	41.0°C	37°C/41°C
LO	2.4×10^6	7.0×10^4	3.4×10^1	5.0×10^5	6.0×10^3	8.3×10^1
LC16	1.0×10^5	2.4×10^4	4.2×10^0	4.0×10^5	-	$4.0 \times 10^5 <$
LC16mO	8.0×10^5	3.0×10^4	2.7×10^1	3.0×10^5	-	$3.0 \times 10^5 <$
LC16m8	1.0×10^5	-	$1.0 \times 10^5 <$	2.0×10^5	-	$2.0 \times 10^5 <$
CV1-78	1.0×10^5	3.5×10^4	2.9×10^0	3.5×10^5	1.5×10^4	2.3×10^1

Titer: PFU/0.2 ml
- : non-detectable per 0.2 ml

The thermal stabilities of the LC16, LC16mO, and LC16m8 viruses at 40°C were almost identical, although the LC16m8 was slightly more heat labile than the other viruses.

Intracerebral Inoculation of the Clone Viruses into Rabbits

Rabbits, weighing about 2.5 kg, were inoculated intracerebrally with $10^{5.7}$ or $10^{6.7}$ $TCID_{50}$/0.5 ml for LO, LC16, and LC16mO; and with $10^{5.7}$ or $10^{6.7}$ PFU/0.5 ml for LC16m8.

The rabbits inoculated with the LO developed clinical signs of encephalitis at 4 to 5 days after inoculation and one of the rabbits inoculated with $10^{6.7}$ $TCID_{50}$ died. No clinical symptoms were observed in any of the rabbits inoculated with the LC16, LC16mO, and LC16m8 viruses.

A 10% rabbit brain homogenate was prepared after sacrifice at 5 or 6 days post-inoculation, or just after the animal died, to assay the virus titers. No significant difference was observed in the rabbits inoculated with the LC16 and LC16mO. In the cases of the LC16m8, only a small amount of virus was detected in the brains, even though the rabbits were inoculated with $10^{6.7}$ of the virus. The LO virus was the most virulent of the clone viruses. It was suggested that the LC16m8 had a lower capacity of multiplication in the rabbit brain than the other clone viruses (Table III).

Intracerebral Inoculation of the Virus into Cynomolgus Monkeys

Previous reports [3,4] showed that CV1-78 virus was highly neurovirulent, Lister virus was slightly less virulent than CV1-78, and the LC16 virus obviously less virulent than the other vaccine strains of vaccinia virus based on from the comparative studies of several vaccinia virus strains by intrathalamic inoculation into cynomolgus monkeys.

TABLE III. Virus recovery from the rabbits inoculated into the cerebrum

Virus strain	Inoculum	Days p.i. dead or sacrificed	Clinical symptom	Virus recovery from the brain
LO	$10^{6.7}$ TCID$_{50}$	5	+++(D)	$10^{5.4}$ TCID$_{50}$
	$10^{6.7}$	5	++	$10^{5.6}$
	$10^{5.7}$	5	+	$10^{5.0}$
	$10^{5.7}$	6	+	$10^{5.6}$
LC16	$10^{6.7}$	6	−	$10^{4.6}$
	$10^{5.7}$	6	−	$10^{2.0}$
	$10^{5.7}$	6	−	$< 10^{0.2}$
LC16m0	$10^{6.7}$	5	−	$10^{4.8}$
	$10^{6.7}$	5	−	$10^{3.2}$
	$10^{5.7}$	5	−	$10^{2.4}$
	$10^{5.7}$	6	−	$10^{0.4}$
LC16m8	$10^{6.7}$ PFU	5	−	$< 10^{0.2}$ PFU
	$10^{6.7}$	5	−	$10^{2.0}$
	$10^{5.7}$	5	−	$10^{1.2}$
	$10^{5.7}$	5	−	$10^{1.0}$

(D): Death

Neurovirulence of the LC16m0 and LC16m8 was compared by the same method as in the previous report [4]. Two monkeys for each group were inoculated intrathalamically with 0.5 ml of $10^{8.0}$ PFU of the LC16m8 or $10^{8.0}$ TCID$_{50}$ of the LC16m0 virus. One monkey in each group was sacrificed on the 6th day and other was sacrificed on the 14th day after inoculation for histological examination and for virus isolation from the CNS.

None of the monkeys did not show any clinical symptoms. In the monkey inoculated with the LC16m0, virus was isolated from the brain following sacrifice on the 6th day after inoculation, and the titer was $10^{3.2}$ TCID$_{50}$/ml. The specimens taken from the monkey inoculated with the LC16m8, which was sacrificed on the 6th day after inoculation, contained only a small amount of virus, $10^{0.3}$ PFU/ml in the cervical cord and $10^{0.2}$ PFU/ml in the lumbar cord.

The histological findings were that all the monkeys inoculated with both viruses showed very mild leptomeningitis, and the changes were localized as compared with the previous results with other vaccinia viruses [4]. The monkey with LC16m8, sacrificed on the 6th day post-inoculation, showed milder changes than the monkey inoculated with the LC16m0, with respect to infiltration of polymorphonuclear leucocytes and edema. The neurovirulence of the LC16mO and LC16m8 was not significantly different from the LC16 when compared with the previous data for that virus (Table IV).

TABLE IV. Virus isolation and histological findings of the CNS of monkeys inoculated with LC16mO and LC16m8.

Strain	LC16mO				LC16m8			
Inoculum		1×10^8 $TCID_{50}$				1×10^8 PFU		
Clinical symptom		-	-			-	-	
Days p.i.		6	14			6	14	
Virus isolation	B :	3.2^a	-		B :	-	-	
	CC:	-			CC:	0.3^a		
	LC:	-			LC:	0.2		
Change in								
Leptomeninges		++	+			+	+	
Choroid plexus		+	-			+	+	
Softening		-	-			-	-	
Perivascular edema		+	-			+	-	
Hemorrhage in brain		-	-			-	-	
Degeneration of nerve cells		-	+			-	-	
Glia proliferation		-	-			-	+	
Perivascular cellular cuffing		-	+			+	+	
Spongy degeneration		-	-			-	+	

B : Brain
CC : Cervical cord
LC : Lumbar cord
a : 10^n/ml

Intraperitoneal Inoculation of the Viruses into Mice

To establish a property of spreading of the virus to the CNS via the blood, groups of mice were inoculated intraperitoneally with $10^{7.3}$ PFU of LC16m8 and $10^{7.3}$ $TCID_{50}$ of either CV1-78, LO, LC16, or LC16mO, and divided into 2 subgroups to either receive, or not receive subcutaneous administration of each 2 mg of cortisone. Five mice of each group were sacrificed every day after inoculation to determine the virus titer in the blood and the brain. The virus titer in the brain and blood is expressed in the Figures as the average titer of the 5 mice.

In the mice inoculated with the LO virus, the viremia was recognized from 1st to 6th day post-inoculation. The virus was detected from the brain on only one day (on the 6th day) for the group that were not injected with cortisone, but on 3 days (on 4th to 6th day) for the group injected with cortisone (Figure 1).

Mice inoculated with CV1-78 virus also had the virus which was isolated from the brain in two groups, i.e. with or without cortisone.

Among the mice inoculated with the LC16 virus, the virus was recovered only from the brain of the mice treated with cortisone and not from the mice which were not injected with cortisone, but the viremia was observed in both groups (Figure 2).

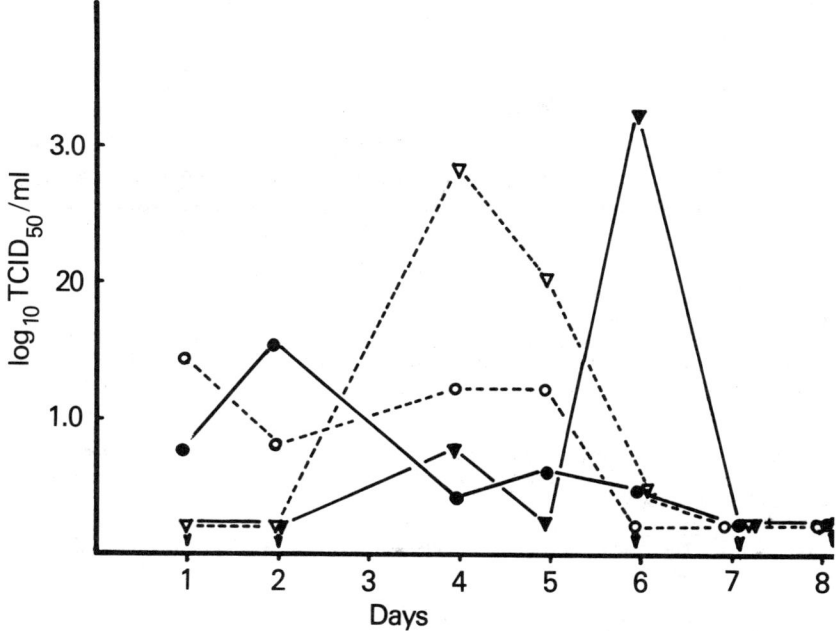

FIG. 1. Virus recovery from the blood and brain of mice which were inoculated intraperitoneally with $10^{7.3}$ $TCID_{50}$ of LO virus and divided into 2 subgroups to either receive, or not, subcutaneously administration of each 2 mg of cortisone. The virus titer is expressed as the average titer of the 5 mice. Symbols ●——●, titer in the blood, without cortisone group; o ----- o titer in the blood with cortisone group; ▼——▼ titer in the brain, without cortisone group; ▽----- ▽ titer in the brain, with cortisone group.

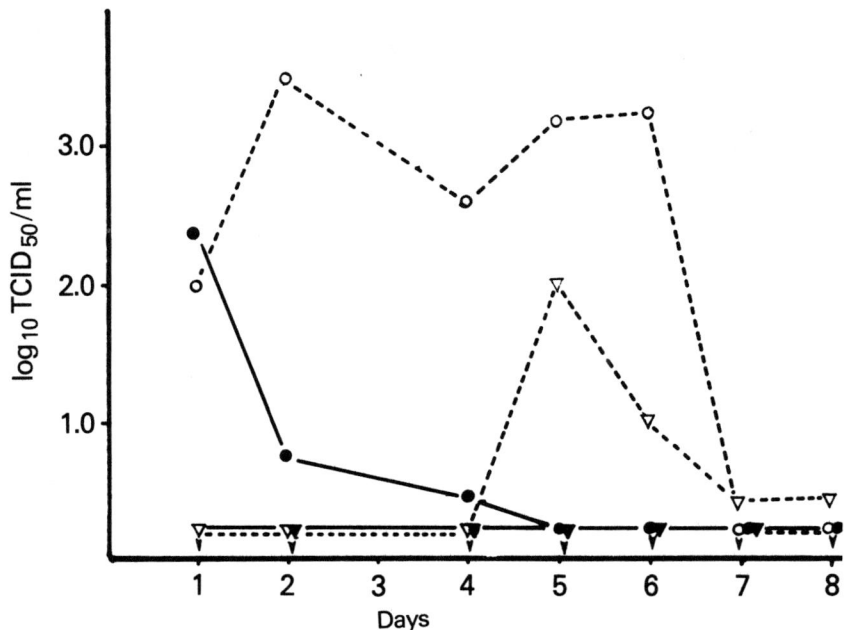

FIG. 2. Virus recovery from the blood and brain of mice which were inoculated intraperitoneally with $10^{7.3}$ $TCID_{50}$ of LC16 virus and divided into 2 subgroups to either receive, or not, subcutaneously administration of each 2 mg of cortisone. The symbols are the same as in Figure 1.

In the groups inoculated with LC16m8, the viremia was observed from 1st to 3rd day post-inoculation in the mice which were not injected with cortisone, but from 1st to 7th day in the mice injected with cortisone. The virus was not recovered from the brain in both groups (Figure 3). The results of the groups inoculated with LC16mO was almost the same as that of the LC16m8 groups.

The Skin Reaction and Antibody Response of Rabbits After Intradermal Inoculation

Serial decimal dilution of each virus, LO, LC16, LC16mO, and LC16m8 was intradermally inoculated in 0.1 ml amounts into rabbits' back skin. Each rabbit received two serial injections; one side was injected in order of decreasing concentration from the shoulder to the rump, and other was from the rump to the shoulder. Four rabbits were used for each virus dilution. The skin reaction, erythema and induration, was measured every day for a week after inoculation. A diameter of the erythema which exceeded 10 mm was scored as a positive reaction and erythema dose (ErD_{50}) was calculated by the Reed and Muench method.

The reaction of the skin inoculated with LC16 was most severe. ErD_{50} of the LO and LC16mO was almost the same and slightly higher than LC16. The LC16m8 showed $10^{3.9}$ ErD_{50}, i.e. the virus had less capacity of producing erythema than the other viruses (Table V).

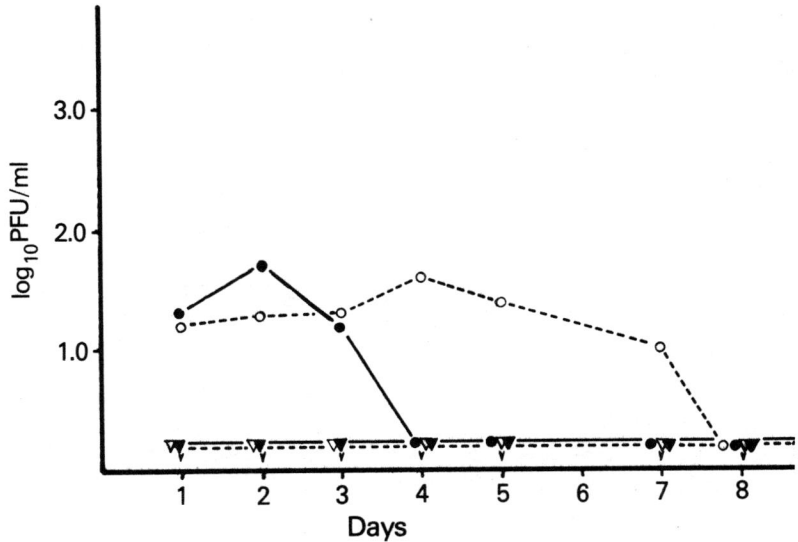

FIG. 3. Virus recovery from the blood and brain of mice which were inoculated intraperitoneally with $10^{7.3}$ PFU of LC16m8 virus and divided into 2 subgroups to either receive, or not, subcutaneously administration of each 2 mg of cortisone. The symbols are the same as in Figure 1.

TABLE V. Skin reaction of rabbits injected intradermally with vaccinia strains.

Inoculum	LO	LC16	LC16mO	LC16m8	CV1-78
10^6	8/8	8/8	8/8	8/8	8/8
10^5	8/8	8/8	8/8	8/8	8/8
10^4	7/8	8/8	8/8	5/8	8/8
10^3	7/8	6/8	8/8	0/8	6/8
10^2	1/8	4/8	0/8	0/8	2/8
ErD_{50}	2.6	2.3	2.5	3.9	2.5

Positive No./Test No.
ErD_{50} : 10^n

Pairs of rabbits were inoculated with $10^{8.0}$ TCID$_{50}$ of the LO and LC16mO, and with $10^{8.0}$ PFU of LC16m8 virus. The hemagglutination inhibition (HI) and neutralizing (NT) antibody response in the rabbits inoculated with LC16mO was the best. The HI antibody response in the rabbits inoculated with LO was better than that of the rabbits inoculated with LC16m8, but the NT antibody response of the rabbits inoculated with LC16m8 was almost the same as that of the rabbits inoculated with the LO virus (Table VI).

TABLE VI. Vaccinia antibody levels after dermal inoculations of LO, LC16mO, and LC16m8 strains.

Weeks p.i.	HI			NT		
	LO	LC16mO	LC16m8	LO	LC16mO	LC16m8
2	$2^{6.5}$	$2^{8.0}$	$2^{4.5}$	$4^{4.9}$	$4^{5.7}$	$4^{4.9}$
4	$2^{6.5}$	$2^{7.5}$	$2^{5.0}$	$4^{4.9}$	$4^{6.9}$	$4^{4.7}$
6	$2^{4.5}$	$2^{7.5}$	$2^{5.0}$	$4^{5.0}$	$4^{6.6}$	$4^{4.6}$
13	$2^{3.5}$	$2^{7.0}$	$2^{5.5}$	$4^{5.0}$	$4^{6.8}$	$4^{4.7}$

LO, and LC16mO: Inoculated 10^8 TCID$_{50}$/animal
LC16m8: Inoculated 10^8 PFU/animal

Clinical Observation of LC16m8 Strain Vaccine

Comparative studies of field trials with Lister, CV1-78, LC16mO, and LC16m8 strain vaccines were carried out by the Smallpox Vaccine Research Committee sponsored by the Ministry of Health and Welfare (1968-1973) [6]. Tables VII to X show the results of those studies. The LC16m8 vaccine exhibited a high rate of take and a low incidence of fever. Table VIII shows local and febrile reactions to LC16m8 strain by age groups. No difference in incidence was observed between any age groups. Many cases of allergic or convulsive constitutions were included among the vaccinees, but no complications were observed among more than 10,000 persons, other than three cases of febrile convulsions and several mild skin complications. In addition to these carefully monitored cases, around 20,000 children were inoculated with the LC16m8 vaccine, and more than 90,000 doses of the vaccine were released in 1974 and 1975, but no reports of severe complications were received.

Table IX shows HI antibody response, and Table X shows NT antibody response, following primary vaccination. The mean HI titer of LC16m8 expressed in terms of log 2 was 3.5 at one to six months after vaccination.

The mean NT titer of the LC16m8 expressed in terms of log 4 was 2.5 at one to 1.5 months after vaccination. The antibody level was slightly lower than that of ordinary strains for HI but the same for NT.

TABLE VII. Local and febrile reactions after primary vaccination by several strains.

Strains	Duration tested	Number observed	Major reaction (Take rate %)	Mean diameter (mm)		Febrile reaction (%)
				Erythema	Induration	
Lister	1968-71	3,662	93.7	17.6	15.3	26.6
CV1-78	1971-73	22,976	92.4	21.1	16.8	8.5
LC16m0	1973-74	829	94.8	19.6	14.5	12.1
LC16m8	1973-74	10,578	95.1	18.4	6.1	7.7

TABLE VIII. Local and febril reaction of LC16m8 vaccine.
(1974, primary vaccination)

Age group	Number observed	Major reaction (%)	Local reaction Mean diameter (mm)		Febrile reaction		
			Erythema	Induration	Febrile (%)	Mean max. temp.	Mean duration[a]
1y	687	97.4	20.8	7.2	10.9	38.5	1.9
2-4y	6,800	95.5	19.0	6.1	7.8	38.5	1.6
5y	2,040	93.1	18.2	6.7	6.6	38.4	1.5
Total/means	9,527	95.1	18.9	6.3	7.8	38.5	1.6

Observed at 9th day.
Surveyed from 4th to 14th day after vaccination.
a = Day

TABLE IX. HI antibodies after the primary vaccination with several strains.

Strains	Months after vaccination	Number of sera examined	HI Titer							Geometric mean titer
			>4	4	8	16	32	64	128	
Lister	1-2	112		4	19	43	27	13	6	4.7
CV1-78	1-2	187	6	11	35	60	47	28		4.1
	3-7	162	12	35	54	46	10	5		3.2
LC16m0	1-2	47			4	23	16	4		4.4
LC16m8	1-2	513	18	100	161	155	72	6	1	3.4
	3-6	19	1	6	3	6	6			3.5

Geometric mean titer : 2^n

TABLE X. NT antibodies after the primary vaccination with several strains.

Strains	Months after vaccination	Number of sera examined	NT Titer							Geometric mean titer
			>$4^{0.9}$	$4^{1.0}$	$4^{1.5}$	$4^{2.0}$	$4^{2.5}$	$4^{3.0}$	$4^{3.5}$	
Lister	1-1.5	5				3	2			$4^{2.4}$
	3-6	12	1	2		2	7			$4^{2.2}$
CV1-78	1-1.5	6	1		2	2		1		$4^{1.9}$
	3-6	11	1	1	4	2	3			$4^{2.0}$
LC16mO	1-1.5	15					6	9		$4^{3.0}$
LC16m8	1-1.5	97		5	10	25	37	18	2	$4^{2.5}$

DISCUSSION

Several strains have been proposed as the best candidate for attenuated smallpox vaccine strain, e.g. CV1-78 derived from New York City Department of Health Laboratory (NYCDHL or NYBH) strain (rabbit testis(RT)/4, chick embryo/34, RT/6, CEF/59, CAM/19); CVII from the same strain (RT/4, CE/31, CEF/180) [7]; MVA by Stickl et al. from Ankara strain (CEF/532) [8,9]. They are mostly obtained through a large number of passages in chick embryo or CEF cells. DIs strain produced by Tagaya et al. [7,10] was a small pock mutant isolated following 13 passages in one-day-eggs.

The cases of polio and measles, attenuated strains especially those with reduced neuropathogenicity were selected from ts mutants and variola minor virus (low virulence wild virus) which has a lower ceiling temperature than that of variola major virus (classical smallpox in Asia, high virulent virus) [11,12]. These results suggest significant correlations between attenuation and ts mutants.

Though the pathogenesis of post-vaccinal encephalitis and encephalopathy (PVE) have yet to be elucidated, the following three points may be agreed upon: (a) most PVE cases are related to the primary vaccination and cases related to secondary or later vaccinations are quite few; (b) administration of vaccinia immune globulin can reduce the incidence of PVE; and (c) morbidity of PVE seems to have some relationship with the virus strain used.

From pathological findings in monkey experiments by Morita et al. [4] and immuno-fluorescence studies by Aoyama et al. in monkey experiments and human PVE cases [4,13], the virus grow primarily in the meninges, choroid plexus, ventricular and vascular walls, but not in the cerebral matrix, and the perivascular infiltration of microglial cells, demyelinations, and other encephalitic findings may appear secondary by immuno-pathological process. This seems to support the hypothesis that PVE occurs by active growth of vaccinia virus in the CNS, rather than that of being primarily caused by the allergic mechanisms.

Three strains of LC16 series were demonstrated to have a remarkably reduced capacity to grow in the CNS. Furthermore, CL16mO and LC16m8 had reduced the activity of transversing the blood-CSF junction in the meninges or choroid plexus in comparison with the LO or CV1-78 virus. The LC16m8 strain had a rather lower immunogenicity than the LC16mO. However, the LC16m8 had an appropriate efficiency of local growth to induce immunity as strongly as calf lymph vaccine of LO strain, and it showed slightly lower neurovirulence than that of the LC16mO in the results of monkey and rabbit experiments. Considering these points, the LC16m8 strain may become the most practically suitable vaccine strain.

REFERENCES

1. M. Mackett, G.L. Smith, and B. Moss, Proc. Nat. Acad. Sci. 79, 7415-7419 (1982).
2. D. Panicali and E. Paoletti, Proc. Nat. Acad. Sci. 79, 4927-4931 (1982).
3. S. Hashizume, M. Morita, H. Yoshizawa, S. Suzuki, M. Arita, T. Komatu, H. Amano and I. Tagaya, Internal Symposium on Smallpox Vaccine, Bilthoven; Symp. Series Immunobiol. Standard 19, 325-331 (1973).
4. M. Morita, Y. Aoyama, M. Arita, H. Amano, H. Yoshizawa, S. Hashizume, T. Komatu and I. Tagaya, Arch. Virol. 53, 197-208 (1977).
5. J.H. Nakano in: Poxvirus: Diagnostic Procedures for Viral, Rickettsial and Chlamydial Infections, 5th ed., pp. 257-308 (1979).
6. M. Yamaguchi, M. Kimura and H. Hirayama, Clin. Virol. 3, 269-278 (in Japanese) (1975).
7. R. Wokatsch in: Vaccinia Virus, Strains of Human Viruses, M. Majer and S.A. Plotkin, eds. (S. Karger, Basel 1972) pp. 2410247.
8. H. Stickl and V. Hochstein-Mintzel, Munch. Med. Wschr. 113, 1149-1153 (1971).
9. H. Stickl, V. Hochstein-Mintzel and C. Huber, Internal Symposium on Smallpox Vaccine, Bilthoven, Symp. Series Immunobiol. Standard 19, 275-279 (1973).
10. I. Tagaya, T. Kitamura and Y. Sano, Nature 192, 381-382 (1961).
11. M.D. Nizamuddin and K.R. Dumbell, Lancet i, 68-69 (1961).
12. K.R. Dumbell, H.S. Bedson and E. Rossier, Bull. Wld. Hlth. Org. 25, 73-78 (1961).
13. T. Kurata, Y. Aoyama and T. Kitamura, Japan J. Med. Sci. Biol. 30, 137-147 (1977).

IMMUNOGENICITY OF VACCINIA VIRUS: RESPONSES TO VACCINATION

J. DONALD MILLAR

*Director, National Institute for Occupational Safety and Health Centers for Disease Control, Atlanta, Georgia 30333

It is very difficult for me to communicate adequately my appreciation for the invitation to be here. Eighteen years ago this month, November 1966, I was appointed Director of the CDC Smallpox Eradication Program, just after Dr. D. A. Henderson went to Geneva as Director of the WHO Smallpox Eradication Unit. My major responsibility was to implement the West and Central African Smallpox Eradication and Measles Control Program. Field operations in Africa were expected to begin early in 1967; vaccine, equipment, and people had to be sent to Africa as rapidly as possible, a thousand-and-one other logistical problems had to be solved before field operations could begin. Though frequently hectic, the next 4 years as Director of that unprecedented regional health assistance program were the most fulfilling of my professional career ...then in April 1970, on the very eve of final victory over smallpox in West and Central Africa, my "commanding officer," Dr. David J. Sencer, then Director of CDC, asked me to relinquish the Smallpox Eradication Program, and take charge of a new organization combining all the domestic disease control activities of CDC. While I was greatly flattered by his confidence in me, I felt, as Shakespeare put it, from my "mother's womb Untimely ripp'd."** With mixed feelings, I turned away from smallpox eradication and assumed my new assignment.

Since then, Drs. Henderson (both D. A. and Ralph), Foege, Lane, Mack, Neff, Wulff, and other compatriots have marched to glory in global smallpox eradication; meanwhile, my professional path meandered instead through programs such as urban rat control, fluoridation, and swine flu immunization, to more contentious spheres of environmental and occupational public health.

To be sure Dr. Sencer, perhaps expiating feelings of guilt, released me for three further brief stints of duty with smallpox eradication, in India (1975, as a field epidemiologist during the last days of smallpox there), and for WHO International Commissions for the Certification of Smallpox Eradication in South America (1973) and in Somalia (1979). However, in a very important way, this Workshop is my attempt to return to a love lost long ago.

Hence, I make no pretense of being expert in any aspect of the immunogenicity of vaccinia virus. On the contrary, the sciences of immunology and virology have virtually exploded in the last 25 years, and I was left, fire-blinded, in the cratered ashes of my outdated knowledge. Today, much like Rip Van Winkle, I am blinking awake in a virologic world many years ahead of me!

All of this I told to your Program Chairman when he invited me here; I offered to attend this meeting as an old warrior and sit quietly in the corner. However, he insisted that I speak, so here I am, not at all comfortable on an agenda devoted to space-age issues of molecular virology.

As a coping mechanism, I have reverted to my past personal experience, dusted off some golden memories and old reprints, and tried to reacquaint myself with the lost love. My presentation is an attempt to summarize

---
**(Shakespeare, W.; Macbeth, Act V, Sc. viii, spoken by MacDuff).

Published 1985 by Elsevier Science Publishing Co., Inc.
VACCINIA VIRUSES AS VECTORS FOR VACCINE ANTIGENS, Quinnan, Editor

broadly the results of CDC's work with vaccinia virus, in which I was personally involved. My conclusion is simple, and I state it at the outset: Vaccinia virus is a remarkably effective immunogen which has changed the history of mankind.

Studies of Smallpox Vaccination by Intradermal Jet Injection: 1963-1972

Beginning in 1963, we at CDC conducted a series of studies of smallpox vaccination (Table I). Our major interest was the interruption of smallpox transmission by mass vaccination, and we were specifically interested in evaluating technologic innovations which offered hope of improved campaigning in the field. Executing these studies led us to an ever-deeper involvement in, and commitment to, the eradication of smallpox from the world. These studies culminated in the CDC-directed, USAID-financed, WHO-sponsored West and Central African Smallpox Eradication and Measles Control Program which, in my opinion, was the most spectacularly successful foreign aid program in health ever undertaken by the United States. During those years, we looked very often and very closely at the behavior of vaccinia virus as an immunogen in humans.

An important impetus for our work was the development by the United States Army of a mechanical device for performing inoculations by intradermal jet injection. Specifically, the device was a nozzle developed by Mr. Aaron Ismach at the U.S. Army Research and Development Laboratory, Fort Totten, New York. Jet injector guns had been available in one form or other since World War II. However, existing models had nozzles that directed the stream of inoculum straight into subcutaneous and intramuscular spaces, and were of no use for smallpox vaccination, which required intracutaneous inoculation. To be sure, Drs. Harry Meyer and Bennett Elisberg experimented with an adapter cuff which raised the nozzle from the skin, permitting a greater than ordinary amount of the inoculum to be trapped in the dermal layers. Ismach, with strong encouragement from Colonel Abram S. Beneson (well known to many of you) conceived a specific solution to the problem. He designed a nozzle which bent the stream of inoculum, directing it into the dermis. In collaboration with Ismach, we explored the utility of this nozzle for smallpox vaccination and for fungal skin testing [8].

To evaluate the intradermal nozzle for smallpox vaccination, we established a study plan which involved tests of intradermal jet injection vaccination in study populations of varying age, and with varying degrees of pre-existing immunity to vaccinia virus. We planned our progress so as to generally move from smaller to larger numbers of subjects as we developed increasing knowledge of the efficacy and safety of the procedure. We began by testing adult male revaccinees in Georgia, making close and frequent observations and documenting the results. Opportunities led us to Jamaica, for studies of primary vaccination in school children; to Tonga, for a large scale trial in an unvaccinated and smallpox-free population; and finally to Amapa, Brazil, for a large scale trial in a smallpox-endemic territory of a major smallpox-endemic country.

Though smallpox vaccination was 200 years old when we began these studies, we documented some clinical and immunological events following vaccination, in ways never previously done. We compared results of intradermal jet injection with those of the traditional multiple pressure method of inoculation; employed various log dilutions of smallpox vaccine by jet injection to determine dose-response relationships; and collected a lot of information on operational aspects of mass vaccination campaigns in the developing world. We systematically observed, and documented with

TABLE I: Studies of smallpox vaccination by intradermal jet injection: 1963-1972. Centers for Disease Control, Atlanta, Georgia

Date	Place	Subjects Number	Subjects Type	Serologic findings reported	Comments	Reference
1963	Georgia, USA	156	Adult male "distant" revaccinees	Yes	Various doses compared	1
1964	Jamaica	636	Unvaccinated school children	Yes	Various doses compared	2
1964	Georgia, USA	140	Adult male "recent" revaccinees	Yes	Various doses compared	3
1964	Tonga	44,000	Unvaccinated general population	Yes	Field trial, smallpox-free area; various doses compared	4
1965	Amapa, Brazil	48,000	General population	No	Field trial, smallpox-endemic area; various operational methods compared	5
1967-72*	21 Nations, West and Central Africa	120,000,000	General population	No	Smallpox eradication campaign	6,7

*Though, obviously the West and Central African Smallpox Eradication/Measles Control Program was not "a study," the ongoing assessment component of the program included systematic, periodic documentation of "take rates."

photography, the evolution of cutaneous results of vaccination and revaccination, comparing results produced by jet injection with those by the traditional multiple pressure method. We collected and tested sera for serologic evidence of response using both neutralizing and hemagglutination inhibition tests.

Ultimately, we joined together with the ministries of health of 21 countries in West and Central Africa and, using the operational advantages of jet injection and epidemiologic intelligence, executed a highly successful regional smallpox eradication program. During the course of that effort, we made millions of systematic observations of the results of vaccination in individuals. Moreover, in Africa we thoroughly documented the success of vaccination in interrupting the transmission of smallpox in a large and important segment of the smallpox-endemic world. All of these things were accomplished a decade ago, and the results were long-since published.*

Major Conclusions of the Studies by CDC

One could consume hours presenting the detailed results of these studies. There seems very little reason to do so, in light of their prior publication and the pressing contemporary issues which ought to command our attention during these two days. Therefore, I will broadly summarize our major findings (and provide the references to the published papers which may be consulted for details):

1. Commercially produced (Wyeth Laboratories) lyophilized calf lymph smallpox vaccine with a titre of $10^{8.5}$ $TCID_{50}$/ml inoculated by the multiple pressure method, produced cutaneous and serologic evidence of vaccinial infection in virtually 100% of primary vaccinees and revaccinees previously vaccinated more than 10 years before. Among subjects previously vaccinated less than 10 years previously, the same inoculation produced "major reactions" (WHO definition) in about 70%, and significant neutralizing antibody responses in approximately 70% of those with initial titres less than 160.

2. Intradermal jet injection of 0.1 ml of diluted vaccine with a titre of $10^{7.0}$ $TCID_{50}$/ml produced cutaneous and serologic results equal to or better than, those observed with the multiple pressure method using undiluted vaccine. The cutaneous reactions following jet injection vaccination differed little from those seen after the traditional method.

3. Jet injection technology offered distinct operational advantages for rapid mass vaccination of a large population.

4. Smallpox vaccination, appropriately applied among populations, is capable of eliminating the transmission of smallpox.**

Jet injection seemed especially well adapted to West and Central Africa where (particularly in Francophone countries, and in Ghana) there were rich traditions of mobile health services, and where the gathering

---

*Dr. Roberto's report on the experience in Tonga is detailed only in his dissertation for the academic post graduate diploma in tropical public health at the University of London, London School of Hygiene and Tropical Medicine on file in the CDC Library.
**Indeed, the 23rd World Health Assembly, on May 8, 1980, declared that global smallpox eradication has been accomplished.

together of the population for various reasons was an important cultural value. The use of jet injection vaccination in "collecting points" was uniquely appropriate in this setting, making possible rapid execution of mass vaccination campaigns across the region.

The West and Central African Smallpox Eradication and Measles Control Program exerted a distinct influence on the remainder of the global program by discovering an important alternative to mass vaccination as the foundation of eradication. Epidemiological information developed principally by Foege [9] in Nigeria, led us to the conclusion that active surveillance of smallpox coupled with epidemiologically-directed field operations (vaccinations targeted so as to specifically exploit seasonal and geographical vulnerabilities in the transmission of smallpox) was a faster and more efficient way to interrupt transmission than was mass vaccination. Hence, "surveillance-containment" operations replaced mass vaccination campaigns as the principal tactic of smallpox eradication. This development in West and Central Africa became the backbone of smallpox eradication efforts elsewhere in the world.

The bifurcated needle, a brilliant, yet simple and inexpensive invention by Dr. B. A. Rubin of Wyeth Laboratories, became the principal inoculating device used in the global program beyond West and Central Africa. This virtually fool-proof device in hands of limitless numbers of indigenous personnel produced the successful vaccinations that stopped the transmission of smallpox in the rest of the world.

During the course of this exciting era, literally millions of systematic observations of vaccination produced overwhelming evidence that in all kinds of settings, in all kinds of populations, in all kinds of delivery systems, and in the hands of all kinds of vaccinators, vaccinia virus proved to be a highly effective immunogen. It produced readily interpretable cutaneous results, and predictable serological results reasonably consistent with the cutaneous findings and reasonably well correlated with protection. For me, the net result of this massive experience is the conviction stated at the outset, "that vaccinia virus is a remarkably effective immunogen which has changed the history of man."

In a textbook chapter [10] on smallpox and other pox virus infections, Dr. James Nakano and I wrote "over the years, vaccinia virus vaccine has proved to be one of the most effective and safest of immunogens...in every sense smallpox vaccine deserves the title 'noble' agent."

That this "noble agent," which has eliminated one major scourge of mankind, should now become a vehicle through which to conquer other plagues, is a prospect most exhilarating to this aging warrior. I eagerly anticipate the discussions which will occur here.

REFERENCES

1. J.D. Millar, R.R. Roberto, H. Wulff and D.A. Henderson, Bull. Wld. Hlth. Org. $\underline{41}$, 749-760 (1969).
2. R.R. Roberto, H. Wulff and J.D. Millar, Bull. Wld. Hlth. Org. $\underline{41}$, 761-769 (1969).
3. J.M. Neff, J.D. Millar, R.R. Roberto and H. Wulff, Bull. Wld. Hlth. Org. $\underline{41}$, 771-778 (1969).
4. R.R. Roberto, Dissertation submitted for the Academic Post Graduate Diploma in Tropical Public Health, University of London, London School of Hygiene and Tropical Medicine, June 1965.
5. J.D. Millar, L. Morris, A. Macedo Filho, T.M. Mack, W. Dyal and A.A. Medeiros, Trop. Geogr. Med. $\underline{23}$, 89-101 (1971).

6. J.D. Millar and W.H. Foege, J. Inf. Dis. 120(6), 725-732 (1969).
7. W.H. Foege, J.D. Millar, and D.A. Henderson, Bull. Wld. Hlth. Org. 52, 209-222 (1975).
8. J.D. Millar, F. Tosh, A. Ismach, L. Morris, and T.F. Sellers, Jr., Am. Rev. Resp. Dis 100, 542-549 (1969).
9. W.H. Foege, J.D. Millar, and J.M. Lane, Amer. J. of Epid. 94(4), 311-315 (1971).
10. J.D. Millar and J.H. Nakano in: Infectious Diseases, 3rd Ed., Paul D. Hoeprich, M.D., ed. (Harper and Row Publishers, Philadelphia, 1982), pp. 867-875.

DISCUSSION

Dr. Halstead: I would like to express some misgivings about vaccinia. You quite correctly characterized vaccinia as a remarkable immunogen, as a live virus vaccine. It is not only a remarkable live virus vaccine, but it has some characteristics that are quite unique. With most viral vaccines, it appears that we have recapitulated the same phenomenon that we see with wild viruses, and that is the permanent production of sustained antibody and, apparently, sustained protection. It has been widely accepted that the degree of protection afforded by vaccinia infection as compared to variola infection, is nowhere near as complete. I am not sure this is as scientific as it ought to be, but certainly it was part of conventional wisdom. Whether it is part of the scientific record, that vaccinia in fact does lead ultimately to a loss of protective state and the possibility of a repeat viremic infection is something that certainly needs to be worked out.

If one then takes an immunogen that has those attributes and adds to it some other DNA, are we not going to produce the same type of immunity, that is, an immunity that apparently has some attributes of short-term nature? I wonder if the model that Dr. Buller described of ectromelia virus in mice is really an appropriate model for vaccinia in man. As far as I know, vaccinia doesn't generalize even to regional lymph nodes. Where are the antibodies made following the intradermal inoculation of vaccinia? Is it local? Is it regional? Is it in the spleen? Is that going to be important in terms of inserting measles or hepatitis genomes into these agents? Do we need to have antibody at some certain site or at some certain level in order to provide protection against some of the viruses that we would like to insert onto this? I think these are key questions that have to be answered before we go full tilt into the use of vaccinia as a carrier to substitute for living virus genomes that have highly desirable attributes. I don't think we want to give up a remarkable immunogen for one that may have less than remarkable properties.

Dr. Ada: Dr. Fenner has written some things that may be relevant to that point, in his chapter on the pathogenesis, pathology, and immunology of smallpox and vaccinia. He states that vaccinia virus occurs in enveloped and non-enveloped forms. There are two types of neutralizing antibodies to these. The envelope virus spreads better than the non-enveloped virus. The antibody to non-enveloped virus is less effective at passive protection than antibody to the enveloped virus. Inactivated vaccine does not protect against vaccinia. There is a short-lived IgM response and a persistent IgG response to both types of virus. After vaccination neutralizing antibody has been detected for up to 20 years. Inactivated antigen induced delayed-type hypersensitivity (DTH) but no cytotoxic T cell response. The active virus gives both DTH and a cytotoxic T cell response.

He claims there are three types of antibody produced, one which is involved in neutralization, one which relies on the presence of complement, and those which form immune complexes. He is not at all sure how important antibody is in recovery from infection. Passive antibody can prevent infection, but is much less effective in modifýding the course of the disease. Antibody produced after infection with live virus is more protective than antibody produced by immunization with inactive virus. Cell-mediated immunity is almost certainly more important.

In model systems with both ectromelia and vaccinia in the mouse, after intravenous injection, cytotoxic T cells are first detected about day four and rise to maximum titer at about day six. DTH can also be measured at day six. Mice treated with antithymocyte sera die from a sublethal dose of virus, even though neutralizing antibody and interferon might be present.

Dr. Blanden did cell transfer studies in the ectromelia system. He showed that this was a very quick and rapid way of reducing virus titers. Within 12 hours he detected a difference in virus titers in liver, and within 24 hours titers of virus in liver were down by three to four logs, which is a very rapid effect of cytotoxic T cells indeed.

Another point I can mention is that in children with immune deficiency states, vaccinia replicated without restriction, progressive primary lesions occurred, and death was often the outcome. Patients with defects in antibody production were able to mount a cell-mediated immune response and usually reacted normally to vaccination.

Dr. McIntosh: The incidence of fever in children undergoing primary vaccination was approximately 40-50 percent. This rate is higher than virtually any other vaccine that we now give. It would be surprising if such febrile reactions could occur purely as a result of epidermal or dermal reactions. Also, local lymphadenopathy is extremely common, if not universal. Attempts to isolate virus from blood during febrile reactions have been, as far as I know, almost universally unsuccessful. However, we isolated virus from the throat in a surprising number of infants who had severe reactions to vaccinia in our study.

Dr. Moss: The reason you can revaccinate and get a response is that you are giving a high dose of virus, and it is replicating right at the site of inoculation. That is the reason that you get a revaccination response, not because the animal has lost immunity. If you try to do the same thing with herpes virus, for example, even though the animal is immune, you also get replication. If you do it with foot-and-mouth disease virus, I think you will also see it happen. If you do it with vesicular stomatitis virus, it is a common phenomenon if the virus is replicating at the site of inoculation.

Dr. Halstead: The issue that needs resolution is whether vaccinia provides lifelong immunity against viremic reinfection with variola. With rubella and rubeola there is a "reinfection phenomenon" in people who are systemically protected. The pharynx or gastrointestinal tract can become infected. Virus can be present in the throat or excreted in the stool, even though there is no risk of developing clinical rubeola or rubella. It used to be the conventional wisdom that, after a period of three to five or so years, systemic reinfection was possible with vaccinia. If that is not true, it would be comforting.

Dr. D.A. Henderson: In trying to determine the duration of immunity following vaccinia virus inoculation we encountered enormous difficulties.

Prior to 1967, vaccine potency was rarely in excess of seven or seven and a half logs of virus, and there were many who had vaccination scars that were probably the result of a septic process rather than a vaccinial proliferative process. So it was difficult to measure how many people have been successfully vaccinated.

The issue was complicated by people in endemic areas having subclinical infections with variola. Whether these were viremic infections or not, I don't know. I suspect they probably were, but it is not very clear.

So it was very difficult to measure what was the duration of protection, but I think duration of protection for an individual vaccinated with a high titer of vaccinia virus vaccine and exposed subsequently was very high for a long period of time. In support of this assessment, we found that people who were in more remote areas and were vaccinated with known, high-titered vaccines, did not come down with the disease when smallpox was introduced. To quantitate the level and duration of protection was just impossible. So my guess is, it does protect for a very long period of time.

With regard to protection against vaccinia virus proliferation at the inoculation site, it obviously depends very much upon the titer of the vaccine. With the Russian vaccine which had nine-and-a-half logs of virus per ml, you could get what nearly amounted to primary takes in people vaccinated one and two years before. I think these people clearly were protected against viremic smallpox.

Dr. Neff: I think the studies performed by Dr. Thomas M. Mack (previously with the C.D.C.) were a little purer. They were able to show during smallpox importation into European countries, that if a person had been vaccinated at least once in their lifetime, even though they could get a modified case, it was very, very rare to find a death. You really did decrease the mortality just by having one bone fide vaccination in your lifetime.

SMALLPOX VACCINE IN VIVO PRODUCTION AND TESTING

DON P. METZGAR*

*Connaught Laboratories, Inc., Swiftwater, Pennsylvania 18370

INTRODUCTION

Early supplies of "lymph" used for smallpox vaccination were obtained from "spontaneous outbreaks" of cowpox in cattle from local farms or from primary human immunization--harvested "scabs"--with vaccination carried out until the supply was exhausted. By 1842, vaccine pulp or "lymph" was being produced in Italy by direct passage and propagation in cows. Up until 1980, this was the primary means of manufacturing smallpox vaccine.

The basic manufacturing process has remained virtually unchanged for the last 140 years or so. Certainly refinements in standardization, testing requirements and vaccine presentation have been made during that time, but animal propagation of vaccinia virus has been the primary source of smallpox vaccine. While other animals such as sheep and rabbits have been used to produce the vaccine, the calf has remained the animal of choice. Not only because large quantities of vaccine pulp could be produced from a single animal, but also the calf could be easily housed and controlled during the incubation phase.

It is interesting to note that in the early years, manufacturers used to rent calves from farmers and then return them when vaccine production was completed. Only small areas of the calf were used and only the formed scabs were harvested. More extensive use of the animals' productive areas in later years required sacrificing the animal.

The manufacture of smallpox vaccine by propagation of vaccinia virus in calves is a unique process. It is quite different from the ordinary tissue culture or fermentor-derived product. Only a very few people have actually manufactured the vaccine and few in the scientific community have witnessed the process. For this reason, a major portion of this presentation will be a film, produced by Connaught Laboratories Limited. The film portion will run for about 15 minutes and will cover the preparation, inoculation, and harvest phases of smallpox vaccine manufacture. The process to be described will be production of smallpox vaccine in calves. It is recognized that vaccinia virus can be propagated in other species but most of the vaccine produced in the past has been produced in bovines.

METHODS OF MANUFACTURE

The Calves

The manufacture of smallpox vaccine in calves is a "clean process" not a sterile process. The resulting product is often sterile and process precautions can result in a sterile product about 80% of the time.

The production animal is a heifer (female) between 6 months and 1 year of age with black marking of no greater than 50% of the scarification area and weighing 400 to 500 pounds.

The animal should be in overt good health, free of detectable skin infections and negative for tuberculosis.

The animal is quarantined (isolated) in the production facility for a period of 14 days before use. During the last 7 days of the quarantine, the animal must maintain a normal rectal temperature (102-103°F).

Animal Preparation

The injection sites of the calf are closely clipped and washed using an alcoholic-based soap such as tincture of green soap. The calf is then transferred to the production unit. From this point on, sterile hospital operating room conditions are exercised.

The clipped and washed calf is strapped to a vertical operating table which hydraulically lifts the calf to a horizontal position. The areas to be scarified are washed with soap and then shaved with a straight razor. The total animal is then rinsed with sterile water for injection.

The areas for scarification include: exposed back and side; limbs to the knee (first joint); entire ventral surfaces. The head, neck, shoulders, udder and umbilicus are not included.

Scarification

The entire washed, exposed area is scarified using a suitable instrument. The scarification tool should provide continuous skin lesions spaced about 1/8 to 1/4 inch apart. The scarification should be deep enough to penetrate the epidermis, but not the corium.

The excess blood is removed with sterile absorbent cloth and the entire area is bathed with smallpox seed. The application is allowed to dry and the animal is transferred to a holding stall.

The 7 days between scarifications and pulp harvest are critical to the quality of the final product.

The animal must be immobilized and is not allowed to lie down. Feces and urine must be collected and disposed of without animal and quarters contact. This is usually done by ceiling suspensions and bag collection.

The animal is monitored daily for temmperature and general conditions with a veterinarian in attendance.

Harvest of Pulp

After 7 days, the vesicle formation is complete and the animal is again transferred to the operating room where it is strapped to the horizontal hydraulic lift table. The animal is sacrificed and exsanguinated.

The infected areas are washed with a disinfectant and rinsed with sterile water and covered with sterile dressing.

The vesicles are harvested with sterile curettes and placed in collection jars and stored at -20°C or lower.

This constitutes the completion of the infection and harvest stage. The amount of pulp and the quality of the pulp harvested depend upon the size of the animal, the extent of the "take" and the skills of the technician. The average yield should be in the range of 250 to 350 grams of vaccine pulp, with an ultimate yield of several hundred thousand doses of final vaccine.

Preparation of Vaccine

The crude vaccine pulp is ground in an "eppenback" mill, blender, or over stone or glass beads with a suitable diluent such as glycerinated saline or saline alone. The extraction fluid may contain phenol or brilliant green as a bacteriostatic agent. The pulp may undergo several extractions or grinding procedures and the final bulk vaccine is devoid of the spent pulp, which is discarded. The spent pulp is removed by low speed centrifugation or screening.

The final vaccine presentation can be either a fluid, glycerinated product, which is applied by needle scarification, or a freeze-dried product that can be administered by jet gun or needle scarification.

The requirements for product specifications for smallpox vaccines set by the United States Food and Drug Administration and the World Health Organization are listed in Table I. They were really quite simple.

TABLE I. Product specifications for smallpox vaccines

Characteristic	Specification
1. Potency	A minimum of 1×10^8 viable particles as measured by titration of the chorioallantoic membrane of chicken embryos, as compared to the U.S. standard
2. Viable bacteria	No more than 200 viable organisms per ml
3. Coliforms	No allowance
4. Hemolytic strep	No allowance
5. Coagulase + staph	No allowance
6. Anaerobes	No allowance
7. Phenol content	No more than 0.5%

REFERENCES

1. CFR 21, Part 630, Sub-part H; U.S. Government Printing Office, 1984.
2. C.W. Dixon, Smallpox. (J.A. Churchill, Ltd., London, 1962).
3. Connaught Laboratories, Inc., Swiftwater, PA 18370.

TISSUE CULTURE SMALLPOX VACCINE

ANTON C. HEKKER*

*Rijksinstituut voor de Volksgezondheid, Bilthoven, The Netherlands

Our attempts to make smallpox vaccine in tissue culture started in 1964. Before that I worked in the laboratory of polio vaccine where I was responsible for safety and potency testing of inactivated poliovirus vaccine. I brought with me to the smallpox vaccine laboratory a number of years of experience with cell culture. The method of smallpox vaccine production on the skin of living animals had not changed for several decades. We were of the opinion at that time that the more modern methods of virus vaccine production could also be applied to this vaccine.

The first question to answer was what cell substrate to use. We decided not to use the CAM of the embryonated chicken egg because during that period Van der Noordaa [1] in the Amsterdam University had just finished a study on smallpox vaccine made on CAM. Potency and stability of this vaccine did not meet WHO minimum requirements. A second possibility was to use chicken embryo monolayer cultures. However, at that time it was not possible for us to have at our disposal a flock of chickens known to be free from fowl leucosis virus. Finally we chose primary rabbit kidney cells, because for other reasons we had already gained some experience with this type of cells, and during that time it was generally thought that the laboratory rabbit was a rather clean animal as far as adventitious agents were concerned. The discussions on the virus strain to be used ended up in the Elstree strain of vaccinia virus. This strain was also in use in our laboratory for the production of calf lymph.

A number of attempts to make smallpox vaccine in tissue culture or cell culture had already been published. These publications were from Frenkel and Kapsenberg [2], Wesslen [3], Herrlich and Mayer [4], Bonitz and Seeleman [5], Subramanyan and co-workers [6], and the abovementioned study of Van der Noordaa and co-workers [1]. All these experimental tissue culture smallpox vaccines, however, were not acceptable for general use because potency, stability, nor immunogenicity met the requirements for a regular satisfactory primary vaccination or revaccination. One of the things these vaccines had in common was that the vaccinia virus had at least a number of passages in cell culture before the vaccine was made. Therefore we were careful to use vaccinia virus with not more than one passage in tissue culture. In this way the seed virus used for the production of the tissue culture vaccine was the same as that used for the production of calf lymph. The scheme of the production is given in Table I.

This vaccine meets the WHO potency and stability requirements. This means that the vaccine had a log potency of at least 8 pock-forming units per ml, also after one month storage at 37°C. Stability data are given in Table II and Table III. It is self-evident that it does not contain bacteria.

With this vaccine field studies have been conducted in The Netherlands. No differences as regards the development of vaccination illness, the take rate and antibody-inducing capacity were observed between the tissue culture vaccine and calf lymph vaccine in approximately 1600 persons subjected to either primary vaccination or revaccination. In order to supplement and confirm these results on a larger scale under

TABLE I. Production, safety- and potency-testing of tissue culture smallpox vaccine.

Specific pathogen-free rabbit
↓
Trypsinization of kidneys or perfusion of the kidneys via carotid artery
↓
Production of monolayers in so-called Povitsky bottles
↓
Homogenization of seed virus suspension (= $Li^{II}K^{II}$ calf lymph)
↓
Inoculation of the monolayers with 100 ml seed virus suspension
↓
Incubation during 1 hour at room temperature
↓
Addition of 400 ml medium 199 with 0.1% proteose pepton
↓
Three days incubation at 36.5°C
↓
Storage at -70°C
↓
Thawing under streaming tap water and shaking the ice clumps in order to get the cells loosened from the bottom
↓
Pooling via 3 liter bottles into 10 or 20 liter bottles
↓
Storage at -4°C
↓
Homogenization in 400 ml quantities in continuous flow Sorval omnimixer at 0°C
↓
10x concentration in Amicon Hollow Fiber Filter (HIDX 50)
↓
Addition of equal quantity of McIlvaine's buffer with 10% pepton and 2% sorbitol
↓
Storage at 4°C
↓
Lyophilization
↓
Vaccine

---

field conditions the Island of Lombok, Indonesia was chosen for the mass vaccination of 50,000 children below 15 years of age with the tissue culture vaccine. The take rate and adverse reactions were observed. For comparative purposes 10,000 children were vaccinated with calf lymph vaccine. Both vaccines were produced in the RIV, were freeze-dried and had a log potency of 8.5 pock-forming units per ml. The studies were conducted in May and June 1973 with the assistance of the WHO SE Unit and the Indonesian government.

TABLE II. Titer of tissue culture smallpox vaccine after storage during 4 weeks at 37°C.

Batch No.	Titers in ^{10}log pfu/ml	
	-4°C	after 4 weeks storage at +37°C
74-kn-1	8,3	8,2
	8,3	8,2
74-kn-2	8,4	8,4
	8,4	8,3
	8,7	8,4
74-kn-3	8,3	8,2
	8,3	8,2
	8,5	8,5
75-kn-8	8,4	8,4
	8,6	8,5
75-kn-9	8,4	8,3
	8,7	8,6
75-kn-11	8,4	8,1
	8,4	8,4
81-01	8,4	8,1
81-02	8,5	8,3
81-03	8,6	8,5
81-04	8,6	8,5
84-01	8,4	8,3
84-03	8,5	8,1

TABLE III. Stability of tissue culture smallpox vaccine at -4°C

Batch No.	Number of years storage at -4°C								
	0	1	2	3	8	9	10	14	17
67-kn-1	8,3	8,2	8,6	-	-	-	-	-	8,6
GV-1	8,7	-	-	-	-	-	-	8,6	-
GV-2	8,7	-	-	-	-	-	-	8,4	-
70-kn-1	8,3	-	-	-	-	-	-	8,4	-
74-kn-1	8,2	8,3	-	8,3	-	8,4	8,4	-	-
74-kn-2	8,4	8,4	-	8,7	-	8,2	8,5	-	-
74-kn-3	8,2	8,3	-	8,5	-	8,0	-	-	-
75-kn-8	8,4	-	8,6	8,9	8,3	8,4	-	-	-
75-kn-9	8,4	-	8,6	8,7	-	8,6	-	-	-
75-kn-11	8,3	-	8,4	8,7	-	8,4	-	-	-
81-01	8,3	-	8,2	8,3	-	-	-	-	-
81-02	8,4	-	8,2	8,4	-	-	-	-	-
81-03	8,6	-	8,4	8,5	-	-	-	-	-
81-04	8,7	-	8,2	8,6	-	-	-	-	-

Titers in ^{10}log pfu/ml

    Similar results were obtained with both vaccines in primary vacinees and in revaccinees as regards the take rate, pock reactions and serious secondary reactions. It was about that time that smallpox was eradicated. I went into virus diagnostic work and the laboratory of smallpox vaccine was rebaptized into a laboratory for live virus vaccine and started production of measles, rubella and mumps vaccine.

REFERENCES

1. J. van der Noordaa, F. Dekking, J. Posthuma and B.J.W. Beunders, Archiv fur die gesamte Virusforschung 22, 210-215 (1967).
2. H.S. Frenkel and J.G. Kapsenberg, Nederlands Tijdschrift voor Geneeskunde 98, 991-996 (1954).
3. T. Wesslen, Archiv fur die gesamte Virusforschung 6, 430-438 (1956).
4. A. Herrlich and A. Mayr, Archiv fur die gesamte Virusforschung 7, 284-296 (1957).
5. K. Bonitz and K. Seeleman, Archiv fur die gesamte Virusforschung 10, 236-253 (1960).
6. P. Subramanyan, S. Divakaran and P. Vinodraj, Bulletin of the World Health Organization 25, 33-40 (1961).

CAPABILITY OF DEVELOPING COUNTRIES TO PRODUCE VACCINIA VECTOR VACCINE

ISAO ARITA*

*Chief Medical Officer, Smallpox Eradication, World Health Organization, Geneva, Switzerland.

INTRODUCTION

The vaccinia vector vaccine has four major advantages: easy production, easy administration, heat stability and low cost. The first advantage is related to the fact that smallpox vaccine production is the oldest in the history of biologicals. The second advantage derives from the fact that unlike most other vaccines, vaccinia virus can be administered by scarification and does not require a syringe and needle. Use of the bifurcated needle, introduced during the smallpox eradication campaign, simplified the procedure even further. The heat stability of freeze-dried vaccine means that there is no need for a cold chain. Finally, the average cost of 465 million doese donated to WHO between 1967 and 1983 was only US$0.02 per dose. It is thus very much cheaper than other vaccines.

In this meeting I would like to expand on the first advantage, easy production, and comment on its relevance to vaccine production in developing countries. In doing so I am going to make a statement that you, as scientists, may find surprising--namely that for the production of a vaccinia virus vaccine, scarification of the animal skin may still be the method of choice in developing countries. As Hekker et al. [2,3] have shown, potent heat-stable vaccinia virus vaccine can be produced in cultured cells. However, the advantage of this mode of production, namely that the vaccine is bacteriologically sterile, is really only an "aesthetic" advantage. Occasional non-pathogenic bacteria were always present in vaccines made in animal skin (cattle, sheep and water buffaloes), but they never caused problems of any kind during the hundreds of millions of vaccinations carried out in the global smallpox eradication campaign.

During the first three years of the intensified smallpox eradication programme, which started in 1967, we concentrated our efforts on the investigation of the vaccine production situation throughout the world, with the aim of improving the quality of the vaccine being produced. My discussion will be based on this experience, which is fully described in a forthcoming book [1]. In this paper, "vaccine" means freeze-dried vaccine unless otherwise specified.

Improvement of Vaccine Quality

In a worldwide survey of vaccine producers made in 1967, 59 replies, from a total of 77 identified vaccine producers, revealed a most disappointing picture, since only one-third of them appeared to be satisfied with their own testing results (Table I). "Satisfactory" batches were those which met the standards established by the biological standardization section of WHO in 1965 [4], for initial potency, heat stability and bacterial content.

In the same year, we independently tested samples from 20 selected producers whose vaccine was being used or was intended for use for the eradication campaign (Table II). Only about one-third of the batches met WHO standards, unsatisfactory batches being produced by laboratories both in industrialized countries (for donation) and in developing

TABLE I. WHO Survey 1967: Three production lots of vaccine: Stability after 4 weeks at 37°C.

	Number of producers reporting	All 3 lots satisfactory	Some lots satisfactory	No lots satisfactory	No report
Africa	8	2	1	3	1
Americas	13	2	2	3	5
Asia & Oceania	16	5	3	1	6
Europe	22	7	5	5	3
Total	59	16	11	12	15

countries (for local use). Since there would have been further deterioration in the field, it was concluded that at that time only about 10%-15% of the vaccine actually being used met WHO standards of potency and stability.

TABLE II. Independent testing by WHO

	For use in the eradication campaign			Experimental production for donation		
	Producers	Batches tested	Batches unsatisfactory	Producers	Batches tested	Batches unsatisfactory
Americas	1	1	1	-	-	-
Africa	1	1	0	5	21	19
Asia	2	11	9	3	6	4
Europe	2	22	12	6	12	2
Total	6	35	22	14	39	25

Two measures were taken to improve the situation. Firstly, advisory services were organized by WHO to assist producers, and secondly, a system of international quality control of production batches, covering some 67 laboratories throughout the world, was established.

Advisory services. In 1968, a vaccine producers' seminar was held to prepare a practical and simple manual for production and assay methods, since no such information was available either in textbooks or publications. This manual was widely distributed to all laboratories producing freeze-dried smallpox vaccine, in both developed and developing countries (SE/68.3 Rev. 2 Methodology of Freeze-Dried Smallpox Vaccine Production, WHO). In addition, a WHO Collaborating Centre for Smallpox Vaccine at the National Institute of Public Health, Utrecht (under the direction of Dr. Anton Hekker) produced secondary seed lot vials and a working reference vaccine. These were sent upon request to laboratories, mainly in developing countries, which had difficulty maintaining a seed lot system or a working reference vaccine. Since the end of the smallpox eradication campaign these two products have also been stored in four

WHO Collaborating Centres for Orthopoxvirus Research, in Atlanta, USA; Moscow, USSR; Paris, France; and Tokyo, Japan for use if needed in an emergency.

Quality Control. Two laboratories were set up as WHO reference centres for vaccine testing, the Connaught Laboratories Ltd, Toronto, Canada and the National Institute of Public Health in Utrecht, Netherlands. The former tested vaccine from producers in the Americas and the latter batches of vaccine from the rest of the world. Testing involved assay of the initial potency after reconstitution of the freeze-dried vaccine, heat stability and bacterial content. It was agreed by the countries and laboratories involved that all vaccine used in the global smallpox eradication campaign, whether destined for local use, for donation through WHO, or for donation in a bilateral aid programme, should be subjected to these quality control tests.

Implementation of these two services was reinforced by frequent visits to vaccine production laboratories by staff of the Smallpox Eradication Unit in WHO as well as members of a panel of sixteen consultants who were expert in vaccine production. Advice was given for the solution of any and all problems which occurred in production laboratories, from either a technical or managerial point of view.

The results were gratifying (Figure 1). Between 1969 and 1972, the vaccine quality improved dramatically and by 1973 the acceptability rate reached well over 80% and after 1976, over 90%. Considering that

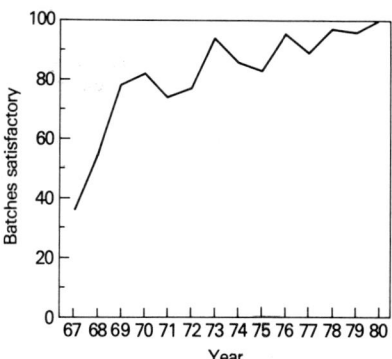

FIG. 1. WHO quality control of 2578 batches of smallpox vaccine from 67 laboratories.

a half of the 67 producers were in the Third World, this was a major achievement, which assured the availability of high quality vaccine for the global programme.

I would now like to discuss the production capability for vaccinia virus vaccine produced in animal skin in various developing countries, based on this experience.

The Performance of Producers in Six Geographic Regions

In 1967, there were altogether 34 producers in developing countries; 7 in Africa south of the Sahara, 11 in South America and 16 in Asia. WHO established the policy that countries planning to use less than 10 million conventional doses a year would be ill-advised to produce the vaccine themselves. This amount of vaccine could be produced within a few months, so that investment and maintenance of laboratory space, freeze-driers and other equipment was not economical. Further, results of WHO quality control testing reminded producers that resources invested for vaccine production were not worth maintaining if the product was not up to standard, because it had then to be discarded. Because of these circumstances, nine laboratories (five in Africa, two each in South America and in Asia) discontinued production of the freeze-dried vaccine between 1967 and 1970. If it was required for local smallpox eradication programmes, they were supplied with good quality vaccine by WHO.

In this manner we were able to identify 41 producers whose vaccine was being donated or used locally for the global smallpox eradication programme. Twenty-five were in developing countries situated in Africa south of the Sahara, South America and Asia, and 16 were in Europe or North America or Oceania. All these producers submitted samples for WHO quality control testing. Table III presents the results of quality control testing from 1971 to 1974 of batches of vaccine from these 41 producers. Since some laboratories did not submit samples each year during this period, the table is not comprehensive, but illustrates the capability for vaccine production in the developing countries.

TABLE III. Quality control of vaccine in use for the Intensified Smallpox Eradication Campaign--results of tests carried out by geographic region.

	Producers	Number of Batches			
		1971 Tested (Satisfactory)	1972 Tested (Satisfactory)	1973 Tested (Satisfactory)	1974 Tested (Satisfactory)
Americas	11	24 (14)	58 (29)	30 (28)	33 (17)
Africa	2	5 (5)	32 (28)	2 (2)	24 (21)
Middle East	3	11 (4)	67 (54)	54 (49)	29 (29)
South East Asia	8	107 (103)	120 (108)	253 (245)	86 (83)
Western Pacific	4	6 (6)	6 (6)	9 (9)	- -
Europe	13	27 (21)	17 (15)	29 (27)	42 (38)
Total	41	180 (153)	300 (240)	377 (360)	214 (188)
% Satisfactory		85%	80%	95%	88%

South America. Brazilian laboratories, except for one in San Paolo, produced vaccine in eggs and had a problem with heat stability. In fact, smallpox eradication was achieved in Brazil by employing vaccine considered substandard by WHO norms. This is probably explained by the fact that jet injection was used and refrigeration facilities were relatively advanced. Other laboratories in South America--Argentina, Colombia, Equador, Peru, and Venezuela--produced good vaccine. On the whole, production of smallpox vaccine was entirely within the capability of laboratories in South America to meet the regional requirements. After eradication of smallpox resulting in discontinuation of routine vaccination programmes, smallpox vaccine production was stopped by all producers in South America during the 1970s.

Africa. Two producers--Kenya and Guinea--produced vaccine of good quality for local use and donation to the smallpox eradication programme in Africa. All the batches submitted by Kenya consistently met WHO requirements. The Guinea laboratory was assisted by a WHO technician and the production ceased, in the early 1970s. Kenya stopped production in 1979. In addition, South Africa produced satisfactory vaccine.

Middle East. Iran, Iraq, and Syria developed good production capability by 1974, but had ceased production by 1981.

South-East Asia. Individual laboratories in Bangladesh, Burma, Indonesia, and Thailand, and four laboratories in India consistently produced vaccine of excellent quality. At one time, the total amount of vaccine produced annually by these eight laboratories reached 160 million doses while their total annual production capacity was estimated to exceed 200 million doses. They all stopped production between 1977 and 1980 except that the Patwadangar laboratory, one of the four laboratories in India, stopped production in 1982.

Western Pacific Region. China (Taiwan Province), the Philippines and Vietnam produced good quality vaccine. The People's Republic of China eliminated smallpox in the 1960s, in a campaign operated independently of WHO. In view of the large population of China, I would like to refer to available data on the smallpox vaccine production situation which was obtained by Dr. F. Fenner and Dr. J. Breman during their visit there in 1979 (F. Fenner and J. Breman, personal communication, 1979). At that time, there were eight production laboratories, one producing tissue culture vaccine, two tissue culture and calf lymph vaccine, and five only calf lymph vaccine. Both freeze-dried and liquid vaccine were produced. Take rates as well as WHO testing results of production lots in 1969 and in 1976 suggested that the vaccine was of good quality. The Temple of Heaven strain was used, and in 1970 Chinese virologists developed an attenuated strain by testing plaque-purified Temple of Heaven virus in children. This was used for the vaccination of some three million children, but no information is available to WHO on its immunogenicity or on complications. Beginning in 1980, China decided gradually to discontinue smallpox vaccination programmes but in 1984 a laboratory produced 5 million doses of freeze-dried vaccine for the national vaccine reserve.

Producers in industrialized countries. Table III also includes data on producers in industrialized countries, thirteen in Europe, two in North America and one in the Western Pacific, all of which produced vaccine of a good quality in animal skin. Although it was quickly improved when deficiencies were found, samples of vaccine from Canada, USA, the USSR and Switzerland occasionally showed unsatisfactory results.

About half of the producers in developed countries have now stopped production.

The Potential Capability for Vaccinia Vector Vaccine Production in Developing Countries

I would like now to comment on the potential capability for vaccinia vector vaccine production in developing countries, assuming that virus would be produced in animal skin and that the laboratories having produced a quality vaccine in mid 1970s would willingly revive their past production resources both in personnel and facilities.

Some 17 developing countries in South America, Middle East, South-East Asia, and the Western Pacific, as mentioned in the preceding section, should be able to produce their own vaccine if provided with genetically-engineered seed vaccines needed for local use (Figure 2). In South America, Brazilian producers may encounter problems with heat stability if they decide to use egg vaccine. In the Western Pacific, China would require a large amount of vaccine but the country would be able to produce good quality vaccina vector vaccine made either on calf skin or cultured cells.

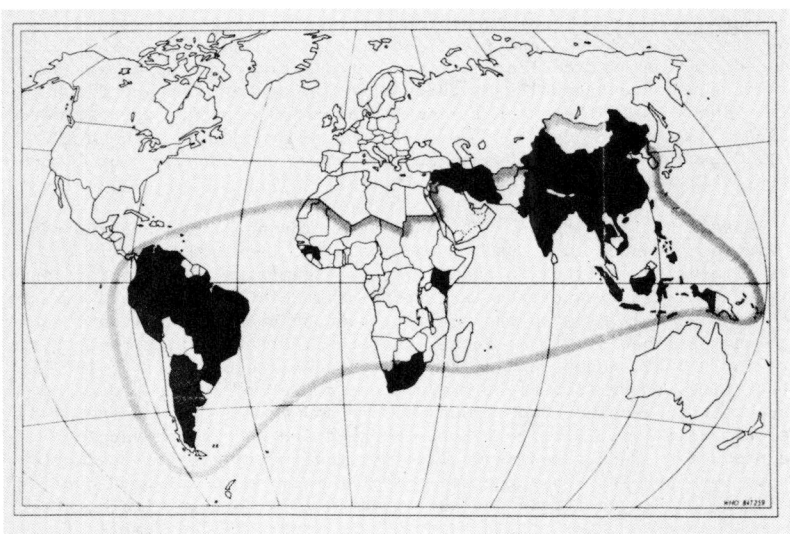

FIG. 2. Developing countries with capacity for smallpox vaccine production.

In Africa south of the Sahara, the number of laboratories able to produce vaccine may be still limited. Special arrangements would probably be necessary, in the form of the provision of special funds to two good candidate laboratories. During the smallpox eradication programme, WHO provided Kenya with the funds necessary for vaccine production. The Kenyan Government in return donated 15 million doses of vaccine to WHO's Special Account for Smallpox Eradication--an amount in fact sufficient to vaccinate 60 million persons using the bifurcated needle. A strategy similar to this would be worth examining for vaccinia vector vaccines, bearing in mind possible international assistance. There would be no problem for South Africa to produce the vaccine.

Production capability for smallpox vaccine was developed through WHO's intensive involvement in terms of an advisory service and quality control. Similar international measures should be reestablished if vaccinia vector vaccine proves to be an important public health tool. Some laboratories which once stopped vaccine production because they could not meet WHO standards, might wish to attempt vaccinia vaccine production again. It is important that no vaccination programme should be put in jeopardy because of poor quality vaccine. The reestablishment of international measures, as mentioned above, would help to ensure that unsatisfactory vaccines were not used.

If producers in developing countries are to reactivate their vaccinia virus production, countries will have to reorganize their facilities and personnel since many laboratories have converted to other purposes, and there would need to be refresher courses for laboratory personnel.

CONCLUSION

WHO's experience in the promotion and quality control of smallpox vaccine production during the global eradication programme in the 1970s was reviewed and it is concluded that production of vaccinia vector vaccine would be well within the capability of the producers in many developing countries. The reestablishment of international quality control of such vector vaccine prodution, however, would ensure that unsatisfactory vaccine was not used. The development of vaccinia vector vaccine may open the way for many developing countries to be able to meet their national requirements through their own vaccine production, not needing to rely on supplies from the industrialized countries.

ACKNOWLEDGEMENT

I am most grateful to Dr. Frank Fenner for his review and advice on the preparation of this paper.

REFERENCES

1. F. Fenner, D.A. Henderson and I. Arita (in association with Z. Jezek and I.D. Ladnyi), Geneva, World Health Organization (in preparation), 1987.
2. A.C. Hekker, J.M. Bos, and L. Smith, J. Biol. Stand. $\underline{1}$, 21-32 (1973).
3. A.C. Hekker, J.M. Bos, N. Kumara Rai, J. Keja, G. Cuboni, W. Emmet and J. Djalins, Bulletin of the World Health Organization $\underline{54}$, 279-284 (1976).
4. WHO Technical Reports Series, No. 323. Requirement for Biological Substances. Report of WHO Expert Group, Geneva, 1966.

DISCUSSION

Dr. Schild: Dr. Arita, I presume the World Health Organization would see the establishment of procedures for good control of vaccines as being an essential part of technology transfer. Approximately what proportion of countries, particularly developing countries, would have facilities for testing these vaccines?

Dr. Arita: Asia, India, Burma, and Thailand have control facilities, and they are reasonably good. Some independent sample testing may still be required in those cases. In Africa, Kenya previously had a good control facility as did countries in South America. However, all these laboratories, except for the one in India, were incorporated into the production facilities, and were not independent national control laboratories.

Dr. Furesz: Quality control is a very important part of the cost of vaccines. In developing countries, having quality control laboratories is just as big a problem as producing vaccines. The problem is not confined to developing countries. The ability of vaccines from many countries to meet requirements improved during the program, but at the beginning there were even some vaccines from Europe that failed. With recombinant vaccinia virus vaccines the quality control testing will be much more costly and complex than with ordinary vaccinia virus vaccines.

Dr. D.A. Henderson: With regard to capabilities of national control authorities, I think there are additional concerns that need emphasis. Smallpox vaccine was clearly the easiest vaccine of all to produce. Yet it was not all that simple. There are important potential roles for an international testing facility and for early agreement on standards. In 1959 the standards for smallpox vaccine were set. By 1967, we found only two or three laboratories in the world that were using a seed lot system. Most were sequentially passing the vaccine virus. When the virus did not grow well enough, it was passed in rabbit testes to increase yield, then passed back in the calf again. It was a primitive system. All of the vaccines ostensibly were being tested by national control authorities, which were usually the production laboratories themselves. Dr. Arita is the one who should be credited for stimulating the laboratories to send in their vaccines for test, and indeed there were some vaccines tested by national authorities in which we could not find any virus at all. From another point of view, the situation in the United States was not wholly satisfactory either. Until 1970 the regulations in the United States for the testing of smallpox vaccine called for a rabbit scarification test. All other industrialized countries were using the chorioallantoic test which gave much more precise results. Establishment of standards early should help avert such problems.

Dr. R. Henderson: The Expanded Program on Immunization has benefited from the experience of the smallpox eradication program. The World Health Assembly adopted a resolution saying that all vaccines used in the Expanded Program on Immunization would meet World Health Organization requirements. As a result we are now in a far more favorable position to assure that all vaccines used in developing countries do get independent testing when that country requires it, or if that vaccine is provided by a donor, such as UNICEF or others.

I think the smallpox experience has also changed our standards for vaccine acceptability. I would guess that if a new vaccinia vaccine were to be used, that there would be few national controller authorities that would accept the old method of production. They will probably require tissue culture vaccines. If so, establishment of production capabilities in developing countries will be a whole new issue. There will have to be the same kind of careful attention given to adequacy of quality control, staff training, and production facilities.

The World Health Organization has encouraged vaccine production in developing countries. However, it has focused on those countries whose domestic production would satisfy domestic needs and has not attempted to set up production facilities in any country that would serve several countries surrounding it. In practice this means that countries with populations above 20 million have had support in establishing vaccine production and quality control facilities, and there are very few of those large countries. Most of them are already well along in their vaccine production capacities.

PART III

EXPERIMENTAL RECOMBINANT VACCINIA VIRUS VACCINES

Chairpersons: R. Chanock and W. Dowdle

VACCINIA VIRUS RECOMBINANTS AS LIVE VACCINES AGAINST HEPATITIS B VIRUS
AND MALARIA

GEOFFREY L. SMITH* ** AND BERNARD MOSS*

*Laboratory of Virus Diseases, National Institute of Allergy and Infectious Diseases, Bethesda, Maryland 20205. **Present Address: Division of Virology, Department of Pathology, University of Cambridge, Laboratories Block, Addenbrooke's Hospital, Hills Road, Cambridge, United Kingdom.

ABSTRACT

Infectious vaccinia virus recombinants have been constructed that express genes from Plasmodium knowlesi, Plasmodium falciparum and hepatitis B virus (HBV). Tissue culture cells infected with the recombinant viruses synthesise discrete sized foreign polypeptides that are detectable with specific antisera. Dermal vaccinations of rabbits with the live viruses result in production of antibodies against the foreign polypeptides. Chimpanzees vaccinated with a recombinant vaccinia virus expressing hepatitis B virus surface antigen (HBsAg) were protected against subsequent intravenous challenge with HBV. These data demonstrate the potential of vaccinia recombinants as live vaccines against HBV and malaria.

INTRODUCTION

The molecular biology of vaccinia virus and the detailed method for construction of recombinant viruses is discussed in another chapter of this volume (Moss, B.) and in previous reviews [1,2]. Consequently, only a brief outline of essential features is given here.

Vaccinia virus is a large complex virus, that possesses virus-specific transcriptional enzymes [3]. These enzymes recognise vaccinia virus transcriptional regulatory DNA sequences (promoters) but not promoters from cells or other viruses [4]. Consequently, expression of foreign genes in vaccinia virus is dependent upon linking foreign protein coding sequences to vaccinia virus promoters [5,6]. This linkage should be precisely engineered to ensure correct usage of the translational initiation codon of the foreign gene. Such a chimaeric gene is assembled in a plasmid vector so that it is flanked by vaccinia virus DNA taken from a nonessential region of the virus genome. The foreign gene is inserted into the vaccinia virus genome by homologous recombination in cells infected with vaccinia virus and transfected with the recombinant plasmid DNA. Commonly the foreign DNA is inserted into the vaccinia thymidine kinase (TK) gene since this allows selection of the recombinant virus by virtue of its TK⁻ phenotype [5]. The viruses described below were constructed in this manner. For simplicity the recombinant viruses expressing HBsAg and circumsporozoite (CS) proteins of Plasmodium species are considered separately.

Vaccinia Recombinants Expressing Malaria Genes

A vaccine against malaria is greatly needed but its development faces formidable problems. The disease is caused by Plasmodium species which have a complex life cycle, great heterogeneity, and which seem capable of rapidly developing resistance to new drugs. Moreover, attempts to control malaria by eradication of the insect vector have largely failed due to the emergence of insecticide-resistant mosquitoes. Malaria still kills more than one million children in Africa each year. Recently, the application of recombinant DNA technology for isolation and studies of malaria genes has been an encouraging development. Genes coding for surface antigens from several stages of the malaria parasite have been cloned and analysed [7-12]. One striking and unusual feature that has emerged is the presence of tandemly repeated short amino acid sequences that can comprise up to 90 percent of the polypeptide.

Knowledge of the primary structure of the antigens and possession of the cloned genes can be applied to vaccine development in several ways. One method is to engineer the genes into expression vector systems to produce large amounts of polypeptides which, after purification, can be used as immunogens. Alternatively, peptides representing the repeating epitopes can be synthesised chemically, linked to carrier molecules and also used as immunogens. Due to the highly repeated nature of these epitopes, synthetic peptides may be particularly attractive in this case. A third approach and the subject of this paper, is the expression of malaria genes in vaccinia virus [13]. This has the advantage that the infectious recombinant virus simultaneously synthesises the foreign polypeptide and delivers it to the host's immune system. Obviously this avoids the necessity for expensive polypeptide purification. Additionally, since vaccination in this manner occurs as a live infection, both cellular and humoral immune mechanisms may be stimulated [14-16]. Here the properties of vaccinia recombinants which express the CS protein of Plasmodium knowlesi and Plasmodium falciparum are described.

The CS gene of Plasmodium knowlesi was cloned into E. coli and identified by use of monoclonal antibody directed against the repeating epitope of the polypeptide [7]. Inspection of the nucleotide sequence of the CS gene revealed that digestion of cloned DNA with restriction endonuclease Aha III would excise the gene as a 1.6 kilobase pair (Kbp) DNA fragment. The putative translation initiation codon of this gene was then approximately 300 base pairs from the end of the DNA fragment and no other ATG was present in the 300 bp upstream. This DNA fragment was cloned into plasmid insertion vector pGS20 [6] so that the malaria gene was under control of a vaccinia promoter. Since the vaccinia promoter had been engineered without a translational start site the first downstream ATG was that of the malaria gene. The resultant plasmid, pGS39, was used to generate TK⁻ recombinant virus v39. This was grown and purified and the genomic DNA analysed by restriction endonuclease digestion, gel electrophoresis and Southern blotting [17]. These experiments showed the Plasmodium knowlesi CS gene to be correctly inserted within the vaccinia TK gene and no other genomic rearrangements were detectable [13].

To test for expression of the CS gene, tissue culture cells were infected with recombinant virus v39 and cell extracts screened with a monoclonal antibody 2G3 which recognises the repeating epitope of this protein. Solid phase radioimmunoassay demonstrated the presence of immunoreactive material in cells infected with recombinant virus but not in uninfected cells, or in cells infected with wild type virus. The specificity of this reaction was proved by the ability of a synthetic peptide representing the repeating epitope to block binding to monoclonal 2G3. The nature of the immunoreactive polypeptide(s) was analysed by immunoprecipitation of radiolabelled infected cell extracts followed by polyacrylamide gel electrophoresis. These analyses together with immunoblotting [18] demonstrated the presence of two polypeptides of 53 and 56 kD [13]. These were larger than the polypeptides present on sporozoites (42 kD and 50 kD) and the differences are most likely attributable to the different type or extent of proteolytic processing.

The ability of the recombinant virus to stimulate specific immunological responses against the foreign polypeptide was tested by vaccination of rabbits. Following a single intradermal inoculation of 10^8 plaque forming units (pfu) of recombinant virus, a typical local vaccinial lesion appeared within 4 days. This subsequently healed and disappeared within 2 weeks. Antiserum from vaccinated animals was taken weekly and tested for antibodies against the CS protein (anti-CS). Such antibodies were detected by three methods: (1) indirect immunofluorescence on whole sporozoites, (2) immunoblotting, and (3) solid phase radioimmunoassay. Antiserum from a control rabbit, vaccinated with wild type virus, was negative in all these tests.

These experiments demonstrate that the CS gene of Plasmodium knowlesi was expressed in vaccinia virus and the recombinant virus stimulated production of anti-CS in vaccinated animals [13]. A similar set of experiments and results have now been completed with the CS gene of Plasmodium falciparum (G.L. Smith, R.S. Nussenzweig, V. Nussenzweig and B. Moss, unpublished). While these results are encouraging they represent only a step towards a malaria vaccine. One reason for this is that the different life stages of the malaria parasite are immunologically distinct. Consequently immunity to sporozoites is ineffective against merozoites or gametocytes. Similarly, immunity against merozoite antigens offers no protection against sporozoites or gametocytes, and so on. Effective malaria vaccines will probably need to stimulate immunity to antigens representing all the life stages of the parasite. In this regard vaccinia virus is well suited since its great capacity for foreign DNA [19] will enable the simultaneous expression of many foreign genes.

Another problem facing development of a malaria vaccine is the great species and strain polymorphism. Analogous antigens from different strains or species may be immunologically non-cross-reactive because they possess different immunodominant repeating epitopes. However, comparison of other regions of the proteins can demonstrate remarkable conservation. An example is the CS protein of Plasmodium knowlesi and Plasmodium flaciparum [8]. These proteins both cover the sporozoite surface and possibly are responsible for the liver tropism of the invading sporozoites. Despite having unrelated repeating epitopes, regions of high conservation have been found before and after the repeats. If immunity could be directed against these conserved regions it may prove cross-reactive among different strains and/or species.

Vaccinia Recombinants Expressing HBsAg

Like malaria, hepatitis B virus (HBV) remains a serious global health problem. Over 200 million people are chronically infected with HBV and some of these patients will subsequently develop hepatocellular carcinoma. HBV is a small DNA virus that has been intensively studied and its genome cloned and sequenced. The development of a HBV vaccine has been hampered by the inability to propagate the virus in tissue culture. However, safe and effective subunit vaccines have been developed and licensed [20,21]. These are made by purifying HBsAg from the plasma of chronically infected patients, but their expense and limited availability make them unavailable to most third world countries where the majority of HBV infection exists. Other approaches to HBV vaccines include production of HBsAg in genetically engineered mammalian or yeast cells [22,23] and synthesis of peptides representing regions of HBsAg [24,25]. Vaccinia virus recombinants expressing HBsAg have also been constructed [26,27]. The construction and properties of one such virus, vHBs4, is described below.

The genome of HBV strain adw has been cloned [28]. Inspection of the nucleotide sequence of a closely related strain indicated that a DNA fragment encoding the surface antigen (S) could be excised with restriction endonuclease BamHl. This left approximately 120 bp upstream of the translational initiation codon of the S gene. The DNA fragment was cloned into the insertion vector pGS20 [6] and a plasmid isolated that contained the HBsAg gene correctly orientated with respect to the vaccinia promoter [26]. The plasmid pHBs4 was transfected into cells infected with wild type vaccinia virus to generate TK⁻ recombinant virus vHBs4. DNA extracted from the purified recombinant virus possessed the predicted genomic structure and the virus was stable upon serial passage.

Expression of HBsAg was demonstrated by AUSRIA II radioimmunoassay (Abbott Laboratories). Extracts from cells infected with vHBs4 contained HBsAg while uninfected cells, or cells infected with wild type virus did not. A characteristic of patients chronically infected with HBV is the presence of HBsAg in their serum as 22 nm lipoprotein particles. It was therefore of interest to find that HBsAg was also present in the culture medium of vHBs4-infected cells. This was a result of specific excretion and not cell lysis since 90 percent of infectious virus remained cell associated while approximately 70 percent of total HBsAg was excreted. Purification of HBsAg from the culture medium by sucrose and CsCl density gradient centrifugation and analysis by electron microscopy, showed the HBsAg to be present as 22 nm particles with the same bouyant density and sedimentation rate as HBsAg excreted from Hepatoma cells [26]. Immunoprecipitation of ^{35}S-methionine-labelled infected cell extracts demonstrated the presence of two polypeptides Pl and P2 which comigrated with HBsAg from hepatoma cells. P2 is a glycosylated derivative of Pl.

The ability of recombinant virus vHBs4 to stimulate immune responses against HBsAg was tested first in rabbits. Eight days after a single intradermal vaccination with 10^8 pfu of vHBs4, antibodies to HBsAg (anti-HBs) were detected. No anti-HBs were detected in a control rabbit vaccinated with wild type virus. Subsequently the anti-HBs titres increased to up to 10 international units (IU)/ml. Revaccination with vHBs4 5 months later resulted in a 5-fold increase in anti-HBs titres [29].

To determine if virus vHBs4 could confer protective immunity to HBV, chimpanzees were intradermally vaccinated with 10^8 pfu of vHBs4 or WT virus and subsequently challenged intravenously with $10^{3.5}$ chimpanzee ID_{50} units of live HBV subtype ayw (Figure 1) [30]. One chimpanzee (A-98) received WT vaccinia virus, while two chimpanzees (66 and 67) received recombinant virus vHBs4. Following vaccination, weekly serum samples from the chimpanzees were tested for serological evidence of exposure to HBV antigens and biochemical evidence of liver disease. With the exception of one weakly positive anti-HBs sample 8 weeks after vaccination of chimpanzee 67 all sera were negative. Fourteen weeks after vaccination the animals were challenged with HBV. Chimpanzee A-98 then developed typical hepatitis B. HBsAg appeared in the serum 4 weeks after challenge and persisted at high levels for 15 weeks. Antibodies to HBV core polypeptide (anti-HBc) and biochemical evidence of hepatitis occurred after 8 and 9 weeks, respectively.

This typical hepatitis B contrasted with the response of chimpanzees 66 and 67 that were vaccinated with recombinant virus. No HBsAg or biochemical evidence of hepatitis was detected. Instead anti-HBs appeared 4 to 7 weeks after challenged and persisted at high levels for

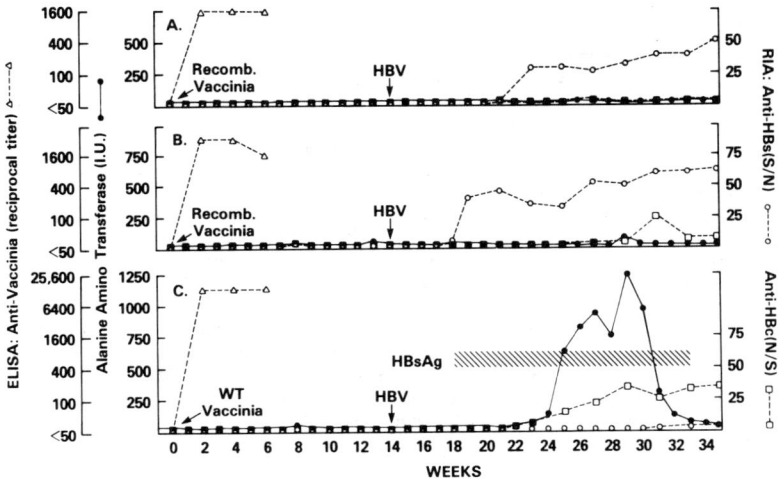

FIG. 1. Effects of intradermal vaccination of chimpanzees with recombinant virus vHBs4 (top and centre panel) or wild type virus (bottom panel) followed by intravenous challenge with live HBV. Antibodies to vaccinia are expressed as reciprocal dilutions, anti-HBs and anti-HBc are expressed as the ratio of sample cpm to mean negative control cpm (S/N) and the negative control cpm to sample cpm (N/S), respectively. Cross-hatching indicates positive HBsAg values of P/N >2.1. Alanine aminotransferase activity is expressed in IU/L. Reprinted by permission from Nature vol. 311, No. 5981, pp. 67-69, Copyright (c) 1984, Macmillan Journals Limited.

the duration of the experiment. Both chimpanzees did develop low levels of anti-HBc 21 or 27 weeks after challenge indicating that they had experienced mild HBV infections. Liver biopsies 11 months after challenge showed no evidence of acute or chronic hepatitis [30].

These results demonstrate that chimpanzees receiving a single intradermal vaccination with recombinant vaccinia virus expressing HBsAg were protected against hepatitis after challenge with HBV of a heterologous sub-type. The failure of the chimpanzees to develop significant anti-HBs levels following primary vaccination contrasted with the response of rabbits, but is consistent with the relatively poor response of primates to a single dose of HBsAg without adjuvants. It is hoped that use of stronger vaccinia virus promoters that express higher levels of HBsAg will result in production of anti-HBs following primary vaccination. Additionally, as demonstrated with rabbits, revaccination of animals already "immune" to vaccinia virus can still result in boosts in antibodies against the foreign polypeptide. Similar observations have been made following revaccination with vaccinia recombinants expressing the influenza virus haemagglutinin, and the herpes simplex virus type 2 glycoprotein D and the vesicular stomatitis virus glycoprotein.

SUMMARY

Here we report that vaccinia virus recombinants expressing the CS genes of Plasmodium knowlesi and Plasmodium falciparum and the surface antigen of HBV can be used to immunise animals against the respective foreign polypeptide. Additionally, primates challenged intravenously with HBV were protected against hepatitis B. The reintroduction of vaccinia virus as a live vaccine against diseases other than smallpox is controversial. However, there are many advantages to this type of live vaccine. These include (1) the ability to mass produce the vaccine cheaply, (2) the stability of the freeze dried vaccine in the absence of refrigeration, (3) the cheap and simple method for mass immunisation under non-sterile field conditions, (4) the ability of the virus to stimulate both humoral and cellular immunity, and (5) the capacity of the virus for simultaneous expression of multiple foreign antigens. The complications of smallpox vaccination are well documented [31]. While these remain a serious consideration, from an overall public health point of view the advantages of vaccinia recombinants which could immunise against hepatitis B and malaria seem to greatly outweigh the risks of complications. Moreover, as described in another chapter of this volume [RML Buller et al.] the vaccinia genome can be manipulated to construct more attenuated and safer viruses. For example, inactivation of the TK gene markedly reduces the pathogenicity of the virus in mice and the dermal lesion size in primates.

The goals for development of future recombinant vaccinia virus vaccines are: the identification of stronger vaccinia promoters; the construction of viruses which have desirable degrees of attenuation while retaining their potency as an immunising vehicle; and the simultaneous expression of suitable combinations of foreign antigens in one virus.

ACKNOWLEDGMENTS

The work described above was performed in the National Institute of Allergy and Infectious Diseases, Bethesda, Md 20205, USA. We thank M. Mackett, B. Murphy, R.H. Purcell, J.L. Gerin, V. Nussensweig, R.S. Nussensweig, and J. Barnwell for their contributions to the work; B. Hoyer, G.N. Godson and J. Dame for generously providing cloned DNA; and to Mrs. M. Wright for typing the manuscript.

REFERENCES

1. B. Moss in: Human Viral Diseases, B.N. Fields, R. Chanock, R. Shope and B. Roizman, eds. (Raven Press, New York 1984) in press.
2. G.L. Smith and B. Moss, BioEssays 1, 120-124 (1984).
3. B. Moss in: Gene Amplification and Analysis, J.G. Chirikjian and T.S. Papas, eds. (Elsevier, North-Holland 1981) pp. 254-266.
4. C. Puckett and B. Moss, Cell 35, 441-448 (1983).
5. M. Mackett, G.L. Smith and B. Moss, Proc. Natl. Acad. Sci. USA 79, 7415-7419 (1982).
6. M. Mackett, G.L. Smith and B. Moss, J. Virol. 49, 857-864 (1984).
7. J. Ellis, L.S. Ozaki, R.W. Gwadz, A.H. Cochrane, V. Nussenzweig, R.S. Nussenzweig and G.N. Godson, Nature 302, 536-538 (1983).
8. J.B. Dame, J.L. Williams, T.F. McCutchan, J.L. Weber, R.A. Wirtz, W.T. Hockmeyer, W.L. Maloy, J.D. Haynes, I. Schneider, D. Roberts, G.S. Sanders, E.P. Reddy, C.L. Diggs and L.H. Miller, Science 225, 593-599 (1984).
9. E. Vincenzo, J. Ellis, F. Zavala, D.E. Arnot, A. Asavanich, A. Masuda, I. Quakyi and R. Nussenzweig, Science 225, 628-629 (1984).

10. R.L. Coppel, A.F. Cowman, K.R. Lingelbach, G.V. Brown, R.B. Saint, D.J. Kemp and R.F. Anders, Nature 306, 751-756 (1983).
11. R.L. Coppel, A.F. Cowman, R.F. Anders, A.E. Bianto, R.B. Saint, K.R. Lingelbach, D.J. Kemp and G.V. Brown, Nature 310, 789-791 (1984).
12. M. Simmons, D.L. Hope, I.A. Mackay, M. Scaife, J. Merkli, R. Richle and J. Stocker, Nature 311, 379-380 (1984).
13. G.L. Smith, N.G. Godson, V. Nussenzweig, R.S. Nussenzweig, J. Barnwell and B. Moss, Science 224, 397-399 (1984).
14. G.L. Smith, B.R. Murphy and B. Moss, Proc. Natl. Acad. Sci. USA 80, 7155-7159 (1983).
15. J.R. Bennink, J.W. Yewdell, G.L. Smith, C. Moller and B. Moss, Nature 311, 578-579 (1984).
16. T.J. Wiktor, R.I. Macfarlan, K.J. Reagan, P.J.C. Dietzschold, W.H. Wunner, M.-P. Kieny, R. Lathe, J.-P. Lecocq, M. Mackett, B. Moss and H. Koprowski, Proc. Natl. Acad. Sci. USA 81, 7194-7198 (1984).
17. E.M. Southern, J. Mol. Biol. 98, 503-517 (1975).
18. H. Towbin, T. Staehelin and J. Gordon, Proc. Natl. Acad. Sci. USA 76, 4350-4354 (1979).
19. G.L. Smith and B. Moss, Gene 25, 21-28 (1983).
20. W. Szmuness, C.E. Stevens, E.J. Harley, E.A. Zany, W.R. Oleszko, D.C. William, R. Sadovsky, J.M. Morrison and A. Kellner, New Engl. J. Med. 303, 833-841 (1980).
21. J. Crosnier, P. Junger, A.M. Courvouce, A. Laplanche, E. Benhamou, F. Degos, B. Lacour, P. Prunet, Y. Cerisier and P. Guesry, Lancet i, 455-459 (1981).
22. P. Valenzuela, A. Medina, W.J. Rutter, G. Ammerer and B.D. Hall, Nature 298, 347-350 (1982).
23. M.F. Dubois, C. Pourcel, S. Roussel, C. Chany and P. Tiollais, Proc. Natl. Acad. Sci. USA 77, 4549-4553 (1980).
24. G.R. Dressman, Y. Sanchez, I. Ionescu-Martin, J.T. Sparrow, H.R. Six, D.L. Peterson, F.B. Hollinger and J.L. Melnick, Nature 295, 158-160 (1982).
25. R.A. Lerner, N. Green, H. Alexandra, F.-T. Liu, J.G. Sutcliffe and T.M. Shinnick, Proc. Natl. Acad. Sci. USA 78, 3403-3407 (1981).
26. G.L. Smith, M. Mackett and B. Moss, Nature 302, 490-495 (1983).
27. E. Paoletti, B.R. Lipinskas, C. Samsonoff, S. Mercer and D. Panicali, Proc. Natl. Acad. Sci. USA 81, 193-197 (1984).
28. A.M. Moriarty, B.H. Hoyes, J.W.-K. Shih, J.L. Gerin and D.H. Hamer, Proc. Natl. Acad. Sci. USA 78, 2606-2610 (1981).
29. B. Moss, G.L. Smith, J.L. Gerin and R.H. Purcell in: Viral Hepatitis and Liver Disease, G.N. Vyas, J. Dienstag and J. Hoofnagle, eds. (Grune and Stratton, Orlando 1984) pp. 293-305.
30. B. Moss, G.L. Smith, J.L. Gerin and R.H. Purcell, Nature 311, 67-69 (1984).
31. J.M. Lane, F.L. Ruben, J.M. Neff and J.D. Millar, New Engl. J. Med. 281, 1201-1208 (1969).

DISCUSSION

Dr. Chanock: Was the monoclonal antibody used to identify and to quantitate production of the sporozoite antigen the monoclone that has been shown to neutralize infectivity of sporozoites? Certain monoclones neutralize infectivity in experimental animals.

Dr. Smith: I don't know specifically with regard to this monoclonal antibody, but I believe all monoclonal antibodies of this class do.

Dr. Chanock: I think that bodes well for this approach. Another problem is the polymorphism of the merozoite antigens. Do you have plans to address this problem in production of a polyvalent vaccine for malaria?

Dr. Smith: The antigens have very large repeating epitopes which, as you point out, have extreme polymorphism. In addition, there are conserved regions of these polypeptides. One thing that has been done is to construct a malarial gene from which these epitopes have been deleted, then look to see whether the conserved regions of the polypeptide are immunogenic, and produce protective immunity.

Dr. Chanock: My third question is, what plans do you have to increase the expression of the hepatitis B surface antigen to a level that will result in satisfactory antibody responses in primates?

Dr. Smith: One approach is to look at more vaccinia promoters. There are 200 genes. Thymidine kinase was the first one we looked at. We used the promoters which code for the major structural polypeptides of the virus, and got significantly increased levels of expression.

A second method might be to put in multiple copies of the gene. Again, the capacity of the virus for that is adequate.

Dr. Obijeski: What dose was used to immunize the rats and chimpanzees, and did you attempt to measure surface antigen in the vesicle that formed in the chimpanzee? A single dose of 20 micrograms of some vaccines will seroconvert all the animals to a very high titer, and there are some very sensitive methods that could be used to measure surface antigens as vesicles.

Dr. Smith: We did not look at the level of antigen which was produced in the local lesion following vaccination. The virus was administered by intradermal inoculation at a single site of 10^8 plaque forming units.

Dr. Warren: How many repeats of the malaria genes did you put in each case?

Dr. Smith: We put in the whole gene which, in the knowlesi case is 12 repeats and, in the falciparum case, 41 repeats.

Dr. Warren: In the case of hepatitis, did you express the pre-S region? There is some recent evidence to suggest that antibodies to epitopes of that region may be very important in preventing initial infection.

Dr. Smith: We are engineering recombinant viruses which contain that region. I think it is expressed in HBV. Because vaccinia has its own RNA polymerases, it can express large and small peptides.

VACCINIA VECTORED VACCINES

ENZO PAOLETTI, MARION E. PERKUS, ANTONIA PICCINI, SUSAN WOS AND BERNARD R. LIPINSKAS*

*New York State Department of Health, Wadsworth Center for Laboratories and Research, Albany, New York 12201

INTRODUCTION

Vaccinia virus has been used for almost 200 years, since its introduction by Edward Jenner, for the immunoprophylaxis of smallpox. The success of vaccinia as a vaccine is attested to by the recent declaration of the World Health Organization that smallpox, as a human disease, has been eradicated from the world. It has been proposed that if one were to modify the vaccinia vaccine virus by incorporating foreign genetic material into the genome of infectious vaccinia virus that live recombinant vaccines could be produced directed against a variety of heterologous infectious diseases. This would be accomplished by the expression of the foreign genetic information into an appropriate antigen under vaccinia virus regulation such that on inoculation with the recombinant vaccinia virus an immunological response would ensue directed against the foreign antigen rendering that vaccinated individual immune to the heterologous infectious pathogen. This hypothesis has been supported by a number of examples wherein foreign genes encoding pertinent antigens have been expressed by vaccinia virus [1,7,9,13,14,16]. When these recombinant viruses were used to inoculate animals, serological evidence was obtained suggesting successful immunization. In some cases, protection of these vaccinated animals against subsequent challenge with the infectious agent has been demonstrated [4,9,16,17].

Published examples of this approach include the expression in vaccinia virus recombinants of the cDNA copy of the RNA segment from Influenza virus encoding the Hemagglutinin [7,16], the gene from Hepatitis B virus encoding the surface antigen [9,14], genes from Herpes simplex virus encoding the glycoprotein D [9], the gene from rabies virus encoding the rabies glycoprotein [1,17], and a malarial antigen from Plasmodium knowlesi [13]. Other examples of expression of foreign genes in vaccinia virus vectors are presented in this volume.

In this chapter we will describe some of the background information setting the stage for the use of vaccinia virus as a eukaryotic cloning and expression vector. We will present examples of expression of foreign genes with particular emphasis on the generation of Hepatitis B surface antigen and Herpes simplex virus glycoprotein D vaccinia vectored vaccines and, lastly, some description of ongoing studies in our laboratory directed toward making an optimal vaccinia vaccine vector. The latter will focus on the use of vaccinia to express multiple genes, the effort to increase the level of expression of the foreign genes resulting in more potent vaccines, and studies on vaccinia virus directed to develop even safer vaccine vectors.

STRATEGY FOR THE INSERTION AND EXPRESSION OF FOREIGN GENETIC ELEMENTS IN VACCINIA VIRUS VECTORS

The ability to introduce endogenous, inactive genomic elements into the genome of infectious vaccinia virus [5,12] suggested a protocol for insertion of foreign DNA sequences into the vaccinia virus genome. This basic strategy is outlined in Figure 1. A foreign genetic element is isolated and inserted at a locus of a cloned subfragment of the

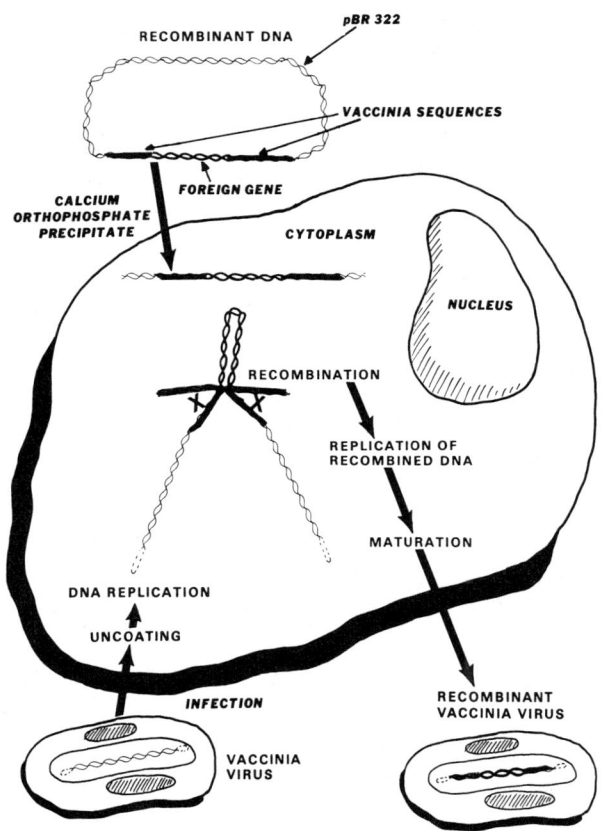

FIG. 1. General Protocol for the Insertion of Foreign DNA into Infectious Vaccinia Virus. Foreign DNA inserted at a locus of a cloned vaccinia subgenomic fragment is introduced into tissue culture cells by transfection procedures. The cell is co-infected with rescuing vaccinia virus. In vivo recombination occurs between the vaccinia DNA sequences flanking the foreign insert and homologous DNA sequences on the replicating vaccinia genome forming a novel recombinant DNA molecule which can in turn be packaged into infectious recombinant vaccinia virus.

vaccinia genome. It is essential that the insertion of the foreign genetic element occurs at a locus of the vaccinia DNA such that the flow of genetic information essential for virus replication is not disrupted. The manipulation of cloned subgenomic vaccinia DNA is necessitated by the fact that the intact vaccinia DNA genome of approximately 180Kb is too fragile to handle as an integral molecule in the test tube. Additionally, finer manipulation of the foreign genetic element is required for optimal expression in vaccinia vectors. Ideally one solely wants the open reading frame of the foreign gene of interest to be flanked by appropriate vaccinia sequences, allowing efficient initiation and termination of transcription. The chimeric construct containing the foreign gene flanked by vaccinia sequences is further amplified in some convenient cloning vehicle such as pBR322 simply to obtain sufficient quantities of DNA for the next step which involves the introduction of donor DNA into tissue culture cells by standard transfection procedures. Since the naked DNA of poxviruses is not by itself infectious, the tissue culture cells must be additionally infected with the rescuing vaccinia virus. This rescuing virus then proceeds through its normal replication cycle. When a DNA molecule generated from the input rescuing virus localizes itself in the cytoplasm in close proximity to the input donor DNA, in vivo recombination can occur between the vaccinia DNA sequences flanking the foreign DNA and the homologous DNA sequences on the replicating vaccinia DNA. This event happens with a frequency of approximately 0.1%. The recombined DNA molecule can itself be replicated and participate in the subsequent maturational steps resulting in infectious progeny recombinant virus. Recombinant vaccinia virus can be identified and prepared as pure virus stocks for subsequent studies by a number of procedures [2,3,7,8,10].

HEPATITIS B VIRUS SURFACE ANTIGEN: EXPRESSION BY RECOMBINANT VACCINIA VIRUS

It is estimated that there are approximately 200 million people that are chronically infected with Hepatitis B. Large numbers of deaths attributed to fulminant hepatitis or to the potential sequelae of chronic Hepatitis B infection, cirrhosis and primary hepatocellular carcinoma, are registered yearly. The inability to cultivate the Hepatitis B virus under laboratory conditions has prevented the preparation of Hepatitis B virus vaccines. A subunit vaccine derived from the Hepatitis B virus surface antigen circulating in the plasma of chronically infected individuals has proven effective, but the cost of the vaccine regimen and the problems in distributing the vaccine to areas of the world where it is most needed speak to the necessity to explore other avenues for a more applicable Hepatitis B vaccine. With this in mind we [9] and others [14] have explored the potential of using recombinant vaccinia virus as a Hepatitis B vaccine. The Hepatitis B virus surface antigen is localized on the surface of the infectious Hepatitis B virus particle. It has been isolated from the plasma of carriers and has been shown to be effective as an immunogen in immunizing individuals. The gene encoding the Hepatitis B virus surface antigen has been expressed in vaccinia virus recombinants. As demonstrated in Table I, the Hepatitis B virus surface antigen as synthesized under virus regulation is secreted from infected tissue culture cells. Hence, more than 75% of the HBsAg is localized extracellularly while more than 90% of the infectious vaccinia virus is still cell-associated. This demonstrates that the HBsAg is truly secreted and not released due to lysis of the cells by vaccinia infection.

When the extracellular material derived from cells infected with the vaccinia virus recombinant expressing the HBsAg was concentrated and banded on CsCl gradients, it was observed that serologically reactive material had a characteristic density of 1.2g/cc similar to authentic HBsAg (Figure 2).

TABLE I. Synthesis and cellular distribution of the HBsAg.

Fraction	Infectivity	Percent infectivity distribution	HBsAg, total ng synthesized	Percent HBsAg distribution
Supernate	10.9×10^5	7	131	76
Cellular	146.0×10^5	93	42	24

CV-1 cells (1×10^6) were infected at 2 pfu per cell with a vaccinia recombinant expressing the HBsAg. The supernate was collected 24 hr after infection and the cells washed with saline and the wash combined with the supernate. The washed monolayer of cells was collected in saline. The fractions were titered for viral plaque forming units to determine the distribution of progeny virus or assayed for HBsAg using the Ausria test kit.

When this serologically reactive material banding at 1.2g/cc on CsCl was negatively stained and visualized by electron microscopy, morphological structures characteristic of the 22nm particles of the HBsAg were observed (Figure 3).

By all biochemical and biophysical criteria applied by our laboratory and others [14], the Hepatitis B virus surface antigen as synthesized by vaccinia virus is indistinguishable from the Hepatitis B virus surface antigen synthesized under native conditions.

When laboratory animals were inoculated with these vaccinia virus recombinants expressing the HBsAg, a very rapid serological conversion was observed and high titers of anti-HBsAg antibodies were obtained. High levels of anti-HBsAg antibodies were present in the sera of these animals more than a year after their inoculation (Table II). Significantly, as is demonstrated in Table II, when these animals were revaccinated with a vaccinia virus recombinant expressing the HBsAg, a booster effect was observed. Revaccination resulted in increased antibody levels not only against vaccinia virus itself but also against the HBsAg. This result is compatible with the interpretation that replication of vaccinia virus occurred on reinoculation with attendant synthesis of additional HBsAg resulting in an anamnestic response. Significantly, when chimpanzees, the only non-human host for Hepatitis B virus, were vaccinated with a vaccinia virus recombinant expressing the Hepatitis B virus surface antigen, they were shown to be resistant to a subsequent challenge with infectious Hepatitis B virus [4].

VACCINIA VIRUS RECOMBINANTS EXPRESSING THE HERPES SIMPLEX VIRUS GLYCOPROTEIN D

Herpes simplex viruses are known to cause both persistent and latent infections in man. Recurrent oral or genital herpetic infections, lethal occurrences in the neonate, and encephalitis are some of the disease states elicited by Herpes simplex virus infections. Approximately 9 million people in the U.S. alone are victims of recurrent genital Herpetic lesions. No vaccine for Herpes simplex is yet available. Herpes simplex viruses elaborate a number of glycoproteins. Of these glycoproteins, glycoprotein D is considered an important antigen in immunity to Herpes simplex. The glycoprotein D, derived from Herpes simplex type 1 (oral herpes), shares antigenic determinants with the

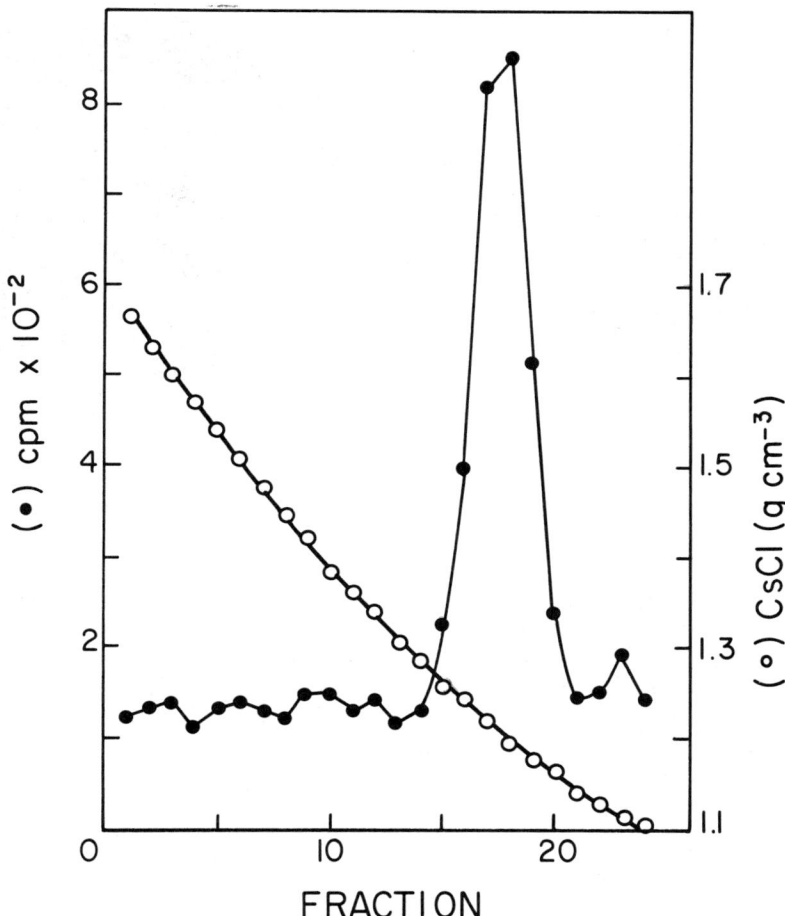

FIG. 2. <u>Equilibrium Density Gradient Centrifugation of HBsAg Synthesized by Vaccinia Virus In Vitro</u>. HBsAg secreted from CV-1 cells infected with a vaccinia virus recombinant was concentrated by high speed centrifugation and banded on CsCl gradients. Serologically reactive material was detected using the commercially available Ausria II test kit (Abbott Laboratories). Densities were calculated from refractive indices.

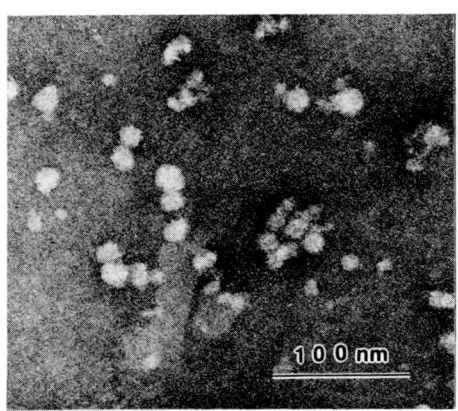

FIG. 3. Electron Micrograph of HBsAg Particles Synthesized by Vaccinia Virus Recombinants. Negatively stained material banding at 1.2g/cc on CsCl density gradients was visualized by electron microscopy. Photograph was generously provided by W. Samsonoff (Wadsworth Center for Laboratories and Research).

TABLE II. Anamnestic response to HBsAg on revaccination of rabbits with recombinant vaccinia virus.

Weeks post inoculation	[a]RIA units/ ml serum	% Vaccinia virus plaque reduction	
		[b]1600	[b]6400
1	0.08	63	12
3	0.36	69	35
6	18.40	82	12
54	6.80	41	0
57	32.70	85	4
62	24.30	90	67

A rabbit inoculated intradermally with 1.8×10^7 pfu of a vaccinia virus recombinant expressing the HBsAg was revaccinated with an equivalent dose of a vaccinia virus recombinant expressing the HBsAg 56 weeks after the initial inoculation. [a]Anti-HBsAg antibody levels were determined using a commercially available RIA kit from Abbott Laboratories and are noted in RIA units ($\times 10^{-3}$) per ml of serum as defined by the manufacturer. Vaccinia virus was mixed with dilutions of antisera and kept at 4°C overnight until titrated on CV-1 monolayers. [b]The percent reduction of plaques obtained on CV-1 monolayers are indicated as the reciprocal of the serum dilution.

glycoprotein D derived from Herpes simplex type 2 (genital herpes), as demonstrated in a number of serological tests, including specific neutralization of viral infectivity.

Vaccinia virus recombinants expressing Herpes simplex virus type 1 glycoprotein D have been constructed and described [9,10]. Serological detection of the glycoprotein D on unfixed infected cells using radiolabeled protein A suggested that the glycoprotein D, as elaborated by vaccinia virus infection, localizes itself on the membrane of the infected cell. This is similar to the localization of the glycoprotein D on the membrane of cells infected with Herpes simplex virus.

Inoculation of laboratory animals with the vaccinia virus recombinant expressing the Herpes simplex virus glycoprotein D resulted in the elaboration of antibodies capable of neutralizing the infectivity of Herpes simplex virus as demonstrated by plaque reduction assays (Table III).

TABLE III. Neutralization of HSV-1 and HSV-2 by rabbit antiserum produced in response to inoculation with the recombinant vaccinia virus expressing HSV-1 gD

Reciprocal of serum dilution	Percent plaque reduction			
	Inactive complement		Active complement	
	HSV-1	HSV-2	HSV-1	HSV-2
320	83	54	95	66
640	59	23	84	37

Herpes simplex virus, type 1 (AA) or type 2 (CURTIS) were mixed with equal volumes of antisera obtained from a rabbit after immunization with a vaccinia recombinant expressing HSV-1 (KOS) gD., and held at 4°C overnight in the presence of 5% inactivated (56°C x 30 min.) or active guinea pig complement. Plaque reduction assays were performed on CV-1 monolayers and results compared with preimmune serum tested at a reciprocal dilution of 40.

As expected, antiserum induced by infection with the vaccinia recombinant expressing the glycoprotein D from HSV type 1 neutralized the infectivity of the heterologous virus HSV type 2 (Table III). The homologous HSV type 1 neutralization appeared to be somewhat more efficient than the neutralization of the heterologous HSV type 2. This may be due to the fact that the antiserum contains antibodies directed against not only the type common but also the type specific antigenic determinants on the HSV type 1 glycoprotein. The antiserum is therefore more effective in neutralization assays with the homologous HSV type 1 than with the heterologous HSV type 2 where the antiserum can react only with the type common determinants. Significantly, neutralization of HSV infectivity was not dependent on the presence of active complement (Table III).

In order to demonstrate the efficacy of the vaccinia virus recombinant expressing the HSV glycoprotein D as a vaccine, we have taken advantage of the susceptibility of the laboratory mouse to herpetic infections. Intraperitoneal injection of infectious Herpes simplex virus into the laboratory mouse results in an encephalitis within 5 to 7 days followed by death within another day or two. The severity of the response is a function of both the genetic makeup of the laboratory mouse and the particular strain of the Herpes simplex virus used as challenge. As demonstrated in Table IV, all of the mice challenged with HSV type 1 survived whereas only 30 percent of the mice inoculated with wild-type vaccinia virus survived the HSV challenge. Other studies have shown 100% protection against HSV type 1 challenge even when as much as 20 times the LD_{50} of challenge virus was used.

TABLE IV. Protection of mice against challenge with HSV by immunization with recombinant vaccinia virus expressing the HSV-gD.

	Immunizing agent	No. of mice	Survivors	% Survival
Exp. A	Wild-type vaccinia	40	12	30
	Recombinant vaccinia	40	40	100
Exp. B	Wild-type vaccinia	80	10	12.5
	Recombinant vaccinia	80	63	78.8

Mice were inoculated intraperitoneally with 5×10^7 pfu of wild-type virus or recombinant vaccinia virus and challenged three weeks later (Exp. A) or six weeks later (Exp. B) with 1×10^4 pfu of HSV type 1 (AA), Exp. A or HSV type 2 (CURTIS), Exp. B.

Similar studies where HSV type 2 virus was used to challenge the mice gave excellent protection (Table IV) when compared to the controls, but not as profound a protection as was obtained with the homologous HSV type 1 as a challenge virus.

Clearly, if one is going to consider a recombinant vaccinia virus as a vaccine against Herpes simplex viruses, then one would want to construct a vaccinia virus recombinant that expressed both the glycoprotein D from HSV type 1 and the glycoprotein D from HSV type 2. Such recombinants have indeed been constructed [10,11]. Success in protecting laboratory mice vaccinated with thse double HSV-gD recombinants against very high doses of HSV challenge virus has been obtained (unpublished data).

USE OF VACCINIA VIRUS RECOMBINANTS FOR THE PRODUCTION OF POLYVALENT VACCINES

One of the advantages of vaccinia virus as a vector is that rather large quantities of foreign DNA can be stably integrated into infectious virus. Already 20-25 Kb of foreign DNA has been inserted in vaccinia viruses [7,15] and additional space for packaging more foreign DNA can be provided by use of viable deletion mutants of vaccinia [6]. The ability to package large quantities of foreign DNA can be taken advantage of in constructing vaccinia virus recombinants expressing multiple foreign genes and thereby be potentially useful as polyvalent vaccines. As noted above, in describing the general protocol for inserting foreign genes into vaccinia virus, foreign DNA must be inserted at loci such that the flow of essential genetic viral information required for replication is not disrupted. Such regions of DNA, missing from viable viral deletion mutants or viral DNA sequences known to encode non-essential functions such as thymidine kinase activity, provide obvious

regions for inserting foreign genetic elements. We have pursued an
active search for loci into which we can insert foreign DNA without
disrupting essential genetic information to provide us with additional
possibilities for constructing recombinant virus expressing multiple
foreign genes. This approach involves the insertion of foreign DNA by
in vivo recombination techniques and empirically ascertaining whether a
viable insertion mutant can be recovered. If so, then another potential
insertion site is discovered which can be further engineered for expression of foreign genetic elements. Such a search for non-essential
insertion loci has demonstrated that more than a dozen loci can be
readily localized within the leftmost 30Kb of the vaccinia genome
(Figure 4). These non-essential insertion sites can in addition be

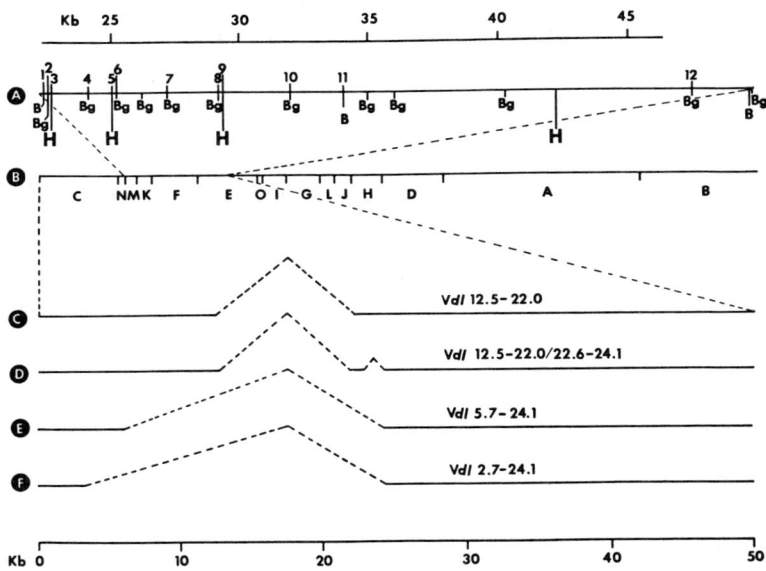

FIG. 4. Insertion and Deletion Mutants of Vaccinia Virus. (B) indicates
the physical map of the L variant vaccinia genome as defined by Hind III
restriction enzyme sites. (A) indicates the location of a dozen viable
insertion mutants of vaccinia virus generated by the site specific insertion of appropriately modified Herpes simplex virus thymidine kinase
coding sequences. A series of viable deletion mutants that have been
derived from the L variant prototypic vaccinia genome are indicated (C-F).
The deletion mutants are indicated as Vdl and assigned map coordinates
based on Kb of DNA deleted referenced to the left terminus of the L
variant vaccinia genome.

used as loci from which viable deletion mutants of vaccinia virus can
be generated. Examples of viable deletion mutants of vaccinia virus
are shown in Figure 4. The generation of viable deletion mutants of
vaccinia virus provides more space for packaging additional foreign DNA
and also indicates one method for eliminating viral DNA sequences that

are not essential for viral replication, but may lead to unnecessary virulence of the virus. This is one approach that may result in more attenuated, and hence safer, vaccinia virus vaccine vectors. Clearly, all the DNA sequences from 2.7Kb to 24.1Kb are not essential since viable deletion mutant (Figure 4/F) can be isolated and therefore any locus within this DNA segment can be used to insert foreign genes.

The construction of vaccinia virus recombinants into which multiple foreign genes have been inserted is shown in Figure 5. This figure demonstrates genomic analysis of a vaccinia virus recombinant wherein the foreign sequences encoding the Hepatitis B virus surface antigen, the Herpes simplex virus glycoprotein D, and the sequences encoding the Influenza virus hemagglutinin are all present within one vaccinia virus genome. Evidence for expression of the three foreign antigens was obtained through a variety of in vitro serological tests and when this triple vaccinia recombinant was inoculated into laboratory animals, immunological reactivity against all three foreign antigens was present in the immune sera (Table V). The ability to express a number of foreign genes in a single vaccinia virus recombinant provides a method

TABLE V. Immunological response to vaccination with a recombinant vaccinia expressing multiple foreign genes.

Weeks post inoculation	Anti-HBsAg RIA units[a]	Anti-HA HI[b]	Anti-HSV[c]	Anti-vaccinia[c]
Rabbit #257				
1	160	160	640	6400
3	160	320	2560	12800
5	1840	640	1280	12800
Rabbit #288				
1	80	20	<40	<40
3	360	40	160	400
5	760	80	160	400

Rabbits were inoculated with 5×10^7 pfu in 0.5 ml either intravenously (#257) or intradermally (#288) with a vaccinia recombinant expressing the HBsAg, HSV-gD and Influenza HA genes and immunological response followed.
[a]Sera was tested for anti-HBsAg antibodies using the commercially available AUSAB radioimmunoassay kit from Abbott Laboratories and titers expressed in RIA units per ml of serum as defined by the manufacturer.
[b]Hemagglutination inhibition tests were performed using 4HA units. Reciprocal of serum dilution is indicated. [c]Plaque-reduction assays monitoring reduction of HSV or vaccinia virus infectivity were performed on CV-1 cells. Reciprocal of serum dilution giving greater than 50% reduction in plaque number is shown.

for eliciting immunity against a number of heterologous pathogens via a live polyvalent recombinant vaccinia virus vaccine. An alternative approach to elicit immunity to multiple infectious diseases is by constructing a cocktail viral inoculum composed of a number of vaccinia viruses each of which is expressing one or more foreign antigens [9].

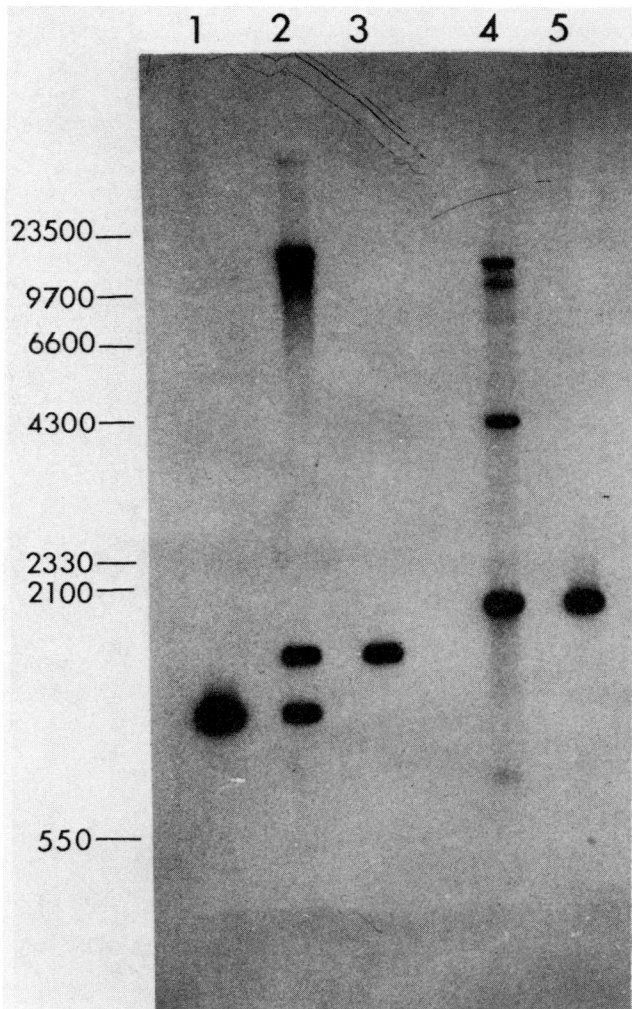

FIG. 5. <u>Genomic Analysis of Vaccinia Virus Recombinants Containing Three Foreign Coding Sequences</u>. Purified vaccinia virus recombinant containing the genes encoding the Hepatitis B virus surface antigen, the Herpes simplex virus glycoprotein D, and the Influenza virus hemagglutinin was prepared, DNA extracted and digested with restriction enzymes. The DNA fragments were separated on agarose gels blotted to nitrocellulose filters and probed with radiolabeled DNA corresponding to the three foreign genes. Lanes 1, 3 and 5 are purified HBsAg, HSV-gD and Influenza HA fragments representing 1,090, 1,338, and 1,780 bp sequences used as markers. DNA from the recombinant virus was digested with either Hind III (lane 2) or Bam HI (lane 4).

ENHANCED EXPRESSION LEVELS OF FOREIGN ANTIGENS

In considering refinement of vaccinia vectored vaccines it is clear that increased levels of expression of the foreign antigen would result in a more potent vaccine. However, in considering polyvalent vaccines it is reasonable to assume that the levels of expression required for optimal responses to each of the foreign antigens involved may not all require the same level of expression. One would have to take into account the relative immunogenicity of the various antigens and possible interferences between them. With these points in mind, we have set out to define vaccinia virus regulatory elements that allow expression of foreign genetic components at defined and manipulatable levels. As shown in Figure 6, different levels of expression of the Influenza virus hemagglutinin, as a test antigen, in vaccinia virus vectors has been obtained by using a variety of regulatory DNA signals to drive the Influenza hemagglutinin expression.

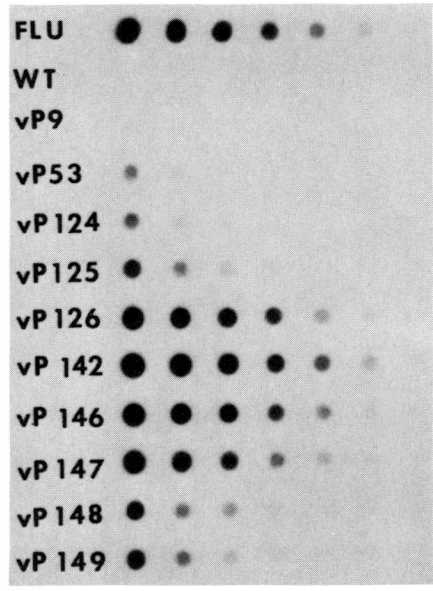

FIG. 6. Expression of Influenza Virus Hemagglutinin by Vaccinia Virus Recombinants. Tissue culture cells infected by influenza virus, wild-type vaccinia virus or a number of vaccinia virus recombinants (noted as vP9 etc.) were fixed to nitrocellulose as twofold serial dilutions. The filter was probed with ^{125}I protein A after exposure to anti-influenza HA serum. A radioautogram showing the relative serologically reactive HA synthesized under these conditions is shown.

MULTIPLE VACCINATIONS

Although a single vaccinia virus vaccination was effective against smallpox, lifetime immunity was achieved by periodic revaccination. In order to better understand the parameters allowed us in the use of vaccinia virus vectored vaccines, it is important to know whether it is possible to induce immunological reactivity in a previously vaccinated individual. To address this question in the laboratory, animals previously vaccinated with a recombinant vaccinia virus, and therefore immune to vaccinia, were revaccinated with a second vaccinia virus recombinant expressing a second novel foreign antigen. As demonstrated in Table VI, the animal responded to the second vaccination by making antibodies to the novel antigen expressed by the second vaccinia virus recombinant. As expected, an increase in antibody titer to vaccinia itself (not shown), but not to the foreign antigen expressed by the first vaccinia virus recombinant (Table VI) was detected. We have gathered a variety of examples of seroconverting animals to novel antigens on subsequent revaccination with novel recombinant vaccinia viruses. Successful results are readily obtained when levels of expression of additional antigens vectored by the second or third recombinant vaccinia virus is high.

TABLE VI. Revaccination with recombinant vaccinia viruses.

Weeks	[a]Anti-HBsAg	[b]Anti-Inf HA
3	0.2	<10
6	16	<10
9	72	<10
40	128	<10
54	72	<10
56	63	160
58	63	160
60	63	640

A rabbit was immunized intradermally with a vaccinia virus recombinant expressing the HBsAg and anti-HBsAg antibodies assayed as described. The same animal was revaccinated at 54 weeks with a novel vaccinia virus recombinant expressing the influenza virus hemagglutinin and anti-Influenza HA antibodies assayed as described.
[a]Anti-HBsAg was assayed using the commercially available radioimmunoassay from Abbott Laboratories and is noted as RIA units (10^{-3}) per ml of serum.
[b]Standard Hemagglutination Inhibition tests using chicken erythrocytes and 4 HA units were performed. Reciprocal of serum dilution is shown.

PROSPECTS

It is clear from the data presented here and throughout this volume that vaccinia vectored vaccines hold considerable promise for combating infectious diseases. The benefit/risk ratio of such vaccines would seem to be in favor of the benefit. A variety of vaccine strains exist with low risk of adverse side reactions. These strains can in turn serve as reagents for additional genetic engineering of the virus, hopefully resulting in even more attenuated vaccine strains. Also, it is important to weigh the relative benefit to be gained by immunizing against a host of infectious diseases, as would be accomplished via a polyvalent recombinant vaccinia virus, versus the risk attendant in a single vaccination dose with the polyvalent recombinant virus.

The generic approach provided here allows the potential to generate vaccines against viral, bacterial or parasitic diseases pertinent to humans. The broad host range of vaccinia, or the manipulation of other members of the Poxvirus family, should allow for the generation of live vaccines, not only for human diseases, and also for disease of veterinary concern.

It will be interesting to follow the development of this technology, to see if indeed the promise of vaccinia is that of the once and future vaccine.

ACKNOWLEDGMENTS

We would like to extend our appreciation to Karen Dombrowski for preparing the manuscript and to all the members of the laboratory who have contributed to this work.

REFERENCES

1. M.P. Kieny, R. Lathe, R. Drillien, D. Spehner, S. Skory, D. Schmitt, T. Wiktor, H. Koprowski and J.P. Lecocq, Nature 312, 163-166 (1984).
2. M. Mackett, G.L. Smith and B. Moss, Proc. Natl. Acad. Sci. USA 79, 7415-7419 (1982).
3. M. Mackett, G.L. Smith and B. Moss, J. Virol. 49, 857-864 (1984).
4. B. Moss, G.L. Smith, J.L. Gerin and R.H. Purcell, Nature 311, 67-69 (1984).
5. E. Nakano, D. Panicali and E. Paoletti, Proc. Natl. Acad. Sci. USA 79, 1593-1596 (1982).
6. D. Panicali, S.W. Davis, S.R. Mercer and E. Paoletti, J. Virol. 37, 1000-1010 (1981).
7. D. Panicali, S.W. Davis, R.L. Weinberg and E. Paoletti, Proc. Natl. Acad. Sci. USA 80, 5364-5368 (1983).
8. D. Panicali and E. Paoletti, Proc. Natl. Acad. Sci. USA 79, 4927-4931 (1982).
9. E. Paoletti, B.R. Lipinskas, C. Samsonoff, S. Mercer and D. Panicali, Proc. Natl. Acad. Sci. USA 81, 193-197 (1984).
10. E. Paoletti, B.R. Lipinskas, S. Woolhiser and L. Flaherty in: Herpesvirus: UCLA Symposia on Molecular and Cellular Biology. F. Rapp, ed. (Alan R. Liss, New York 19) pp.
11. E. Paoletti, M.E. Perkus, A. Piccini, S. Wos and B.R. Lipinskas in: The 1984 International Symposium on Medical Virology, L.M. de la Maza, ed. (The Franklin Institute Press, Philadelphia, in press).
12. C.K. Sam and K.R. Dumbell, Ann. Virol. (Inst. Pasteur) 132E, 135-150 (1981).
13. G.L. Smith, G.N. Godson, V. Nussenzweig, R.S. Nussenzweig, J. Barnwell and B. Moss, Science 224, 397-399 (1984).
14. G.L. Smith, M. Mackett and B. Moss, Nature 302, 490-495 (1983).
15. G.L. Smith and B. Moss, Gene 25, 21-28 (1983).
16. G.L. Smith, B.R. Murphy and B. Moss, Proc. Natl. Acad. Sci. USA 80, 7155-7159 (1983).
17. T.F. Wiktor, R.I. Macfarlad, K.J. Reagan, B. Dietzschold, P.J. Curtis, W.H. Wunner, M.P. Kieny, R. Lathe, J.P. Lecocq, M. Mackett, B. Moss and H.K. Koprowski, Proc. Natl. Acad. Sci. USA 81, 7194-7198 (1984).

DISCUSSION

Dr. Obijeski: In the multiple expression of several antigens, one of which was a surface antigen, do you find any of the antigenicity of either of the other two antigens, associated with the 22-nanometer particle? The reason I ask that question is that the polypeptide backbone of surface antigen has the capability of mobilizing cellular machinery to form a particle, where, in a lot of other cases, proteins will be secreted, or placed in a membrane.

Dr. Paoletti: We haven't looked at that.

Dr. Burke: Are any of the foreign proteins expressed on the surface of the virion, and does that change the tropism of the virus?

Dr. Paoletti: To the extent which we have looked, we cannot detect any significant attachment of the foreign antigens to the surface of virions.

Dr. Chanock: Have you done any work with malarial antigens?

Dr. Paoletti: We are working on malarial antigens, but there is nothing to discuss at this stage.

Dr. Halstead: Does it make any difference what cell culture system you use in terms of the product yielded, and do you have any in vitro correlate of the in vivo cell system in which this virus grows on application by scarification?

Dr. Paoletti: In the limited number of cells lines that we have looked at, there doesn't appear to be any difference in quantity or quality of the antigens expressed. We are still model-building, and that is one of the questions we are going to address.

INFECTIOUS VACCINIA VIRUS RECOMBINANTS EXPRESS HERPES SIMPLEX VIRUS GLYCOPROTEIN D AND PROTECT AGAINST LETHAL AND LATENT INFECTIONS OF HSV

KENNETH CREMER,* CHARLES WOHLENBERG,* MICHAEL MACKETT,** BERNARD MOSS** AND ABNER LOUIS NOTKINS*

*Laboratory of Oral Medicine, National Institute of Dental Research;
**Laboratory of Viral Diseases, National Institute of Allergy and Infectious Diseases, National Institutes of Health, Bethesda, Maryland 20205.

Primary infections with herpes simplex virus types 1 are most commonly manifested as herpetic gingivostomatitis in the oral cavity, while those of herpes simplex virus type 2 usually lead to genital lesions. After infection of epithelial surfaces, HSV often establishes a latent infection in the nervous system which persists for the lifetime of the individual [1,2]. Intermittent reactivation of latent HSV from the trigeminal, lumbosacral and dorsal root ganglia is the hallmark of herpes virus infections. Reactivation can occur despite the presence of high titers of circulating neutralizing antibody against HSV [3]. Our understanding of these viral processes, primary infection, establishment of latent infections, reactivation of latent HSV and recurrent infections, has been aided by the use of a mouse model [4-9]. Upon infection of epithelial surfaces, such as the lips, HSV is taken up by the nerve terminals at the site of inoculation and spreads by axoplasmic transport to nerve cell bodies in the trigeminal ganglia. There, an acute infection occurs for one or two weeks, during which time infectious HSV can be detected in cell-free homogenates of trigeminal ganglia [7]. After two weeks (latent phase), infectious virus can no longer be recovered from cell-free homogenates but can be recovered by explantation of viable ganglia tissues and co-cultivation on sensitive indicator cells (primary rabbit kidney) [7,9]. To prevent the establishment of latent infections, experimental studies in the animal model indicated that vaccination must take place before a primary infection occurs [7].

Herpes simplex virus types 1 and 2 have large double-stranded DNA genomes with molecular weights of $95-100 \times 10^6$ daltons and have the capacity to code for at least 50 different proteins. The viral envelope and infected cell-surfaces bear a number of virus-coded glycoproteins. Four major glycoproteins, termed gB, gC, gD and gE have been genetically mapped on the HSV genome and characterized biochemically [10]. Some antigenic determinants on the homologous HSV-1 and HSV-2 glycoproteins are identical (type common epitopes) while others are non-identical (type specific epitopes). The gD glycoprotein contains mostly type-common antigenic determinants and is a major target for neutralizing antibodies [11,12]. It was demonstrated that gD plays a major role in protecting mice from lethal HSV infections and would therefore logically be included among candidate vaccines. HSV subunit [12] and recombinant DNA-derived HSV proteins [13-15] were also proposed as possible vaccines. The cloned gD gene was biochemically expressed in procaryotic [16] and eucaryotic vectors [17] and in different poxvirus recombinants [15]. None have yet been shown to prevent the establishment of latent infections. In this report, we describe the construction of a live vaccinia virus recombinant that expresses HSV-1 glycoprotein D and its use to immunize mice against lethal and latent HSV infections.

CONSTRUCTION AND CHARACTERIZATION OF RECOMBINANT VIRUSES EXPRESSING HSV-1 gD

We constructed two vaccinia recombinants containing the entire coding sequence of the HSV-1 gD gene (strain KOS), the sequence of which was determined by Watson and co-workers [13]. The cloned gD gene was fused to a vaccinia virus promoter and inserted into the thymidine kinase locus of vaccinia virus [18,19]. The two constructs, vgD28 and vgD52 (Figure 1) contained the viral promoters $P_{7.5}$ and P_{28}, respectively, derived from two different vaccinia virus transcription units [20,21]. $P_{7.5}$ contains both early and late regulatory sequences [19,22], while P_{28} contains only late regulatory signals [21]. In both constructs, the first translation-initiation codon following the vaccinia virus RNA transcription-initiation sequence was from the gD gene, ensuring the synthesis of the intact HSV gD protein.

To determine whether the vaccinia HSV-1 gD recombinant viruses expressed the complete HSV-1 gD polypeptide, tissue culture cells infected with wild-type or recombinant vaccinia viruses were grown in the presence of ^{35}S-methionine or ^{3}H-glucosamine. HSV specific polypeptides were immunoprecipitated with a polyclonal antisera to HSV viral proteins or a monoclonal antisera prepared against the HSV-1 gD protein. The immunoprecipitates were then dissociated with SDS and size separated by polyacrylamide gel electrophoresis. Autoradiographs of the gels (Figure 2) showed that recombinants vgD28 and vgD52 synthesized an HSV polypelptide which co-migrated with the authentic 60,000 dalton gD of HSV-1. The 60,000 dalton polypeptide also incorporated ^{3}H-glucosamine indicating that the recombinant derived protein was glycosylated and processed identically to HSV-1 infected cells.

INDUCTION OF HSV NEUTRALIZING ANTIBODY

To assess the ability of the vaccinia HSV-1 gD to induce neutralizing antibodies, two rabbits were inoculated intradermally with the vgD52 recombinant virus. HSV-neutralizing antibody was detected in sera ten to fourteen days after immunization and reached maximum titers of 1:64 and 1:128 three weeks later (Figure 3). This titer remained constant through the next nine months.

The ability of the vaccinia HSV-1 gD recombinant to induce neutralizing antibodies in Balb/c mice was assessed by immunizing with the vgD52 recombinant by any of three different routes: intraperitoneally, subcutaneously (injection into the rear footpad) or intradermally (scarification on the tail). Other mice were inoculated by tail scarification with wild-type vaccinia, a vaccinia recombinant expressing the hepatitis B surface antigen or with saline. The titer of HSV-neutralizing antibody in sera from vaccinated mice was determined four to six weeks after inoculation by assay in a complement-dependent microneutralization assay for HSV [23]. Neutralizing antibody to HSV was detected as early as seven days after vaccination; three to four weeks later the HSV neutralizing titer ranged from 1:8 to 1:128 (Table I). The geometric mean HSV antibody titers were similar in mice inoculated with the vgD52 recombinant by any of three routes. In comparison, mice vaccinated with wild-type vaccinia virus or a recombinant expressing the hepatitis B surface antigen demonstrated no detectable neutralizing antibody titer to HSV.

PROTECTION AGAINST LETHAL INFECTIONS

To assess the ability of the recombinant virus to induce protective immunity, mice were immunized by tail scarification with vaccinia HSV-1 gD,

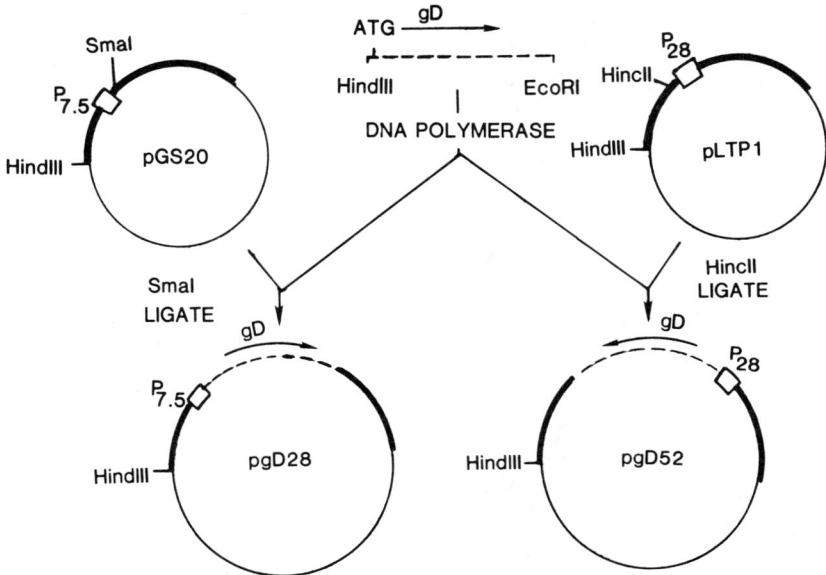

FIG. 1. Construction of vaccinia virus recombinants expressing HSV-1 gD. (Left) Construction of recombinant vgD28. Nucleotide sequence data indicated the presence of a HindIII site within the untranslated leader segment of the HSV gD gene [13]. Plasmid pACP13, obtained from A. Poley (NIH), contained an 8.4 kilobase (kb) HindIII-EcoRI fragment of HSV-1 (strain KOS) DNA including the entire coding sequence of the gD gene. Excess DNA beyond the distal end of the gD gene was removed by cleaving the plasmid with restriction endonucleases SstI and EcoRI, removing the single-stranded ends with T4 DNA polymerase, and recircularizing the plasmid with T4 ligase. The new plasmid, containing a 2.5 kb HSV insert was designated pMM27. Ligation of the 2 blunt ends regenerated an EcoRI site. The HindIII-EcoRI segment of pMM27 was excised, the staggered ends were filled in with Klenow fragment of DNA polymerase, and blunt-end ligated into the unique SmaI site just downstream of the $P_{7.5}$ vaccinia virus promoter in the plasmid pGS20 [19]. The resulting plasmid, containing the $P_{7.5}$ vaccinia promoter and HSV gD gene in the correct orientation, was called pMM28. The HSV gene under control of the vaccinia virus promoter was then inserted into the TK locus of the vaccinia virus genome by homologous recombination [24,18,19] and TK⁻ recombinants were selected and plaque purified. The predicted structure of the recombinant DNA was confirmed by restriction endonuclease digestion and hybridization to appropriate HSV DNA probes. (Right) Construction of recombinant vgD52. The staggered ends of the 2.5 kb HindIII-EcoRI segment of pMM27 were filled in with the Klenow fragment of DNA polymerase and the resulting DNA was blunt-end ligated into the unique HincII site just downstream of the P_{28} vaccinia virus promoter in plasmid pLTP1 [22]. The resulting plasmid having the P_{28} promoter and HSV coding sequences in the correct orientation was named pMM52. Cell-mediated homologous recombination was used to insert the gene into the TK locus of vaccinia virus [18].

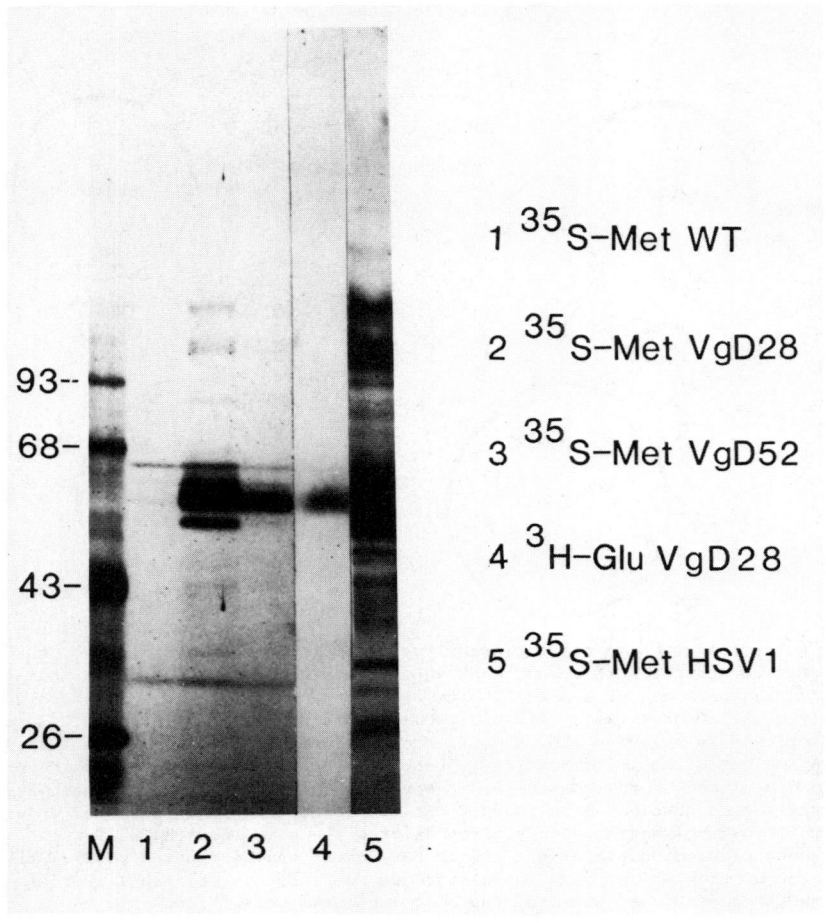

FIG. 2. Expression of HSV-1 gD by vaccinia virus recombinants. Monolayers of CV-1 cells were infected with wild-type vaccinia virus (lane 1), recombinant vgD28 (lanes 2 and 4), recombinant vgD52 (lane 3) or wild-type HSV-1 (lane 5). After 2 hours at 37°C. 1-- uCi of ^{35}S-methionine (1000 Ci/mmole) (lanes 1,2,3,5) or 100 uCi of ^{3}H-glucosamine (100 Ci/mmole) was added and the incubation was continued for approximately 10 hours. Cytoplasmic extracts were prepared and immunoprecipitated with a rabbit anti-HSV antiserum (lanes 1 to 4) or with a monoclonal antiserum against HSV-1 gD (lane 5; obtained from M. Zweig). Immunoprecipitated polypeptides were dissociated with SDS and resolved by polyacrylamide gel electrophoreses [24]. The positions of marker polypeptides (M) are at the left (molecular mass x 10^{-3}). Arrow designates the position of the 60,000 dalton HSV protein.

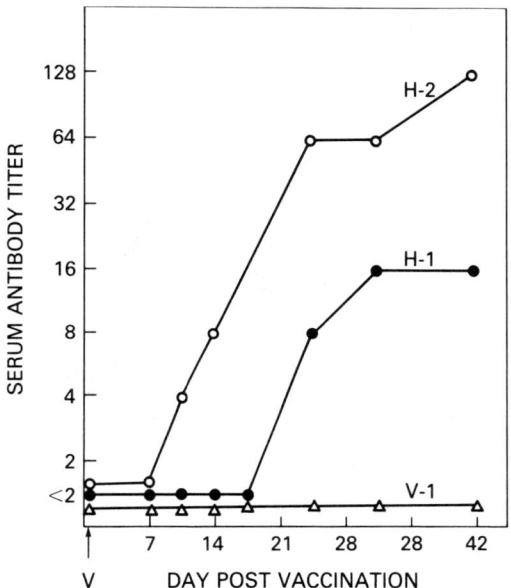

FIG. 3. Production of neutralizing antibody in vaccinated rabbits. Rabbits (H-1, H-2) were inoculated intradermally with 1×10^8 pfu of purified vaccinia HSV-1 gD (vgD52) at four sites or with 1×10^8 pfu of wild-type vaccinia (V-1) at four sites. Serum was prepared on the days indicated and assayed for HSV neutralizing antibody in a complement-dependent microneutralization assay [23]. The endpoint of the assay was expressed as the reciprocal of the highest two-fold serum dilution in which HSV was completely neutralized and no cytopathic effects due to virus infection were visible.

vaccinia expressing the hepatitis B surface antigen or saline. Ten weeks later all mice were challenged with a lethal intraperitoneal infection of HSV-1 (strain MacIntyre). One hundred (100) percent of the mice vaccinated with the vgD52 recombinant survived a lethal HSV-1 infection (Figure 4). In contrast, 10 percent (2/20) and 0 percent (0/20) of mice vaccinated with the hepatitis recombinant or saline, respectively, survived the lethal HSV-1 infection.

To determine whether vaccinia-HSV-1 gD would protect mice against a lethal infection of HSV-2, mice were immunized with a single dose of vaccinia HSV-1 gD, vaccinia HBsAg (expressing hepatitis B surface antigen) or wild-type vaccinia virus injection into a rear footpad or by tail scarification. Ninety-five (95) percent of mice immunized with vaccinia-HSV-1 gD survived a lethal intraperitoneal challenge with HSV-2 (strain G) while less than 5 percent of mice in the control groups survived (Table II). These results, with a single inoculation of vaccinia-HSV-1 gD,

TABLE I. HSV neutralizing antibody in immunized mice.

Immunizing agent	Route of immunization	Antibody titer (range)	(geometric mean)
None	-	<4	<4
Vaccinia	Tail	<4	<4
Vac HBsAg	Tail	<4	<4
Vac HSV-1 gD	IP	8-128	54
Vac HSV-1 gD	Footpad	16-128	75
Vac HSV-1 gD	Tail	8-128	60

Balb/c mice, 6 to 8 weeks old, were vaccinated by different routes with either 1×10^8 pfu of vaccinia HSV-1 gD (vgD52), vaccinia HBsAg (vHBs4) or wild-type vaccinia. Sera for antibody determinations were collected from retro-orbital plexus four weeks after immunization. HSV neutralizing antibody titers were determined in a complement dependent microneutralizing assay [23]. Endpoints were expressed as the reciprocal of the highest two-fold serum dilution which prevented a cytopathic effect by 100 tissue culture infectious doses of HSV. Geometric mean antibody titers were based on data from groups of 15 to 20 mice.

TABLE II. Effect of immunization with recombinant vaccinia HSV-1 gD on lethality of mice challenged with HSV-1

Immunizing agent	Route of vaccination	Dead/Challenged	Mortality (%)
None	-	39/40	98
Vaccinia	Footpad	20/21	96
	Tail	19/21	90
Vac HBsAg	Footpad	18/19	95
	Tail	19/20	95
Vac HSV-1 gD	Footpad	0/20	0
	Tail	1/20	5

Balb/c female mice, 6 to 8 weeks old, were vaccinated with 1×10^8 pfu of vaccinia-HSV-1 gD (vgD52), vaccinia HBsAg (vHBs4) or wild-type vaccinia virus by inoculation into a rear footpad or by tail scarification. Control mice were not vaccinated. Eight (8) weeks later all mice were challenged with an intraperitoneal dose of 2×10^6 pfu of HSV-2 (strain G). Mice were observed for survival during the next 3 weeks.

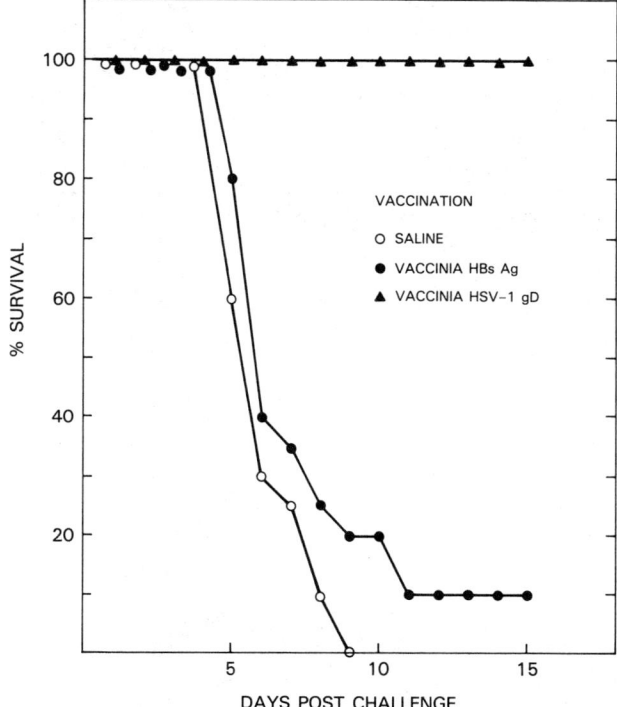

FIG. 4. Protection against a lethal HSV-1 infection. Balb/c mice (20 per group) were vaccinated by tail scarification with either 1×10^8 pfu of purified vaccinia expressing the hepatitis B surface antigen (Vac HBsAg), expressing the HSV-1 glycoprotein D gene (Vac HSV-1 gD) or saline. Ten (10) weeks later all mice were challenged with an intraperitoneal dose of 1×10^7 pfu of HSV-1 (strain MacIntyre). Mice were observed for survival during the next 15 days.

along with experiments of Long et al. [12], with multiple injections of purified HSV-1 gD protein, demonstrated that an immune response against the type common antigenic determinants present on HSV-1 gD was sufficient to protect mice from lethal intraperitoneal infections with HSV-1 or HSV-2.

PROTECTION AGAINST LATENT HSV INFECTIONS

The mouse latency model was used to determine the efficacy of vaccination to prevent the establishment of latent HSV infections in the trigeminal ganglia [7]. Mice were immunized by the intradermal route (tail scarification) with vaccinia-HSV-1 gD or with vaccinia HBsAg (hepatitis B surface antigen) and four weeks later challenged with HSV by the lip route with the KOS strain of HSV. Twenty-four days later the trigeminal ganglia were assayed for the presence of latent virus by explanting viable ganglia tissues and co-cultivating on primary rabbit kidney indicator cells. HSV was recovered from 88 percent (53/60) and 83 percent (50/60) of ganglia from unvaccinated controls or mice inoculated with vaccinia HBsAg, respectively, but from only 27 percent (16/60) of ganglia from mice vaccinated with the HSV-1 gD recombinant (Table III). Thus, 69 percent of the ganglia from mice vaccinated with the recombinant virus were protected from the development of a latent HSV infection. This is the first demonstration that a genetically engineered vaccine substantially prevents the development of a latent HSV infection.

TABLE III. Prevention of latent HSV infection by recombinant vaccine.

Vaccination	Number of mice	Trigeminal ganglia (number positive/ number tested)	% protection
None	30	53/60	0
Vaccinia HBsAg	30	50/60	5
Vaccinia-HSV-1 gD	30	16/60	69

Balb/c female mice were vaccinated with 1×10^8 pfu of vaccinia-HSV-1 gD or vaccinia HBsAg virus by tail scarification. Seven weeks later, the mice were challenged by bilateral labial scarification (i.e., to infect both trigeminal ganglia) with 7.5×10^6 pfu of HSV-1 (strain KOS). Twenty-four days later all animals were sacrificed, trigeminal ganglia were removed and cultured separately on primary rabbit kidney cells for 3 weeks, and observed for cytopathic effects indicating reactivation of latent HSV. Results are expressed as the ratio of the number of positive ganglia to the total number assayed. The percent protection represents the difference between the percent positive trigeminal ganglia from unvaccinated mice compared to the percent positive ganglia from mice receiving vaccinia HBsAg or vaccinia HSV-1 gD, divided by the percent positive from unvaccinated mice.

SUMMARY

A vaccinia virus recombinant expressing the gD protein of HSV-1, inoculated into mice, stimulated the production of HSV neutralizing antibodies and protected mice against a lethal challenge with either HSV-1 or HSV-2. The vaccinated mice also showed substantial protection against the development of a latent ganglionic infection.

REFERENCES

1. J.R. Barringer and P. Swoveland, N. Eng. J. Med. 288, 648-650 (1973).
2. J.R. Barringer, Prog. Med. Virol. 20, 1-26 (1978).
3. A.J. Nahmias, S.L. Shore, S. Kohl, S.E. Starr and R.B. Ashman, Cancer Res. 36, 836-844 (1976).
4. J.G. Stevens and M.L. Cook, Science 173, 843-845 (1971).

5. M.A. Walz, R.W. Price and A.L. Notkins, Science 184, 1184-1187 (1974).
6. R.W. Price, B.J. Katz and A.L. Notkins, Nature 257, 686-687 (1975a).
7. R.W. Price, M.A. Walz, C. Wohlenberg and A.L. Notkins, Science 188, 938-940 (1975b).
8. T. Sekizawa, H. Openshaw, C. Wohlenberg and A.L. Notkins, Science 210, 1026-1028 (1980).
9. H. Openshaw, T. Sekizawa, C. Wohlenberg and A.L. Notkins in: The Human Herpesviruses, A.J. Nahmias, W.R. Dowdle and R.F. Schinazi, eds. (Elsevier, New York 1981) pp. 289-296.
10. P.G. Spear, J. Virol. 17, 991-1008 (1976).
11. W. Chan, Immunology 49, 343-352 (1983).
12. D. Long, T.J. Madara, M. Ponce de Leon, G.H. Cohn, P.C. Montgomery and R. Eisenberg, Infect. Immun. 37, 761-764 (1984).
13. R.J. Watson, J.H. Weis, J.S. Salstrom and L.W. Enquist, Science 218, 381-384 (1982).
14. L.A. Lasky, D. Dowbenko, C. Simonson and P.W. Berman in: Modern Approaches to Vaccines, R.M. Chanock and R.A. Lerner, eds. (Cold Spring Harbor, N.Y. 1984) pp. 189-194.
15. E. Paoletti, B.R. Lipinskas, C. Samsonoff, S. Mercer and D. Panicali, Proc. Nat. Acad. Sci. 81, 193-197 (1984).
16. J.H. Weis, L.W. Enquist, J.S. Salstrom and R.J. Watson, Nature 302, 72-74 (1983).
17. P.W. Berman, D. Dowbenko and L.A. Lasky, Science 222, 524-527 (1983).
18. M. Mackett, G.L. Smith and B. Moss, Proc. Nat. Acad. Sci. 79, 7415-7419 (1982).
19. M. Mackett, G.L. Smith and B. Moss, J. Virol. 49, 857-864 (1984).
20. S. Venkatesan, B.M. Baroudy and B. Moss, Cell 25, 805-813 (1981).
21. J.P. Weir and B. Moss, J. Virol. 51, 662-669 (1984).
22. M. Cochran, C. Puckett and B. Moss, J. Virol., in press (1985).
23. P. Morahan, T.A. Thomson, S. Kohl and B.K. Murray, Infect. Immun. 32, 180-189 (1981).
24. G.L. Smith, M. Mackett and B. Moss, Nature 302, 490-495 (1983).

DISCUSSION

Dr. Neff: Have you taken animals that already had latent infection and looked to see if the vaccine would prevent recurrent infections?

Dr. Karzon: At what level does the vaccine work to prevent latency, at the ganglion, or before?

Dr. Cremer: Those experiments should be done, but we have not done them yet.

Dr. Wallace: Do you get reactivation of latent virus in mice?

Dr. Cremer: The efficiency of the reactivation is about 20 to 25 percent, so you would have to look at large groups of animals to specifically look at whether you can prevent reactivation in the animal. Those would be good experiments to do, but have not yet been done.

Dr. Ada: Have you looked at cell-mediated immunity at all?

Dr. Cremer: We have not looked at cell-mediated immunity yet.

Dr. Bennink: I used the same recombinant, and I tried to look for cytotoxic T cell responses. I found that there were not any responses. Even primed mice did not respond to HSV in vitro, secondarily. However, there was proliferation in response to a secondary restimulation with HSV-1.

INDUCTION OF VIRUS NEUTRALIZING ANTIBODIES AND PROTECTION AGAINST RABIES USING A VACCINIA RABIES GLYCOPROTEIN RECOMBINANT

BERNHARD DIETZSCHOLD,* TADEUSZ J. WIKTOR* AND HILARY KOPROWSKI*

*The Wistar Institute, 36th and Spruce Streets, Philadelphia, Pennsylvania 19104

The glycoprotein of rabies virus which forms the 10 nanometer peplomas (spikes) on the external surface of the virus membrane, is responsible for many of the important biological properties of the virus, including the induction of VNA and the induction of T cells which express helper, suppressor, or cytotoxic activities. It has been associated with antigenic drift and attachment of virus to cell surface receptors. Furthermore, immunization of animals with native glycoprotein can confer protection against a lethal challenge infection with rabies virus. Thus the rabies glycoprotein molecule represents a logical choice for a subunit vaccine against rabies virus infection.

Recently an approach to a new type of vaccine, the so-called second generation type vaccine, has been made. The approach utilizes the expression of a gene encoding for an immunogenic protein in a new host using DNA recombinant methods. A prerequisite of this new strategy in vaccine production is a detailed analysis of the gene structure and consequently the structure of the gene product. In order to analyze the structure of the rabies virus glycoprotein gene we cloned a double-stranded complementary DNA (cDNA) copy of the glycoprotein mRNA into pBR322 [3]. The cDNA copy was inserted into pBR322 at the Pst1 site by dG-dC tailing and the complete nucleotide sequence of the G protein cDNA containing 1650 base pairs determined [1]. The nucleotides sequence allowed us to predict several features of the glycoprotein from the deduced amino acids. An open reading frame beginning with an initial codon (ATG) and ending with a stop codon (TGA) suggested the nucleotide sequence coded for 524 amino acids. However, direct amino acid sequence analysis of purified rabies glycoprotein [8] indicated that the first 19 amino acid residues that precede the amino terminal lysine of G presumably represent a signal peptide. An uninterrupted hydrophobic sequence of 22 amino acids bound by residues 439 and 462 is the proposed transmembrane region. From the presumptive transmembrane domain a cytoplasmic sequence extends to the carboxy terminal lysine. There are three carbohydrate acceptor sequences, N(x)S or N(x)T located on the amino terminal side.

The antigenic structure of the rabies virus glycoprotein has been investigated in detail. An operational map of the rabies virus glycoprotein (G) of the DVS-11 strain was described which delineated three functionally independent antigenic sites based on the grouping of 90 G variant rabies viruses which were resistant to neutralization by one or more of a panel of anti-G monoclonal antibodies [7]. All of the monoclonal antibodies are known to be directed against highly conformational determinants. That is, any treatment of the glycoprotein which even mildly denatures the molecule destroys conformation and activity of these monoclonal antibodies. Therefore, we have concentrated our efforts to express the rabies G gene in a eucaryotic system which allows correct folding and processing of the G molecule.

Recently, experiments have shown that genetically engineered vaccinia recombinant viruses have a potential as vaccines [9,11]. We have used vaccinia virus to express the rabies virus glycoprotein. The construction of the vaccinia rabies G recombinant virus is described

© 1985 Elsevier Science Publishing Co., Inc.

elsewhere [6]. The exogenous coding rabies G sequence was aligned with a functional early vaccinia virus promoter so as to be controlled by this promoter and inserted in vitro at the Bam HI site within the thymidine kinase gene cloned in a suitable bacterial plasmid. The chimeric gene formed in this manner contains the vaccinia RNA start site juxtaposed with the rabies translational initiation codon so as to avoid the production of a fusion protein. This plasmid construct was used to transfect vaccinia virus infected cells to prepare a recombinant virus which contains the rabies G cDNA into the thymidine kinase locus.

Successful expression of a novel rabies G in V-RG1eu8 virus-infected BHK-21 cells resulted in a protein that was metabolically labeled with [^{35}S] methionine and [^{3}H] glucosamine, was immunoprecipitable with polyclonal rabbit anti-G antibodies, but which migrated faster than rabies virion G in NaDodSO$_4$ polyacrylamide gel. Comparison of tryptic peptides of G expressed by V-RG1eu8 and rabies virion G showed a strong similarity of both molecules. However, a panel of anti-G monoclonal antibodies which bind only to native rabies virus G failed to detect the V-RG1eu8 virus-expressed antigen. Moreover, injection of V-RG1eu8 virus into animals failed to induce rabies VNA (Table I) and protect against rabies, suggesting that the protein expressed by V-RG1eu8 virus was not in a native configuration. Direct amino acid analysis of the

TABLE I. Induction of VNA and protection from rabies by vaccinia recombinant viruses.

| Animals, route of inoculation | Vaccine[a] | VNA titers | | | | | Protection[b] |
| | | Rabies | | | | Vaccinia | |
		0d	5d	11d	14d	14d	
Rabbits, intradermal	V-RGpro8	<10	800	10,000	>30,000	250	3/4
	V-RG1eu8	<10			10		
	None	<10			10		0/5
Mice, intradermal	V-RGpro8	<10			>30,000	250	12/12
	V-RG1eu8	<10			10		0/12
	Vaccinia	<10			10	250	0/12
Mice, footpad	V-RGpro8	<10			>30,000	1250	12/12
	V-RG1eu8	<10			10		0/12
	Vaccinia	<10			10	1250	0/12

[a] Vaccine was inoculated on day 0 using 2×10^8 pfu (intradermal) or 5×10^7 pfu (footpad) of virus.
[b] A challenge dose of 2400 or 24,000 mouse LD$_{50}$ of MD5951 rabies virus was given on day 14 to mice and rabbits, respectively, by intracerebral inoculation.

N-terminus of the rabies virus G [4] revealed a discrepancy at amino acid position 8 (Pro) with the predicted sequence (Leu) of the original cDNA clone [1]. By sequencing this entire viral G gene, this amino acid change and one other at position 399 (Leu to Val) were identified (Wunner, unpublished). Assuming that the change near the N-terminus might have a greater impact on the structure formation of nascent G, the cDNA clone was modified by site-directed mutagenesis to rectify the amino acid at position 8 [6].

This modified clone was used to prepare another vaccinia recombinant virus designated V-RGpro8. Infection of BHK-21 cells by V-RGpro8 virus resulted in expression of a rabies G on the cell surface and in cytoplasm detected by immunofluorescence [12]. The protein expressed by this recombinant virus reacted with a panel of anti-G monoclonal antibodies in a pattern identical with native rabies virus G [6].

Inoculation of rabbits and mice with V-RGpro8 virus resulted in a rapid induction of rabies VNA (Table I). In rabbits, rabies VNA titers at 5, 11, and 14 days after inoculation were 800, 10,000, and greater than 30,000, respectively. Vaccinia VNA titers after 14 days were substantially lower. Rabbit serum (day 14) neutralized between $10^{5.3}$ and $10^{6.6}$ tissue culture ID_{50} of ERA rabies virus and three street rabies virus isolates previously shown to differ from the ERA strain in their reactivity with a panel of anti-rabies virus G monoclonal antibodies. Neutralization indices against rabies-related Duvenhage, Lagos bat and Mokola viruses were $10^{6.2}$, $10^{3.1}$, and $10^{3.4}$, respectively. These results, which are comparable to those obtained using anti-ERA rabies virus serum, demonstrate that Duvenhage virus is more closely related to rabies than are rabies-related Lagos bat and Mokola viruses.

Three out of four rabbits vaccinated with V-RGpro8 virus resisted a severe intracerebral challenge with 24,000 mouse LD_{50} of MD5951 rabies virus, whereas all five unvaccinated control rabbits died from rabies after 12 to 15 days (Table I). The one vaccinated rabbit that died from rabies survived until 21 days after challenge.

Inoculation of mice with V-RGpro8 virus, by either scarification or injection into the footpad, resulted in rabies VNA titers of 30,000 or higher after 14 days. All mice were protected against challenge with either HI5 or MD5951 rabies viruses, or with the rabies-related Duvenhage virus. No protection was seen following challenge with Mokola virus. Mice inoculated with wild-type vaccinia or V-RG1eu8 virus did not develop rabies VNA and were not protected against rabies.

A minimum dose of V-RGpro8 virus capable of protecting 50 percent of recipient mice was 10^4 pfu. In this experiment, mice were inoculated in the footpad, and challenged intracerebrally with 2,400 mouse LD_{50} of MD5951 rabies virus after 15 days. Levels of rabies VNA were determined at 7 and 14 days.

Reintroduction of vaccinia virus may be controversial. Therefore, we tested the ability of BPL-inactivated preparations of V-RGpro8 virus to induce an anti-rabies immune response. Extracts of V-RGpro8 virus-infected cell extracts using an affinity column prepared with anti-rabies virus G antibody, were inactivated and inoculated i.p. into mice. The mice were inoculated again after 6 days, and challenged intracerebrally with 240 LD_{50} of MD5951 rabies virus after a further 7 days. All three preparations induced high levels of rabies VNA, and protected against rabies (Table II).

Our experiments have shown that the genetically engineered vaccinia rabies glycoprotein recombinant virus has a great potential as a vaccine. The use of vaccinia recombinant virus might be particularly promising for wildlife immunization because of its wide host range. However, decisions would have to be made concerning the safety of this approach.

Rabies vaccines for human use are administered predominantly in post-exposure treatment of rabies. The exact mechanisms involved in prevention of clinical rabies are unknown. It has been demonstrated that whole virus vaccines have prevented development of rabies when administered in post-exposure situations [2,10]. However, the effectiveness of glycoprotein alone in post-exposure treatment has never been proven. Therefore, any recombinant vaccine based solely on the glycoprotein structure which might be used for post-exposure treatment of humans must be at least as effective as whole virus vaccine.

TABLE II. Induction of VNA and protection from rabies by inactivated preparations from V-RGpro8 rcombinant virus.

Vaccine	PFU/ml (log 10) before inactivation	Protein concentration (ug/mouse)[a]	Rabies VNA titers		Protection[b]
			Day 7	Day 14	
V-RGpro8 virus-infected cell extract	7.5	140	80	8,000	12/12
V-RGpro8 purified virus	8.6	9	270	4,000	12/12
V-RGpro8 virus-infected cell extract	-	50	120	15,000	12/12
Vaccinia virus-infected cell extract	8.6	900	<10	<10	0/12
Unvaccinated controls	-	-	-	<10	0/12

[a] Total protein in two i.p. inoculations given on days 0 and 7.
[b] A challenge dose of 240 mouse LD_{50} of MD5951 rabies virus was given on day 14 to mice by intracerebral inoculation.

Of theoretical concern regarding the use of a vaccinia rabies glycoprotein recombinant virus is the possibility that the rabies virus glycoprotein which has been implicated as one of the factors responsible for the neurovirulence of rabies virus, may be inserted in the vaccinia virus membrane and thereby increase the neurotropism of the virus. Since arginine at position 333 of rabies virus glycoprotein has been identified as the integral part of a site responsible for rabies virus pathogenicity [5], the codon in the rabies glycoprotein cDNA which codes for arginine 333 could be changed by site-directed mutagenesis to a codon which codes for isoleucine instead.

REFERENCES

1. A. Anilionis, W.H. Wunner and P.J. Curtis, Nature 294, 275-278 (1981).
2. M. Bahmanyar, A. Fayaz, S. Nour-Salehi, M. Mohammadi and H. Koprowski, J. Am. Med. Assoc. 236, 1751-1754 (1976).
3. P.J. Curtis, A. Anilionis and W.H. Wunner in: Replication of Negative Strand Viruses, D.H.L. Bishop and R.W. Compans, eds. (Elsevier, Amsterdam 1981) pp. 721-725.
4. B. Dietzschold, T.J. Wiktor, R. Macfarlan and A. Varrichio, J. Virol. 44, 595-602 (1982.

5. B. Dietzschold, W.H. Wunner, T.J. Wiktor, A.D. Lopes, M. Lafon, C. Smith and H. Koprowski, Proc. Natl. Acad. Sci. USA 80, 70-74 (1983).
6. M.P. Kieny, R. Lathe, R. Drillient, D. Spehnert, S. Skory, D. Schmitt, T.J. Wiktor, H. Koprowski and J.P. Lecocq, Nature 312, 163-166 (1984).
7. M. Lafon, T.J. Wiktor and R.I. Macfarlan, J. Gen. Virol. 64, 843-851 (1983).
8. C.-Y. Lai and B. Dietzschold, Biochem. Biophys. Res. Commun. 103, 536-542 (1981).
9. D. Panicalli, S.W. Davis, R.L. Weinberg and E. Paoletti, Proc. Natl. Acad. Sci USA 80, 5356-5368 (1983).
10. R.K. Sikes, W.F. Cleary, H. Koprowski, T.J. Wiktor and M.M. Kaplan, Bull. WHO 45, 1-11 (1971).
11. G.L. Smith, M. Mackett and B. Moss, Nature (London) 302, 490-495 (1983).
12. T.J. Wiktor, R.I. Macfarlan, K.J. Reagan, B. Dietzschold, P.J. Curtis, W.H. Wunner, M.P. Kieny, R. Lathe, J.P. Lecocq, M. Mackett, B. Moss and H. Koprowski, Proc. Natl. Acad. Sci. USA 81, 7194-7198 (1984).

DISCUSSION

Dr. Quinnan: Would you comment on the comparability of the recombinant vaccine to human diploid cell vaccine? The human diploid cell vaccines, when used appropriately, have been associated with 100 percent response rate in thousands of individuals. In the repeated use of vaccinia, you may not achieve a 100 percent response rate. On the other hand, one of the great limitations of the human diploid cell vaccines is their cost, which makes them unavailable to most of the world. How would you compare them in that respect?

Dr. Dietzschold: I would think that the response rate should be 100 percent. With regard to cost, we are studying the possibility of a subunit vaccine produced by infection of human diploid cells with recombinant vaccinia virus. If we can get tenfold more expression of glycoprotein with the vaccinia recombinant, compared with rabies virus, the vaccine might be less expensive.

Dr. Wallace: Have you studied duration of immunity following immunization with the live recombinant virus compared to inactivated vaccine or a purified antigen preparation?

Dr. Dietzschold: Yes, we looked for the duration of immunity after immunization with recombinant vaccine in mice. After six months, they still had high titers of neutralizing antibodies.

INFLUENZA VIRUS SPECIFIC CELL-MEDIATED IMMUNITY TO VACCINIA VIRUS
RECOMBINANTS

JACK R. BENNINK,* JONATHAN W. YEWDELL,* GEOFFREY L. SMITH,** AND BERNARD
MOSS**

*The Wistar Institute, 36th and Spruce, Philadelphia, Pennsylvania 19104.
**Laboratory of Viral Diseases, National Institute of Allergy and
Infectious Diseases, NIH, Bethesda, Maryland 20205.

INTRODUCTION

The construction of vaccinia virus recombinants expressing cloned genes [1-3] encoding immunologically important proteins of unrelated infectious agents [4-10] provided a new approach to the development of live vaccines. These vaccinia virus recombinants have been shown to induce the production of specific antibodies to the cloned gene products in vaccinated animals. Furthermore, animals immunized with recombinants expressing the influenza virus haemagglutinin (HA) [5], the hepatitis B virus surface antigen [11], and type 1 herpesvirus glycoprotein D [8] have been shown to be protected against subsequent challenge with the corresponding virus.

One important effector mechanism of immune responses is mediated by T-cells which lyse histocompatible cells bearing foreign antigens. These cytotoxic T lymphocytes (CTL) are thought to be of particular importance in tumor immunity and in eradicating viral infections [12]. Because poxviruses induce a potent virus specific cell-mediated immune response, they have been extremely useful in studying CTL. In this role, poxviruses (vaccinia in particular) have added greatly to our knowledge of the class I molecule major histocompatibility complex restriction of CTL, the effect of immune response genes on virus specific CTL responses, and CTL repertoire development [12]. The vaccinia virus recombinants add a new dimension to our ability to dissect the specificity of CTL responses. Through their use it is now possible to examine CTL recognition of individual viral components. This knowledge is important for vaccine design, since for many viruses it is likely that the optimal vaccine should stimulate cell-mediated as well as humoral immunity.

In this paper we review our current studies in which we have used vaccinia virus recombinants expressing influenza virus gene products to examine the recognition of individual influenza virus gene products by CTL. To place these studies in the proper context it is necessary to briefly present some background information. The influenza viruses acquire their envelope by budding through the plasma membrane of the host cell. The virion consists of 7 proteins. Two glycoproteins, haemagglutinin and neuraminidase (NA) are integral membrane proteins expressed in large quantities on infected cell surfaces which form a dense layer of spikes on the virion surface. The matrix protein (M1) forms a shell beneath the lipid envelope, and the nucleoprotein (NP) combines with small amounts of the three viral polymerases (PA, PB1, PB2) to form the ribonucleoprotein complex. The serological relationships of viral proteins derived from different type A influenza virus strains reflect their amino acid homologies. HA and NA glycoproteins derived from different influenza A virus subtypes exhibit relatively low homology (30 to 80%) [13] and are largely serologically non-cross-reactive, while the highly conserved internal proteins (over 90% homologous) are antigenically cross-reactive (a difference reflected in the fact that influenza viruses are classified as to which of the 13 known HA and 9 known NA glycoproteins they possess). The finding that most influenza A specific CTL lysed cells infected with any influenza A virus was puzzling [14,15], since at that time it was thought that only the glycoproteins were expressed on infected cell surfaces. The viral antigens recognized by these "cross-reactive" CTL has remained a vexing problem to both immunologists (due to the possibility that CTL may recognize the glycoproteins differently than antibodies) and virologists (due to the possibility that internal virion proteins may be expressed on the infected cell surface). This problem is also of importance from a practical standpoint, since current evidence suggests that CTL plays an important role in reducing the severity of influenza virus infection [16-18]. Thus, identification of the viral antigen(s) recognized by cross-reactive CTL would be extremely useful in producing vaccines which prime for a strong cross-reactive CTL response upon subsequent influenza virus infection. Such a vaccine could potentially confer longer lasting immunity than currently used vaccines, which are designed to optimally induce anti-glycoprotein antibodies and, as such, are inherently limited by the frequent antigenic changes in the glycoproteins.

The availability of cloned viral genes in appropriate eukaryotic expression vectors has finally allowed us and others [19-22] to directly examine which viral proteins are recognized by CTL. What follows is a brief summary of both recently published [20,22] and unpublished work.

RESULTS AND DISCUSSION

Experiments to date have utilized four vaccinia virus recombinants expressing influenza virus genes. These recombinants were made by inserting DNA copies of cloned influenza genes derived from either A/Japan/305(H2N2)(JAP) (kindly provided by M.J. Gething) or A/Puerto Rico/8/34(H1N1)(PR8) (kindly provided by P. Palese) into vaccinia virus (VAC) under the control of an early vaccinia virus promoter as previously described [3,4]. The recombinants were named as follows: H1-VAC (PR8-HA gene); H2-VAC (JAP-HA gene); NP-VAC (PR8-NP gene); and M1-VAC (PR8-M1 gene).

Initial experiments examined whether inoculation with the vaccinia recombinants primed splenocytes for a secondary influenza specific CTL response upon in vitro stimulation with autologous virus infected splenocytes (Table I). First, we established that vaccinia virus alone did not prime for secondary influenza specific T-cell responses. Thus, splenocytes derived from mice primed with JAP but not VAC could be restimulated in vitro with JAP to yield specific lysis of JAP infected target cells. Reciprocally, cells derived from mice immunized with VAC, but not JAP could be restimulated in vitro with VAC to yield specific lysis of VAC infected target cells. When the recombinant vaccinia viruses were similarly tested it was found that H2-VAC and NP-VAC, but not M1-VAC primed for a secondary CTL response upon in vitro stimulation with JAP. While H2-VAC⁻ primed JAP stimulated CTL were largely specific for JAP infected cells, NP-VAC primed CTL lysed cells infected with viruses representing each of the human influenza A virus subtypes (H1N1, H2N2, H3N2). Importantly, stimulation of splenocytes derived from NP-VAC primed mice with PR8 and HK infected cells also generated potent fully cross-reactive CTL (not shown). CTL recognition of HA, NP and M was more directly examined in experiments which tested the ability of various anti-influenza CTL populations to lyse P815 cells (a murine DBA/2 mastocytoma line) infected with vaccinia recombinants.

Preliminary experiments established that: (1) the influenza virus gene products produced by the recombinants were antigenically indistinguishable from the authentic viral protein as determined by the binding

TABLE I. The effect of in vivo priming with recombinant vaccinia viruses.

Virus stimulation		CTL specific lysis of target cells				
Primary in vivo	Secondary in vitro	VAC	JAP (H2N2)	PR8 (H1N1)	HK (H3N2)	UNINF
JAP	JAP	−	+	+	+	−
VAC	JAP	−	−	−	−	−
NP-VAC	JAP	−	+	+	+	−
H2-VAC	JAP	−	+	+/−	−	−
M1-VAC	JAP	−	−	−	−	−
JAP	VAC	−	−	−	−	−
VAC	VAC	+	−	−	−	−
NP-VAC	VAC	+	−	−	−	−
H2-VAC	VAC	+	−	−	−	−
M1-VAC	VAC	+	−	−	−	−

Mice were primed in vivo with 10^7 plaque-forming units of vaccinia virus or 10^2 haemagglutinating units of JAP virus 2 to 4 weeks prior to in vitro stimulation. Secondary cultures consisted of 6×10^7 responder splenocytes and 3×10^7 stimulators infected with 10^3 haemagglutinating units of JAP or 10^8 plaque-forming units of vaccinia virus. The effector populations were harvested for assay after incubation at 37°C for 6 days. Specific lysis of P815 infected and uninfected target cells was measured using a 4 h ^{51}Cr release assay.

of panels of monoclonal antibodies to infected P815 cells, (2) recombinant infected cells produced as much antigenically active influenza virus protein as influenza virus infected cells which were efficiently lysed by the CTL populations used, (3) processes related to vaccinia infection did not interfere with recognition of target cells by anti-influenza CTL.

Summarized in Table II are results obtained regarding the recognition of cloned PR8 gene products by 3 anti-influenza virus CTL populations. All 3 populations contain cross-reactive CTL as evidenced by their ability to lyse cells infected by H1N1 (PR8), H2N2 (JAP), and H3N2 ((A/Hong Kong/107 (HK)) viruses. In addition, the PR8 primary-PR8 secondary and JAP primary-JAP secondary populations are expected to contain H1N1 and H2N2 subtype specific CTL, respectively. The recognition of the individual gene

TABLE II. Lysis of recombinant vaccinia virus infected target cells.

Virus stimulation		CTL specific lysis of target cells						
Primary in vivo	Secondary in vitro	VAC	NP-VAC	H1-VAC	M1-VAC	PR8	HK	JAP
PR8	PR8	−	+	+	−	+	+	+
JAP	JAP	−	+	+/−	−	+	+	+
JAP	HK	−	+	−	−	+	+	+
VAC	VAC	+	+	+	+	−	−	−

See Table I.

products by the various populations is consistent with the priming data presented above. Thus NP-VAC infected cells were efficiently lysed by all 3 CTL effector populations. This provides a direct demonstration that this internal virion protein which is expressed on infected cell surfaces in relatively small quantities [23], can serve as a target antigen for CTL. Furthermore, the efficient lysis of NP-VAC infected cells by CTL induced by heterosubtypic viruses suggests that a substantial proportion of cross-reactive CTL recognize the NP (a point confirmed by additional "unlabeled target" inhibition experiments, and limiting dilution studies). In contrast, H1-VAC infected cells were consistently lysed only by PR8 primed and stimulated CTL. Although low levels of lysis were occasionally observed with JAP-primed and stimulated CTL, these targets were never lysed by CTL primed and stimulated by H3N2 viruses, or CTL primed and stimulated by heterosubtypic viruses (similar results were obtained with H2-VAC infected cells). This indicates that CTL recognition of the HA is largely limited to subtype specific CTL, although it does appear that a minor CTL population which cross-recognizes H1 and H2 HAs does exist. M1-VAC infected cells were not lysed by any of the CTL populations presented in Table II, nor were they lysed by a large number of additional populations tested in subsequent experiments. This finding is consistent with the failure to detect M1 on infected cell surfaces using monoclonal antibodies [23], and in conjunction with the failure of M1-VAC to prime for a secondary CTL response strongly suggests that M1 is not recognized by CTL.

In conclusion, we have shown that recombinant vaccinia viruses containing cloned influenza virus genes are able to prime animals for secondary CTL responses. We have also used these viruses to examine the specificity of anti-influenza CTL and have found that NP is a major target antigen for the cross-reactive components of the CTL response. Experiments are currently in progress to examine the ability of the recombinants to protect animals from influenza virus infection.

SUMMARY

Studies have been done using vaccinia virus recombinants containing DNA copies of individual influenza virus genes. Immunization of mice with either H2-vaccinia (A/JAP/305 haemagglutinin) or NP-vaccinia (A/PR/8 nucleoprotein) primes spenocytes for secondary CTL responses. The fact that vaccinia recombinants stimulate both humoral and cell-mediated immunity makes them good candidates for use as live vaccines. Results using recombinant vaccinia virus infected target cells indicate that cytotoxic T cells capable of recognizing the haemagglutinin molecule are almost entirely subtype specific. Although a small degree of cross-reactivity has been observed between H1 and H2 haemagglutinin it is clear that the haemagglutinin in no way accounts for the major cross-reactive specificity observed in anti-influenza virus cytotoxic T cell populations. Experiments with NP-vaccinia indicate that the nucleoprotein does serve as a type A influenza virus cross-reactive target structure. Cytotoxic T cells appear not to recognize the matrix protein, since M1-vaccinia (A/PR/8 vaccinia) neither primes for secondary influenza cytotoxic T cells nor are target cells infected with M1-vaccinia lysed by anti-influenza cytotoxic T cell populations.

ACKNOWLEDGMENT

This work was supported by NIH grants AI 14162, AI 20338, AI 13989 and NS 11036.

REFERENCES

1. D. Panicali and E. Paoletti, Procl Natl. Acad. Sci. USA 80, 5364-5368 (1982).
2. M. Mackett, G.L. Smith and B. Moss, Proc. Natl. Acad. Sci. USA 79, 7415-7419 (1982).
3. M. Mackett, G.L. Smith and B. Moss, J. Virology 49, 857-864 (1984).
4. G.L. Smith, M. Mackett and B. Moss, Nature(Lond) 302, 490-495 (1983a).
5. G.L. Smith, M. Mackett and B. Moss in: Gene Expression, UCLA Symp. Molec. Cell Biol. New Ser., D. Hamer and M. Rosenberg, eds. (Liss, New York 1983b) Vol. 8, pp. 534-554.
6. G.L. Smith, B.R. Murphy and B. Moss, Proc. Natl. Acad. Sci. USA 80, 7155-7159 (1983c).
7. D. Panicali, S.W. Davis, R.L. Weinburg and E. Paoletti, Proc. Natl. Acad. Sci. USA 79, 1593-1596 (1983).
8. E. Paoletti, B.R. Lipinski, C. Samsonoff, S. Mercer and D. Panicali, Proc. Natl. Acad. Sci. USA 81, 193-197 (1984).
9. G.L. Smith, B.N. Godson, V. Nussenzweig, R.S. Nussenzweig and B. Moss, Science 224, 397-399 (1984).
10. G.L. Smith, M. Mackett, B.R. Murphy and B. Moss in: Modern Approaches to Vaccines, R. Chanock and L. Lerner, eds. (Cold Spring Harbor Laboratory, 1985) in press.
11. B. Moss, G.L. Smith, J.L. Gerin and R.H. Purcell, Nature(Lond) 311, 67-69 (1984).
12. R.M. Zinkernagel and P.C. Doherty, Adv. Immunol. 27, 51-77 (1979).
13. R.A. Lamb in: Genetics of Influenza Viruses, P. Palese and D.W. Kingsbury, eds. (New York. Springer-Verlag, 1983) pp. 21-69.
14. R.B. Effros, P.C. Doherty, W. Gerhard and J.R. Bennink, J. Exp. Med. 145, 557-568 (1977).
15. H.J. Zweerink, B.A. Askonas, D. Millican, S.A. Courtneidge and J.J. Skehel, Eur. J. Immunol. 7, 630-635 (1977).
16. K.L. Yap, G.L. Ada and I.F.C. McKenzie, Nature(Lond) 273, 238-239 (1978).
17. A.E. Lukacher, V.L. Braciale and T.J. Braciale, J. Exp. Med. 160, 814-826 (1984).
18. Y.L. Lin and B.A. Askonas, J. Exp. Med. 154, 225-234 (1981).
19. T.J. Braciale, V.L. Braciale, T.J. Henkel, J.S. Sambrook and M.J. Gethin, J. Exp. Med. 159, 341-354 (1984).
20. J.R. Bennink, J.W. Yewdell, G.L. Smith, C. Moller and B. Moss, Nature(Lond) 311, 578-579 (1984).
21. A.R.M. Townsend, J.J. Skehel, P.M. Taylor and P. Palese, Virology 133, 456-459 (1984).
22. J.W. Yewdell, J.R. Bennink, G.L. Smith and B. Moss, Proc. Natl. Acad. Sci. USA, in press (1985).
23. J.W. Yewdell, E. Frank and W. Gerhard, J. Immunol. 126, 1814-1819 (1981).

DISCUSSION

Dr. Chanock: Your observation that the NP vaccinia recombinant did not confer significant protection against challenge is certainly consistent with what is known of the epidemiology of influenza. Infection with a previous subtype generally does not protect against epidemic influenza.

Dr. Schild: I believe that the Oxford group has found incomplete cross-reactivity of nuclear protein-specific cytotoxic T-cells killing. There is a difference between strains isolated before 1942, which would include PR-8 virus, and those after 1942. It appears there was some antigenic change in the nuclear protein around 1942. Have you compared the PR-8 virus to any later ones, such as A/Hong Kong?

Dr. Bennink: All of the strains we have looked at share complete cross-reactivity in their nuclear proteins.

Dr. Halstead: What was the route of immunization in the mouse experiments?

Dr. Bennink: In general, we give the virus intravenously. We can also give it intraperitoneally. I have tried it subcutaneously, and it does work, but you have to use more virus.

Dr. Ada: Have you tried giving it intranasally?

Dr. Bennink: We haven't tried that yet.

INTRANASAL VACCINATION WITH RECOMBINANT VACCINIA CONTAINING INFLUENZA
HEMAGGLUTININ PREVENTS BOTH INFLUENZA VIRUS PNEUMONIA AND NASAL INFECTION:
INTRADERMAL VACCINATION PREVENTS ONLY VIRAL PNEUMONIA[†]

PARKER A. SMALL, JR.,* GEOFFREY L. SMITH,** AND BERNARD MOSS**

*Department of Immunology and Medical Microbiology, College of Medicine,
University of Florida, Gainesville, Florida 32610; **National Institute
of Allergy and Infectious Diseases, National Institutes of Health,
Bethesda, Maryland 20205.

It has previously been shown [1] that a recombinant vaccinia virus
containing the H2 influenza virus hemagglutinin gene (H2-Vac) can stimulate the production of antibody in hamsters and prevent viral pneumonia
when the animals are challenged with the homologous virus. The mouse
model has previously been used to demonstrate that serum antibody
prevents viral pneumonia [2] but not tracheitis [3] or rhinitis [4].
Prevention of upper respiratory infection has been shown to be a function
of local immunity in the ferret [5]. The work reported in this paper
was undertaken to determine the effect of dermal and nasal immunization
with the recombinant H2-Vac virus on nasal and serum antibody production
and on prevention of influenza of the nose and lung of the mouse.

A recombinant Tk$^-$ vaccinia virus containing the cDNA of the
influenza H1 hemagglutinin gene (10^8 pfu) was administered to mice
either intranasally or by scarification. Control mice were vaccinated
intradermally with either 10^8 pfu of Tk$^-$ vaccinia or 10^8 pfu of Tk$^-$
vaccinia containing the H2 influenza gene. Three weeks later, the four
groups (six mice each) were vaccinated for serum and nasal wash antibody
using a radioimmunoassay (RIA) with either anti-IgG1 (serum) or anti-IgA
(nasal). Another cohort (eight mice each) was anesthetized and challenged
with PR8 (H1N1) influenza virus. Virus shedding from the nose and lung
was determined 1 day after challenge.

As shown in Table I, scarification (scar.) immunization stimulates
the production of serum antibody but not nasal antibody and protects

TABLE I. Response to recombinant vaccinia immunization

Route of Immunization	H1 antibody (RIA titer $\pm$ S.D.)		Virus shedding (log 10 EID50 $\pm$ S.D.)	
	serum	nasal	lung	nose
H1 i.n.	253$\pm$122	70$\pm$148	-0.3$\pm$1.4(2/8)[a]	-0.7$\pm$0.4(3/8)[a]
H1 scar.	326$\pm$160	<2.9	-0.9$\pm$0.3(1/8)[a]	1.0$\pm$0.8
Tk$^-$ scar.	74$\pm$20	<2.9	3.3$\pm$1.5	1.6$\pm$0.7
H2 scar.	76$\pm$11	<3/3	3.7$\pm$0.9	1.9$\pm$0.8

[a] Number of animals shedding virus/total number tested.
In the other five groups, all eight animals were infected.

[†]Reprinted from "Vaccines 85" (R. Lerner, R. Chanock, and F. Brown, eds.)
Cold Spring Harbor Laboratory, Cold Spring Harbor, New York, p. 175
(1985).

Published 1985 by Elsevier Science Publishing Co., Inc.
VACCINIA VIRUSES AS VECTORS FOR VACCINE ANTIGENS, Quinnan, Editor

the lung but not the nose from challenge with homologous virus. In contrast, intranasal (i.n.) immunization elicits both serum and nasal antibodies and protects both sites. Nasal antibody was detected in all mice immunized intranasally but not in the mice in the other three groups.

Additional work (data not shown) has demonstrated that the mice immunized by scarification recovered rapidly from their nasal infection. Bennink et al. [6] have shown that H2-Vac stimulates anti-hemagglutinin cytotoxic T lymphocytes, and these probably play an essential role in the rapid recovery of the mice vaccinated by scarification and infected nasally.

In summary, we conclude that the host defense of the lung is different from that of the nose. Intradermal immunization stimulates only the lung preventative mechanism, but intranasal immunization stimulates both lung and nasal preventative mechanisms. The data are consistent with the lung and nasal preventative mechanisms being serum antibody and IgA nasal antibody, respectively. Perhaps the most surprising observation is that vaccination by scarification does not stimulate local immunity.

ACKNOWLEDGMENTS

We acknowledge the capable technical assistance of Ms. Chrissie Street and Ms. Rosa Hankison. This work was supported by National Institutes of Health grant AI-07713.

REFERENCES

1. G.L. Smith, B.R. Murphy and B. Moss, Proc. Natl. Acad. Sci. 80, 7155 (1983).
2. C.G. Loosi and B.S. Berlin, Trans. Assoc. Am. Phys. 66, 222 (1953).
3. R. Ramphal, R.C. Cogliano, J.W. Shands, Jr. and P.S. Small, Jr., Infect. Immun. 25, 992 (1979).
4. R.M. Kris, R. Asofsky, C.B. Evans and P.A. Small, Jr., J. Immunol. (in press) (1985).
5. W.H. Barber and P.A. Small, Jr., Infect. Immun. 21, 221 (1978).
6. J.R. Bennink, J.W. Yewdell, G.L. Smith, C. Moller and B. Moss, Nature 311, 578 (1984).

DISCUSSION

Dr. McIntosh: Do you see the same protection with either passively transferred antibody, or with conventional inactivated influenza vaccines?

Dr. Small: When you infect nude mice with influenza, they shed virus for more than 60 days, and apparently never recover. If you give them antibody passively, they stop shedding virus and the desquamated epithelium returns to normal for as long as the mouse continues to have antibody detectable in its serum. When the antibody is gone, they shed virus and desquamate their tracheal epithelium once again. So antibody can help with recovery, but is not sufficient to produce permanent recovery.

We have taken normal mice and suppressed them with anti-mu antibody from birth, then infected them with influenza. They recovered from the disease, and never developed any detectable antibody. The recovery took two to five days longer than with normal mice. Cell-mediated immunity is essential for recovery, but that antibody can help.

Dr. McIntosh: My question is an optimistic one. Is it possible that this vaccine may be better than a killed vaccine?

Dr. Small: Yes, it is possible, since it appears to induce cytotoxic T cell responses better than the killed vaccine.

Dr. Dowdle: Could you comment on the dose of recombinant virus used and whether it was optimal?

Dr. Small: We used 10^8 plaque forming units, either intranasally or by scarification. It is impossible to know exactly how much of those doses actually infected the animals when administered by those routes.

Dr. Wallace: In the experiment where you were getting nasal secretion of virus after scarification, could the mouse have infected itself from the scarification procedure intranasally?

Dr. Small: I don't think so. If it had spread the virus from the scarificatrion to its nose, then we would have expected to have seen local antibody production, the way we did when we put the virus directly into the nose.

INFECTIOUS VACCINIA VIRUS RECOMBINANTS THAT EXPRESS THE EPSTEIN-BARR VIRUS
MEMBRANE ANTIGEN gp340

MICHAEL MACKETT AND JOHN R. ARRAND*

*Department of Molecular Biology, Paterson Laboratories, Christie Hospital
& Holt Radium Institute, Withington, Manchester M20 9BX, United Kingdom

SUMMARY

The production and characterization of a vaccinia virus recombinant
which expresses Epstein-Barr virus membrane antigen gp340 is described.
The EB virus gp340 produced by the recombinant is detected at the
surface of infected cells, is approximately the same size as and is
antigenically similar to authentic gp340. Moreover, rabbits vaccinated
with the recombinant produce antibodies that recognize EB virus-containing
lymphoblastoid cells.

INTRODUCTION

Epstein-Barr (EB) virus is the causative agent of infectious mononucleosis and is closely associated with two human malignancies, Burkitt
lymphoma [1] and nasopharyngeal carcinoma [2]. It has been suggested
that a vaccine against EB virus might be an effective means of controlling
these two EB virus-related tumors [3].

EB virus membrane antigen (MA) is detected on the plasma membrane
of virus-producer cell lines and on intact virions. It consists of at
least two high molecular weight glycoproteins (340,000/350,000 and
270,000/220,000 daltons - gp340/gp270) [4-8]. The complete nucleotide
sequence and genomic location of the DNA that codes for gp340 and gp270
have been identified [9,10]. Antibodies raised against the plasma
membranes of producer cell lines or EB virus envelopes have virus
neutralizing activity [11-13]. In addition, monoclonal antibodies or
monospecific antisera which recognize gp340 and gp270 are also virus
neutralizing [14,13,15]. These antibodies also indicate that gp340 and
gp270 share antigenic determinants.

These data suggest that it should be possible to produce an anti-
EB virus vaccine based on gp340/gp270. We have constructed vaccinia
virus recombinants that express the EB virus gp340 and showed that when
rabbits were vaccinated using this recombinant they produced antibodies
that recognize EB virus gp340.

Enzymes

Enzymes were supplied by the companies indicated and used according
to their instructions. Restriction endonucleases were from Bethesda
Research Laboratories, Boehringer Mannheim Biochemicals, P&S Biochemicals
or New England Biolabs. T4 DNA ligase was from Bethesda Research Laboratories. Escherichia coli DNA pol 1, or DNA pol 1 large fragment, and
calf intestine alkaline phosphatase were from Boehringer Mannheim Biochemicals.

Preparation of DNA

Routine procedures were similar to those described in detail by
Maniatis et al. [16]. Recombinant plasmids were prepared using the
vectors pAT153 [17] or pUC9 [18] and purified as described by Birnboim
and Doly [19].

Generation of Recombinants

Recombinants were constructed essentially as outlined previously [20,21]. The EB virus membrane antigen coding sequence was derived from the BamH1 L clone of B95-8 virus DNA [22]. A plasmid vector was constructed which contains a vaccinia virus transcriptional start site upstream of the EB virus membrane antigen coding sequence, inserted into the body of the vaccinia virus TK gene (Figure 1). This plasmid

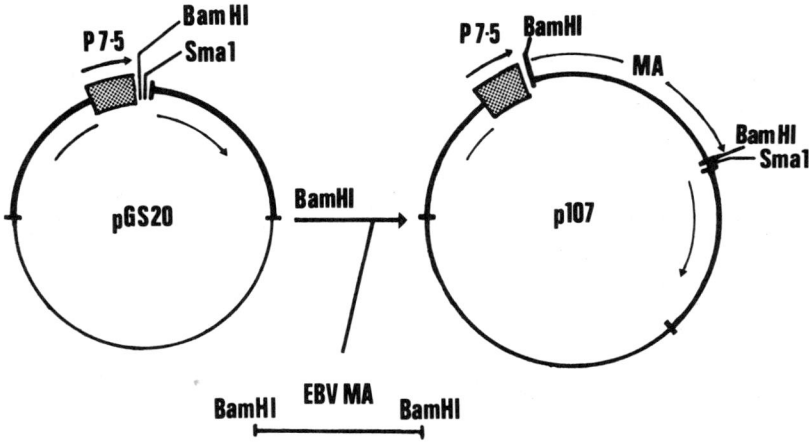

FIG. 1. Construction of a plasmid for the insertion and expression of EB virus membrane antigen in vaccinia virus. A 2.8Kb BamH1 fragment of B95-8 DNA containing the EB virus membrane antigen gp340 coding sequence was inserted into the BamH1 site of pGS20 (Mackett et al. 1984). This places the EB virus membrane antigen under the control of a vaccinia virus early promoter (indicated by P7.5 and the stippled box). The vaccinia promoter EB virus membrane antigen chimera is flanked by sequences derived from the vaccinia virus thymidine kinase (TK) gene. The TK gene coding sequence and direction of transcription are indicated by the internal arrow. The direction of transcription of the promoter P7.5 is also indicated.

was then used to recombine the membrane antigen gene into the vaccinia virus genome in a manner similar to that performed for marker rescue [23]. Briefly, cells were infected with wild-type (TK$^+$) vaccinia virus strain WR at a multiplicity of 0.01 to 0.05 PFU per cell. At 2 hr after infection, calcium phosphate-precipitated chimeric plasmid DNA was added, and cells were harvested at 48 h post infection. TK⁻ recombinant virus was selected from infected cell lysates by plaque assay on TK⁻ 143 cells with 25 ug of 5-bromodeoxyuridine (BUdR) per ml in the agar overlay.

Cells and Virus

Human TK⁻ 143 cells maintained in minimal essential medium (MEM) containing 25 ug/ml BUdR and 5% fetal calf serum (FCS) were used for selection of TK⁻ recombinants. Before use the cells were passaged twice in MEM + 5% FCS without BUdR. CVI monkey kidney cells were passaged in Dulbecco's modified MEM containing 5% FCS. For large stocks of virus HeLaS3 spinner cells maintained in Joklik's suspension medium supplemented with 10% horse serum were used. Raji [24], B95-8 [25] and W91 [26] EB virus-positive lymphoblastoid cell lines, were grown in RPMI 1640 medium supplemented with 10% FCS. B95-8 and W91 are virus-producer cell lines and are EB virus MA gp340 positive whereas Raji contains EB-virus genomes, does not produce virus and is EB-virus MA gp340 negative.

Vaccinia virus strains WR or TK⁻16 [27] were grown and purified essentially as described by Joklik [28].

Antibody Binding to Virus Plaques

Monolayers of monkey kidney CV1 or Human 143 TK⁻ cells were used for plaquing virus. Two days post-infection cell monolayers showing well separated plaques were fixed with cold methanol for 10 min. After washing with phosphate buffered saline (PBS) the monolayers were incubated at room temperature for one hour with 5 mls of 4% Bovine serum albumin (BSA), 0.02% sodium azide on a rocking platform. This was then supplemented with the monoclonal antibody 72A1 [14], which recognizes the EB virus MA gp340/gp270, and incubated on the rocking platform for a further 1 hr. Monolayers were washed 5 times with PBS and incubated for a further 1 hr with a rabbit anti-mouse IgG antiserum in 5 mls of 4% BSA, 0.02% sodium azide. (This step was necessary because 72A1 is an IgG1 class monoclonal antibody and does not bind staphylococcal protein A). Monolayers were again washed 5 times with 10 mls of PBS. Then 5 mls of 4% BSA, 0.02% sodium azide supplemented with 0.5 uCi of ^{125}I staphylococcal protein A (Amersham) was added and incubated for a further 1 hr. Finally after washing 10 times with PBS, the petri dishes were air dried, the rims were removed and the cell monolayers exposed to X-ray film. We have found that 5% Marvel (low-fat dried skimmed milk powder) can substitute for the 4% BSA.

Immunofluorescence Staining

Slides containing air-dried acetone-fixed B95-8, W91 or Raji cells were incubated at 37°C for 1 hr in a humidified atmosphere with serial dilutions of the rabbit sera under test. Slides were washed 3 times in PBS for 30 mins and subsequently incubated with the appropriate dilution of FITC conjugated goat anti-rabbit antibody (Sigma) for 1 hr at 37°C in a humidified atmosphere. After washing 3 times with PBS for 30 mins, fluorescein tagged cells were visualized by excitation at 450-490 nm using an ultraviolet photomicroscope.

RESULTS

Construction of Vaccinia Virus Recombinants That Express EB Virus MA

A BamH1 2.8Kb fragment of EB virus DNA (details of construction to be presented elsewhere) containing the EB virus MA gene, gp340, coding sequence was inserted into the plasmid vector pGS20 [29,30] as illustrated in Figure 1. The resulting plasmid p107 contains the gp340 gene under the control of a vaccinia virus promoter, translocated within the vaccinia virus thymidine kinase (TK) gene.

Cells infected with vaccinia virus were transfected with calcium phosphate precipitated p107. The cells were subsequently harvested and TK$^-$ recombinants isolated by plaque assay on TK$^-$ cells in the presence of BUdR [23]. Selected TK$^-$ viruses were then grown in small monolayers of TK$^-$ cells in the presence of BUdR, and the virus was screened for the presence of the EB virus MA gene DNA by a dot blot hybridization procedure [20]. Virus which was positive for MA coding sequence was plaque purified once more in TK$^-$ cells with BUdR selection, and large stocks were prepared under non-selective conditions in HeLaS3 cells. This recombinant was designated $V_{MA}1$.

Expression of EB Virus MA by a Vaccinia Virus Recombinant

Evidence for the expression of the MA gene and an indication of the purity of the recombinant viruses was obtained by the binding of antibody to virus plaques. The monoclonal antibody 72A1 which binds to EB virus MA gp340/270 was incubated with fixed monolayers containing plaques of $V_{MA}1$ or a TK$^-$ vaccinia virus TK$^-$16 [27] followed by incubation with rabbit anti-mouse antibody and ^{125}I staphylococcal A protein. Binding of 72A1 to virus plaques was visualized by autoradiography where ^{125}I staphylococcal protein A was used (Figure 2). A direct comparison of the stained cell monolayers with the autoradiograph indicated that all recombinant virus plaques had bound 72A1 whereas binding of 72A1 to TK$^-$16 vaccinia virus was not detected. To characterize further the MA gene product produced by the recombinant $V_{MA}1$, cells infected with $V_{MA}1$ or Vaccinia TK$^-$16 were labelled with ^3H glucosamine and the polypeptides analyzed on SDS polyacrylamide gel electrophoresis. A heavily glycosylated high molecular weight protein similar to authentic EB virus MA gp340 was produced by cells infected with $V_{MA}1$ and not by cells infected with TK$^-$16 vaccinia virus (data not shown).

Vaccination of Rabbits

To determine whether the $V_{MA}1$ vaccinia recombinant would elicit an appropriate antibody response in animals, rabbits were inoculated intradermally with 10^8 pfu of $V_{MA}1$ or TK$^-$16 vaccinia virus. Following vaccination the rabbits all developed typical local skin lesions. At 28 days post-vaccination the rabbits were revaccinated intradermally with 10^8 pfu of $V_{MA}1$. On this occasion skin lesions were not observed. Serum taken from the two rabbits vaccinated with $V_{MA}1$ at 4 weeks and 3 months past the initial vaccination had antibody that recognized B95-8 (or W91) cells but not Raji cells as shown by indirect immunofluorescence (Figure 3). Serum from the rabbit vaccinated with TK$^-$16 virus did not bind to B95-8, W91 or Raji cells. (B95-8, W91 or Raji cells are lymphoblastoid cell lines that contain EB virus. Only B95-8 and W91 are positive for EB virus MA).

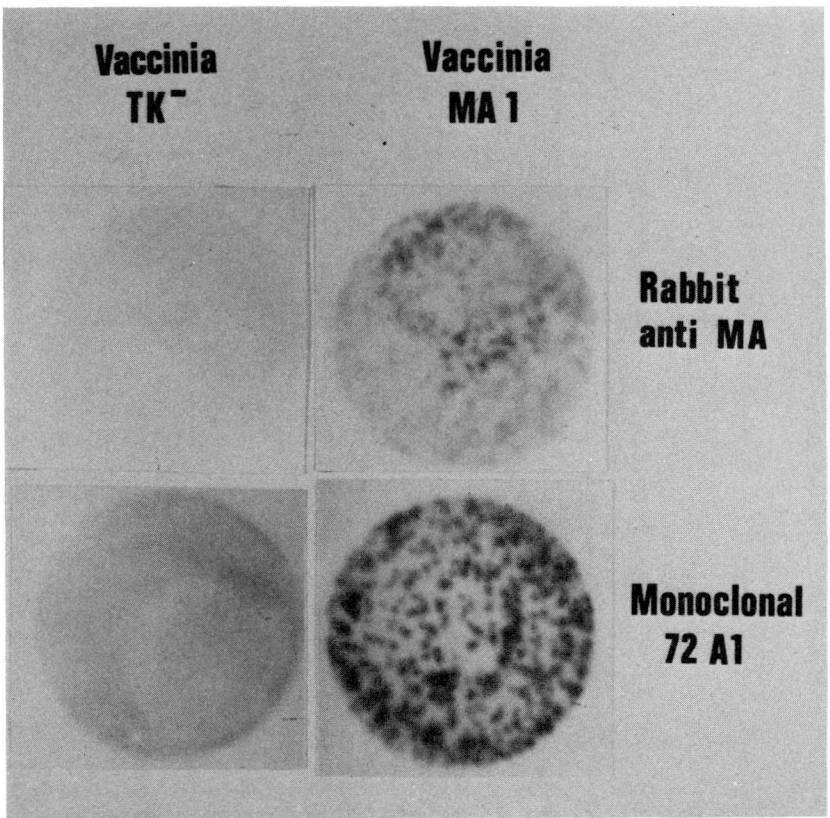

FIG. 2. Detection of the expression of EB virus membrane antigen by individual virus plaques. Duplicate monolayers of CV1 cells containing plaques produced by TK⁻16 vaccinia virus or recombinant virus $V_{MA}1$ are shown. Binding of a polyclonal rabbit anti-MA antiserum or the monoclonal antibody 72A1 (which recognizes EB virus MA) and detection of binding of ^{125}I staphylococcal protein A were carried out as described in the text. After autoradiography, the fixed monolayers were stained with crystal violet. This showed that there were approximately the same number of virus plaques on the cells infected with TK⁻16 virus as on the cells infected with $V_{MA}1$. It also demonstrated that every virus in the cell monolayer infected with $V_{MA}1$ expressed the EB virus membrane antigen.

 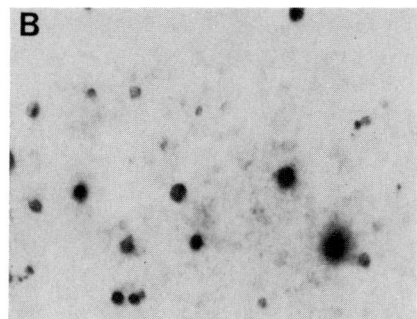

FIG. 3. Indirect immunofluorescence of B95-8 cells using serum from a rabbit vaccinated with $V_{MA}1$. Serum taken from a rabbit 3 months post-vaccination with $V_{MA}1$ was diluted 1:20 with phosphate buffered saline and tested by indirect immunofluorescence on Raji (a) or B95-8 (b) lymphoblastoid cells. It can be seen that rabbit antibodies bound to the EBV membrane antigen (MA) positive cells (B95-8) but not to EBV MA negative cells. Approximately equal numbers of cells are shown in (a) and (b). Similar photographic exposures were used in the two panels.

CONCLUSIONS

We have described a vaccinia virus recombinant which expresses the EB virus MA gp340 gene under the control of a vaccinia virus promoter. The recombinant EB virus gp340 was antigenically similar and corresponded in size to the authentic EB virus MA. Glycoprotein gp340 produced in $V_{MA}1$ infected cells was detectable on the cell surface, the normal subcellular localization of gp340 in lymphoblastoid cell lines containing EB virus. Furthermore, rabbits vaccinated with the recombinant virus produced antibodies that recognized EB virus containing lymphoblastoid cells (presumably by binding to the EB virus MA gp340 on the cell surface).

The cottontop tamarin is the only reliable animal model system which develops a lymphoma when inoculated with EB virus. It remains to be seen whether a vaccinia virus recombinant which expresses gp340 will protect tamarins against EB virus challenge. However, vaccinia virus recombinants expressing foreign genes have protected against other virus infections [29,31-33] and it is anticipated that this recombinant or a similar one expressing higher levels of gp340 will protect the tamarins against EB virus.

Nasopharyngeal carcinoma (NPC) is a serious health problem in southern China and southeast Asia. In males up to 30 new cases of NPC per year per 100,000 population occur in some areas [2]. To control NPC by preventing EB virus infection will require the vaccination of very large numbers of people and in some areas this will have to be done in less than ideal conditions. One of the major factors in the eradication of smallpox was the suitability of vaccinia virus as a vaccine in remote undeveloped areas such as some of those where NPC is prevalent. Presumably vaccinia virus recombinants, e.g. $V_{MA}1$ will, similarly, be suitable for large scale vaccination campaigns. The vaccinia virus recombinant described here could act as a prototype vaccine for the control of EB-virus related malignancies.

ACKNOWLEDGEMENTS

This work has been supported by the Cancer Research Campaign. We would also like to thank Dr. Peter Greenway and Ms. Lynne Francis for vaccinating the rabbits and collecting sera. We are grateful to Dr. G. Miller for the W91 cell line and to Dr. A. Morgan for providing monoclonal antibody 72A1.

REFERENCES

1. G. de Thé, A. Geser, N.E. Day, P.M. Tukei, E.H. Williams, D.P. Beri, P.G. Smith, A.G. Dean, G.W. Bornkamm, P. Feorino and W. Henle, Nature 274, 756-761 (1978).
2. M.J. Simons and K. Shanmugaratnam, eds. The Biology of Nasopharyngeal Carcinoma. UICC Technical report Vol. 71 (1982).
3. M.A. Epstein, J. Natl. Cancer Inst. 56, 697-700 (1976).
4. L.F. Qualtiere and G.R. Pearson, Int. J. Cancer 23, 808 (1979).
5. B.C. Strnad, R.H. Neubauer, H. Rabin and R.A. Mazur, J. Viol. 32, 885 (1979).
6. D.A. Thorley-Lawson and C.M. Edson, J. Virol. 32, 458 (1979).
7. J.R. North, A.J. Morgan and M.A. Epstein, Int. J. Cancer 26, 231-240 (1980).
8. L.F. Qualtiere and G.R. Pearson, Virology 103, 360-369 (1980).
9. M. Biggin, P.J. Farrell and B.G. Barrell, Embo. J. 3, 1083-1090 (1984).
10. M. Hummel, D. Thorley-Lawson and E. Kieff, J. Virol. 49, 413-417 (1984).
11. D. Thorley-Lawson, Nature 281, 486-488 (1979).
12. J.R. North, A.J. Morgan, J.L. Thompson and M.A. Epstein, Proc. Natl. Acad. Sci. USA 79, 7504-7508 (1982).
13. D. Thorley-Lawson and K. Geilinger, Proc. Natl. Acad. Sci. USA 77, 5307-5311 (1980).
14. G.J. Hoffman, S.G. Lazarowitz and S.D. Hayward, Proc. Natl. Acad. Sci. USA 77, 2979-2983 (1980).
15. S.M. Franklin, J.R. North, A.J. Morgan and M.A. Epstein, J. Gen. Virol. 53, 371-376 (1981).
16. T. Maniatis, E.F. Fritsch and J. Sambrook. Molecular Cloning. (Cold Spring Harbor, New York, Cold Spring Harbor Laboratories 1982).
17. A.J. Twigg and K. Sherratt, Nature 283, 216-218 (1980).
18. J. Vieira and J. Messing, Gene 19, 259-268 (1982).
19. H.C. Birnboim and J. Doly, Nuc. Acids Res. 7, 1513-1523 (1979).
20. M. Mackett, G.L. Smith and B. Moss, Proc. Natl. Acad. Sci. USA 79, 7415-7419 (1982).
21. G.L. Smith, M. Mackett and B. Moss, Nature 302, 490-495 (1983a).
22. J.R. Arrand, L. Rymo, J.E. Walsh, E. Bjorck, T. Lindahl and B.E. Griffin, Nuc. Acids Res. 9, 2999-3014 (1981).
23. J.P. Weir, G. Bajszar and B. Moss, Proc. Natl. Acad. Sci. USA 79, 1210-1214 (1982).
24. R.J. Pulvertaft, J. Clin. Pathol. 18, 261-273 (1965).
25. G. Miller and M. Lipman, Proc. Natl. Acad. Sci. USA 70, 190-194 (1973).
26. G. Miller, D. Coope, J. Niederman and J. Pagano, J. Virol. 18, 1071-1080 (1976).
27. J.P. Weir and B. Moss, J. Virol. 46, 530-537 (1983).
28. W.K. Joklik, Virology 18, 9-18 (1962).

29. G.L. Smith, B.R. Murphy and B. Moss, Proc. Natl. Acad. Sci. USA 79, 7415-7419 (1983b).
30. M. Mackett, G.L. Smith and B. Moss, J. Virol. 49, 957-964 (1984).
31. E. Paoletti, B.R. Lipinskas, C. Samsanoff, S. Mercer and D. Panicali, Proc. Natl. Acad. Sci. USA 81, 193-197 (1984).
32. B. Moss, G.L. Smith, J.L. Gerin and R.H. Purcell, Nature 311, 67-69 (1984).
33. M.P. Kieny, R. Lathe, R. Drillien, D. Spehnerd, S. Skory, D. Schmitt, T. Wiktor, H. Koprowski and J.P. Lecocq, Nature 312, 163-166 (1984).

DISCUSSION

Dr. Deinhardt: Is the EBV protein expressed on the virus particle, and did you look to see if there was any change in the ability of the virus to infect different cells?

Dr. Mackett: We haven't looked at those questions yet, but we are planning to.

Dr. Obijeski: Was it the gp220 or the gp350 that was expressed?

Dr. Mackett: As you point out, some cell lines express both gp350 and 220. B95-8 cells, from which the gene was cloned, express only the gp350. The gp350 was expressed in the virus.

VACCINIA VIRUS RECOMBINANTS EXPRESSING VESICULAR STOMATITIS GENES IMMUNIZE MICE AND CATTLE

TILAHUN YILMA,* MICHAEL MACKETT,** JOHN K. ROSE*** AND BERNARD MOSS**

*Department of Veterinary Microbiology and Pathology, Washington State University, Pullman, WA 99164-7040; **Laboratory of Viral Diseases, National Institute of Allergy and Infectious Diseases, Bethesda, Maryland 20205; ***The Salk Institute, San Diego, California 92138-9216.

ABSTRACT

Vesicular stomatitis is a contagious viral disease of cattle, pigs, and horses, occurring mainly in North, Central, and South America. Complementary DNA copies of mRNAs for the G or N proteins of the New Jersey or Indiana serotypes of vesicular stomatitis virus (VSV) were engineered and inserted into the genome of vaccinia virus. Infectious recombinants synthesized polypeptides of the correct size and antigenicity under regulatory control of early and late vaccinia virus promoters. After a single intradermal vaccination, mice produced antibodies to the G protein and were protected against a rabies-like lethal encephalitis upon intravenous challenge with VSV. In cattle, the degree of protection against challenge with intradermal injection of VSV in the tongue was closely correlated with the level of neutralizing antibody produced following two successive vaccinations with live recombinant vaccinia virus.

INTRODUCTION

Vaccinia virus as an infectious eukaryotic cloning vector [1-3] provides a novel alternative to whole virus or subunit vaccines. Heterologous genes, including hepatitis B virus surface antigen [4-6], influenza virus hemagglutinin [7,8], herpesvirus glycoprotein D [6], malaria sporozoite surface antigen [9], rabies glycoprotein [10], and vesicular stomatitis virus (VSV) glycoprotein and nucleoprotein genes [11] have been expressed in this vector system. In several cases, vaccination has protected experimental animals against challenge with the corresponding pathogen. Perhaps because of the historical use of vaccinia virus as a smallpox vaccine, attention has focused on human applications. We envision considerable potential for veterinary use as well, considering the origin of vaccinia virus from cowpox or a related virus and its ability to infect a variety of domesticated animals.

Vesicular stomatitis is a contagious viral disease of cattle, pigs, and horses. The disease is characterized by vesicular lesions on the tongue and other areas of the oral mucosa. In cattle and swine, lesions may develop along the coronary band and in the interdigital space of the foot. Vesicles often appear on the snout in pigs and the teats of the cow.

Outbreaks of vesicular stomatitis have a major economic impact on the livestock industry. The disease causes serious problems for the Animal and Plant Health Inspection Service (APHIS) of the United States Department of Agriculture (USDA) in recognizing and controlling outbreaks of more devastating vesicular diseases, such as foot-and-mouth disease. During the winter of 1982-83, severe outbreaks of vesicular stomatitis in the United States produced substantial economic losses. It is also a public health concern since humans can be infected with the disease, which causes influenza-like symptoms [12]. Since the disease is endemic in Mexico and parts of Central and South America, and the virus may be

Published 1985 by Elsevier Science Publishing Co., Inc.
VACCINIA VIRUSES AS VECTORS FOR VACCINE ANTIGENS, Quinnan, Editor

spread by insect vectors [13,14] there is a danger of continued introduction of the disease to the United States.

Experimental attenuated and inactivated VSV vaccines have been developed, but vaccination for the disease is usually prohibited by the USDA because vaccinated animals cannot be distinguished from naturally infected animals. It is possible to distinguish, by serology, animals vaccinated with the subunit preparation from those that have had the clinical disease or that have been vaccinated with whole virus [11,15]. This ability is an essential consideration for epidemiological studies, disease control, and establishment of quarantine programs. The advantages of both subunit and live vaccines might be combined by constructing vaccinia virus recombinants that express specific VSV proteins. The recombinant has the potential to combine the advantages of antigen amplification of whole virus vaccines and the safety of subunit vaccines. The safety issue is of considerable importance for pathogens that are transmitted by arthropod vectors. There is a danger that attenuated live virus vaccines will revert to virulent forms after passage through the vector.

RESULTS

Construction of Vaccinia Virus Recombinants

The strategy for using vaccinia virus as a vector involves the formation of chimeric genes containing a translocated vaccinia virus promoter region linked to the coding segment of a foreign gene [2,3]. The chimeric gene is then incorporated into the vaccinia virus genome by homologous recombination in cells that have been transfected with a plasmid and infected with vaccinia virus. Although any non-essential region of the vaccinia virus genome can be used as the site of insertion, the thymidine kinase (TK) locus provides some advantages. The TK$^-$ phenotype of such recombinants distinguishes them from wild-type TK$^+$ virus. This phenotype provides a simple method of selection [2] and also serves to attenuate viral pathogenicity [16].

VSV, a member of the rhabdovirus family, contains a single-stranded RNA genome with a minus polarity and encodes 5 known mRNAs and 5 proteins. Complementary DNA copies of mRNAs for the G, M, N, and NS proteins of VSV have been cloned and sequenced [17-20] and the G and N genes of the Indiana serotype (VSV$_I$) have been expressed in eukaryotic cells [21,22]. The entire coding sequence of the G and N genes can be excised from recombinant plasmids with restriction endonuclease XhoI. To facilitate the cloning of XhoI-cut DNA fragments into vaccinia virus, the plasmid vector pGS20 [3] was modified [11] to contain a unique XhoI site downstream of a promoter and RNA start site translocated from a vaccinia virus gene encoding a 7,500 kilodalton (7.5 kd) protein. Into this plasmid, designated pMM34, we placed the G or N genes from VSV$_I$ so that the vaccinia virus transcriptional and VSV translational start sites were juxtaposed, and the resulting chimeric gene was flanked by segments of the vaccinia virus TK gene. The G protein gene from the New Jersey strain of VSV (VSV$_{NJ}$) was modified [11] so that it also could be inserted into the XhoI site of pMM34, as well as into the unique SalI site of the plasmid vector pLTP1, which contains the promoter region of a vaccinia virus gene encoding a protein of 28 kd [23]. As will be discussed later, the promoter regions of the 7.5-kd and 28-kd protein genes operate under different regulatory control mechanisms.

Recombinant vaccinia viruses containing the chimeric genes were prepared as described above. After selection in TK$^-$ 143 cells in the presence of 5-bromodeoxyuridine (BudR), individual virus plaques were picked and used to infect 2-cm^2 monolayers under selection conditions [2]. The presence of recombinant virus was confirmed by hybridization of a ^{32}P-labeled VSV DNA probe [2] and by binding of VSV antibodies and ^{125}I-staphylococcal A protein to lysate material immobilized on nitrocellulose [8,11]. For the VSV$_{NJ}$ G protein gene recombinants, both procedures were used. In one case, 18 out of 24 TK$^-$ plaques were positive by both assay procedures; in another case, 10 out of 24 were positive. Recombinant viruses were purified by at least 2 plaque assays in the presence of BudR, and virus stocks were prepared without selection in HeLa S-3 cells. Correct insertion of the chimeric genes was verified by digestion of genomic DNA extracted from purified virus with at least 2 appropriate restriction endonucleases, followed by agarose gel electrophoresis, transfer to nitrocellulose, and hybridization to ^{32}P-labeled VSV and vaccinia virus DNA probes. Figure 1 shows the chimeric gene structures, flanking DNA, and the code numbers of the recombinant viruses.

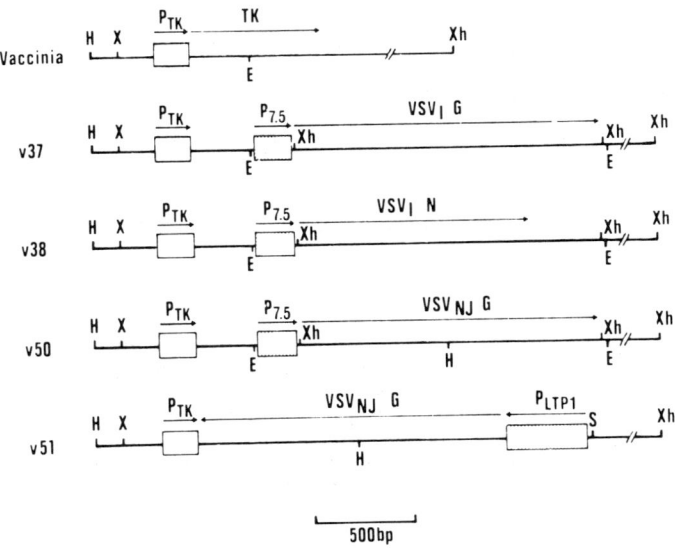

FIG. 1. Representation of chimeric VSV genes in vaccinia virus recombinants. A 2,000 base pair segment from the left side of the HindIII J fragment of vaccinia virus [28,29] is shown on the top line. Lines below that contain chimeric VSV genes inserted into the body of the TK gene. Recombinants v37, v38, v50 were constructed by insertion of the indicated VSV gene into the unique XhoI site of pMM34, and v51 was constructed by inserting the VSV gene into the unique SalI site of pLTPl. The promoter regions of vaccinia virus genes encoding polypeptides of 7.5 kd and 28 kd are indicated as P7.5 and P28. Abbreviations for restriction endonuclease sites are H, HindIII; B, BamHI; E, EcoRI; S, SmaI; X, XbaI; Xh, XhoI.

Recombinants v37, v38, and v50 contain genes for VSV_I G, VSV_I N, and VSV_{NJ} G proteins, respectively, under control of the vaccinia virus promoter for the 7.5-kd protein gene. Recombinant v51 contains the gene for the VSV_{NJ} G protein under control of the vaccinia virus promoter for the 28-kd protein gene.

Expression of VSV Genes

Evidence for expression of the VSV genes and for the purity and stability of the recombinant viruses was obtained by binding antibody directly to virus plaques. Antiserum to VSV_I or VSV_{NJ} was incubated with fixed monolayers containing plaques of recombinants or wild-type virus, and binding of IgG was detected with ^{125}I-staphylococcal A protein followed by autoradiography (Figure 2). Direct comparisons of stained cell monolayers and x-ray film indicated that all v50 and v51 plaques bound antibody raised against VSV_{NJ}. In contrast, VSV antibody did not bind to plaques of wild-type vaccinia virus. As expected, all plaques bound antibody to vaccinia virus. Similar results were obtained when v37 and v38 plaques were incubated with the appropriate VSV_I or VSV_{NJ} antibody (not shown).

Characterization of VSV Polypeptides

Cells infected with recombinants v37, v38, v50, and v51 were pulse-labeled with ^{35}S-methionine, and the polypeptides immunoprecipitated by anti-VSV sera were dissociated with sodium dodecyl sulfate and resolved by polyacrylamide gel electrophoresis. Fluorographs revealed that v50 and v51 synthesized similar amounts of a specifically immunoprecipitable polypeptide of approximately 65 kd that co-migrated with G protein produced in cells infected with VSV_{NJ} (Figure 3). Similarly, v37 and v38 expressed immunoprecipitable polypeptides of approximately 67 kd and 45 kd that co-migrated with authentic VSV_I G and N proteins, respectively (Figure 3). The correct sizes of the G proteins produced by the recombinants suggest that the extent of glycosylation is similar to that occurring in cells infected with VSV.

Localization of the G Protein

In cells infected with VSV, the G protein is transported through the Golgi apparatus to the cell surface. Double-label immunofluorescence of cells infected with recombinant vaccinia viruses v50 and v51 showed clear cell surface labeling of the VSV_{NJ} G protein, Internal labeling of the same cells showed strong fluorescence of the G region, which is typical of normal G protein [21]. Virtually all cells were infected with v50 or v51 and showed similar levels of staining. In contrast, there was no surface staining of cells infected with wild-type vaccinia virus, although there was faint non-specific staining within permeabilized cells (not shown).

Regulation of Chimeric Gene Expression

A rapid antibody-binding procedure was used to investigate the regulation of synthesis of the VSV_{NJ} G protein made in cells infected with v50 and v51. Cells were harvested at 2, 6, or 12 hr after infection with recombinant or wild-type vaccinia virus. Serial 2-fold dilutions of the extracts were spotted onto a nitrocellulose filter, which was then incubated successively with VSV_{NJ} antisera and ^{125}I-labeled staphylococcal A protein [11].

191

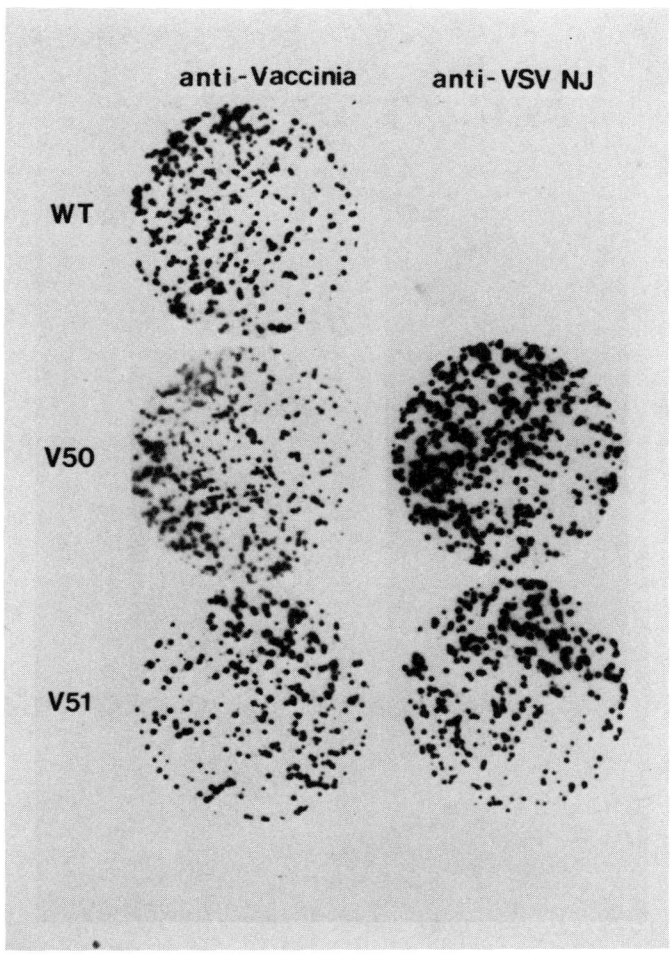

FIG. 2. Expression of VSV_{NJ} G protein by individual virus plaques. Duplicate monolayers of CV-1 cells containing plaques produced by wild-type vaccinia virus (WT) or recombinant viruses v50 or v51 were fixed to petri dishes [8,11]. Binding of antiserum to vaccinia virus or VSV_{NJ} was followed by incubation with ^{125}I-staphylococcal A protein [8,11]. Autoradiographs are shown.

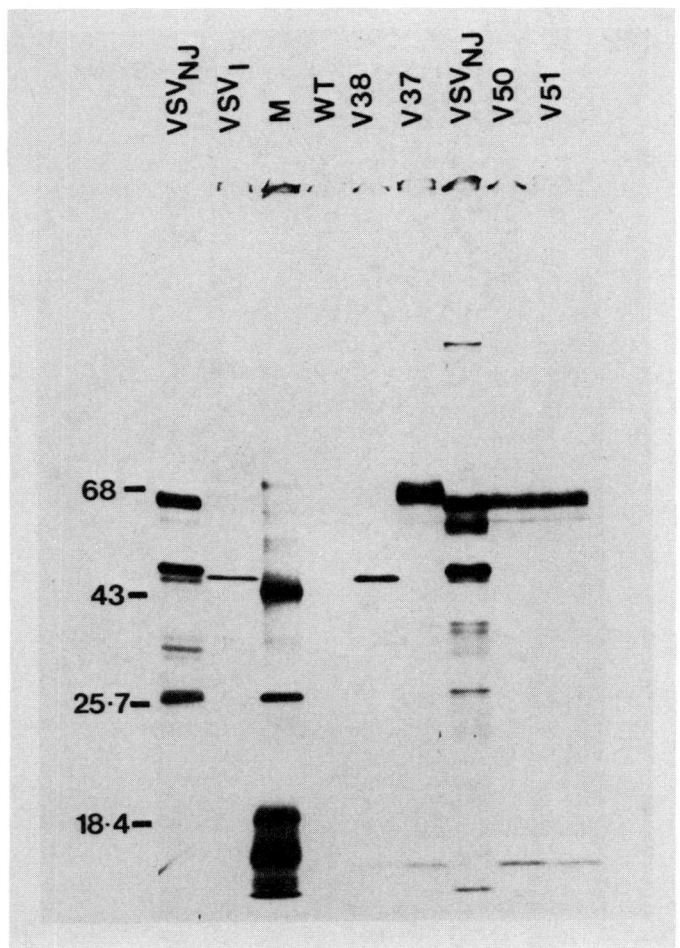

FIG. 3. Characterization of VSV polypeptides made by vaccinia virus recombinants. Monolayers (25cm^2) of CV-1 cells were infected with 30 PFU/cell of wild-type or recombinant vaccinia virus in medium containing 0.01 mM methionine. After 2 hr at 37°C, 100 uCi of ^{35}S-methionine (1000 Ci/mmol) was added and the incubation was continued for an additional 10 hr. The preparation of cytoplasmic extracts, immunoprecipitation, and polyacrylamide gel electrophoresis was similar to that previously described [4]. Antiserum to VSV$_{NJ}$ was used to precipitate polypeptides from cells infected with v50 and v51 whereas antiserum to VSV$_I$ was used for polypeptides from cells infected with v37 and v38. Molecular weights of standards are indicated in daltons X 10^{-3}.

Examination of autoradiographs indicated that in cells infected with v50, G protein was made within 2 hr and was abundant by 6 hr (Figure 4). In contrast, G protein synthesis was first detected at 6 hr after infection with v51. These results are consistent with previous

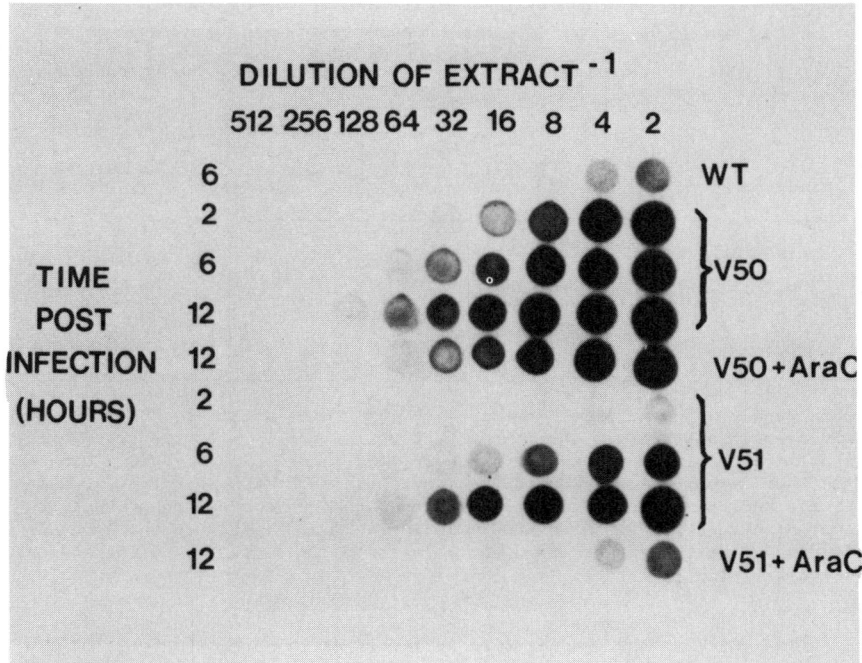

FIG. 4. Regulation of expression of chimeric genes. Monolayers of CV-1 cells were infected with 30 PFU/cell of wild-type (WT) vaccinia virus or recombinants v50 or v51 in the presence or absence of 40 ug/ml of cytosine arabinoside (AraC). Two-fold serial dilutions were made of cytoplasmic extracts and 20 ul volumes were spotted on nitrocellulose and the dot blot was incubated successively with antiserum to VSV_{NJ} and ^{125}I-staphylococcal A protein [11]. An autoradiograph is shown.

data indicating that the promoter of the 7.5-kd protein gene (used for v50) is active at both early and late times after infection [3] whereas the promoter for the 28-kd protein gene (used for v51) is active only at late times [23]. The effect of cytosine arabinoside, an inhibitor of DNA replication, on expression of G protein in cells infected with v51 provides further evidence that the fidelity of regulation of these chimeric genes is maintained.

Immunization of Mice

To protect against VSV infection, the appropriate VSV gene must be expressed during replication of the recombinant vaccinia virus in the inoculated animal. Of the 5 known proteins of VSV, only the antibody to the G protein has been shown to be protective in mice and cattle [15,24]. After mice were injected intradermally in the caudal fold of the tail with 10^5 PFU (plaque-forming units) of purified infectious v50, significant VSV neutralization titers were detectable by day 14 and increased over a 42-day period (Table I). Half of the mice were given a booster vaccination on day 28, which resulted in a 7- to 8-fold increase in serum VSV neutralization titers.

TABLE I. Serum neutralization titers of vaccinated mice and response to challenge with VSV_{NJ}

Group	Day 6	Day 14	Day 28	Day 42	No. Mice Challenged	Died
vHBs4	0	0	0	0	11	7
v50	10	20	420	760	15	1
v50(2X)				5220	16	0

Mice were vaccinated intradermally with 10^5 PFU of purified vHBs4 or v50 at a single site in the caudal fold of the tail. All mice received a primary vaccination on day 0 and half (designated 2X) received a booster vaccination on day 28. Neutralization titers of pooled sera are expressed as the reciprocal of the dilution of serum that gave complete protection against cytopathic effect of 100 $TCID_{50}$ of VSV_{NJ}. Mice were challenged 44 days after the primary vaccination with 10^8 PFU of VSV_{NJ} by intravenous administration in the tail vein.

The VSV challenge was carried out by injecting approximately 10^8 PFU of VSV_{NJ}, isolated from the vesicular fluid of an infected cow, into the tail vein of each mouse. This produces an acute encephalitis that causes death in 6 to 12 days. For control purposes, one group of mice had been vaccinated 44 days earlier with vHBs4 [4], a vaccinia virus recombinant that contains the hepatitis B virus surface antigen gene in place of the VSV G protein gene. When this control group was challenged, 7 out of 11 animals died of encephalitis. By contrast, only 1 out of 15 mice that received a primary vaccination with v50 died. None of the 16 mice that received 2 vaccinations died (Table I).

Immunization of Cattle

Cattle vaccinated intradermally with either v50 or vHBs4 developed typical pox lesions in 4 days (Figure 5). The lesions were confined to the sites of inoculation and were characterized by papules that gradually changed to pustules with a small umbilication. Two weeks post-vaccination, the lesions dried up and were covered by dry scabs, which eventually fell off and left unscarred surfaces. In cattle vaccinated with v50, VSV neutralization titers were significant on day 7 and reached values of 80 to 480 by day 28 (Table II). At that time, a second vaccination was given after which the titers increased several fold. On day 44, the cattle were challenged by injection of 10^2 and 10^3 PFU of VSV_{NJ} into the 2 upper and 2 lower quadrants of the tongue, respectively. Preliminary experiments indicated that unvaccinated cattle challenged in this manner developed vesicular lesions within 2 days (Figure 6).

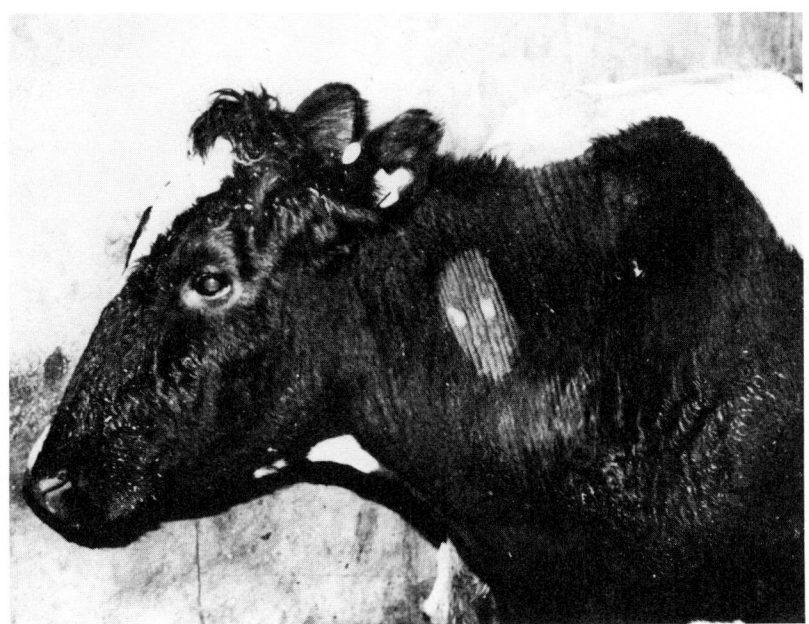

FIG. 5. A cow vaccinated with v50 at 2 sites on a shaven area of the neck. The lesions were localized to the vaccination sites.

Both cows (23Y and 26Y) vaccinated with the recombinant expressing the hepatitis B virus surface antigen and 2 cows vaccinated with v50 developed typical vesicular lesions at the 10^2 PFU and 10^3 PFU VSV injection sites (Table II). The remaining 4 cows (24Y, 27Y, 28Y, and 29Y) that were vaccinated with v50 had no lesions at the 10^2 PFU VSV injection sites, although they all developed lesions at the 10^3 PFU sites. In one case (cow 28Y), the VSV lesion at the 10^3 PFU site remained localized, whereas in all others it generalized to the remaining surface of the tongue.

A striking correlation was observed between antibody titers and protection to challenge with 10^2 PFU of VSV. All animals with neutralizing antibody titers of 1280 or greater were protected, whereas those with titers of 640 or lower were sensitive.

DISCUSSION

Rhabdoviruses are responsible for vesicular stomatitis and rabies, diseases with important veterinary and medical implications. In this communication, we described the construction of vaccinia virus recombinants that express genes from 2 VSV serotypes, Indiana and New Jersey. Although the diseases caused by the 2 VSV serotypes are similar, they are immunologically distinct and are found in separate enzootic areas within the Western Hemisphere. Since the New Jersey strain has been responsible for the recent VSV outbreaks in the western United States, the animal

TABLE II. Serum neutralization titers of vaccinated cattle and response to challenge with VSV_{NJ}

Cow No.	Vaccine	Pre-challenge titers							Vesicular lesions	
		Day 0	Day 7	Day 14	Day 21	Day 28	Day 35	Day 44	10^2PFU	10^3PFU
12Y	none	-	-	-	-	-	-	-	+	+
18Y	none	-	-	-	-	-	-	-	+	+
23Y	vHBs4	0	0	0	0	0	0	0	+	+
26Y	vHBs4	0	0	0	0	5	5	30	+	+
17Y	v50	0	10	120	120	160	320	640	+	+
24Y	v50	0	160	480	480	320	960	2560	-	+
25Y	v50	0	30	160	240	80	320	480	+	+
27Y	v50	0	80	80	80	80	960	1920	-	+
28Y	v50	0	80	160	240	320	640	1280	-	+
29Y	v50	0	160	160	160	160	1280	2560	-	+

Cows were vaccinated intradermally with 4 X 10^8 PFU of purified vHBs or v50 at 4 sites on day 0 and day 28. They were then challenged 44 days after the primary vaccination by intradermal inoculation of 10^2 and 10^3 PFU of VSV_{NJ} on the 2 upper and 2 lower quadrants of the tongue, respectively. Serum neutralization titers are expressed as the reciprocal of the dilution of serum that gave complete protection against cytopathic effect of 100 $TCID_{50}$ of VSV_{NJ}.

studies described here were carried out with VSV_{NJ}. We have demonstrated that the polypeptide products expressed by the recombinant viruses are similar or identical in size and antigenicity to the authentic VSV proteins. In addition, the G glycoprotein was transported to the cell surface, which may be important for the immunogenicity of the vaccine. In mice, 1 or 2 intradermal injections of a recombinant vaccinia virus that expresses the G glycoprotein protected against a lethal VSV challenge. Without vaccination, the animals succumb in 6 to 12 days to a rabies-like encephalitis.

The ecology and method of transmission of VSV_{NJ} to domesticated animals is not well understood and may involve insect vectors [13,14]. For this reason, the design of animal models is difficult, and it is likely that the challenge used in our study is more severe than that occurring naturally. Ordinarily, the incubation period is from 2 to 4 days, whereas vesicles appear within 2 days of direct injection of VSV into the tongue. Nevertheless, 2 successive vaccinations provided protection for two-thirds of the animals inoculated with 100 PFU of VSV. Protection was closely correlated with neutralizing antibody titers,

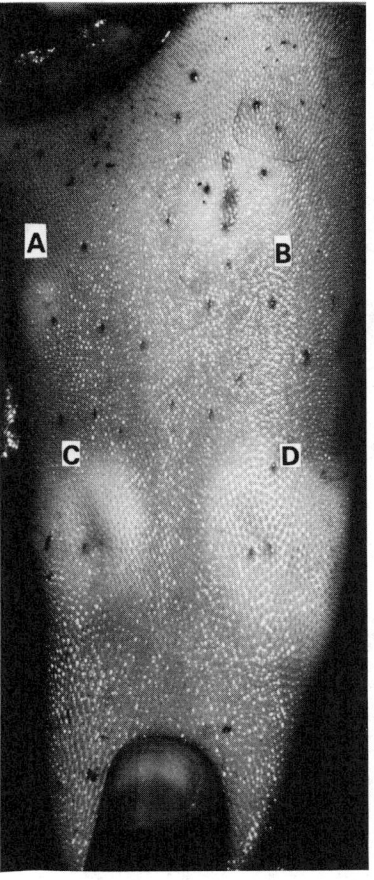

FIG. 6. Four vesicular lesions on the tongue of an unvaccinated cow 48 hr after challenge by intradermal injection of VSV_{NJ} (A and B, 10^2 PFU; C, 10^3 PFU; D, 10^4 PFU). The lesions generalized after an additional 24 hr.

although other factors, including cell-mediated immunity, may be involved in protection. Since the engineering of vaccinia virus vectors for improved expression capability is just beginning, we can reasonably expect that recombinants synthesizing considerably more G glycoprotein will be available in the future.

Since the duration of immunity is not yet known, the ability to boost antibody levels by secondary vaccination is important. In this study, we demonstrated that antibodies to VSV G glycoprotein were boosted only 28 days after primary vaccination of mice and cattle. In other experiments, boosting of antibodies to influenza virus hemagglutinin and hepatitis B virus surface antigen occurred after secondary vaccination of rabbits [25]. Evidently, sufficient replication of recombinant vaccinia virus must occur in order to permit antigen production even in the presence of neutralizing antibodies to vaccinia virus.

Previous experience with smallpox vaccine suggests that there would be numerous advantages to the development of vaccinia virus or other poxvirus recombinants as veterinary vaccines. Vaccinia virus can be economically produced in the skin of cattle or in tissue culture and stored in a heat-resistant lyophilized form. Since the vaccine can be administered to humans with a bifurcated needle or on a mass scale with a jet gun, equally efficient methods should be possible with domesticated animals. The ability of recombinant vaccinia virus to stimulate a cytotoxic T-cell response specific for a foreign surface glycoprotein [26] may be a significant advantage over subunit or inactivated whole vaccines, which, in general, do not prime effectively for cell-mediated immunity. The large capacity of vaccinia virus for the insertion of foreign DNA [27] also raises the possibility of multivalent vaccines for different serotypes of the same virus, or vaccines against entirely different pathogenic agents.

Despite these possible advantages, the introduction of live recombinant poxviruses into the environment requires considerable thought and further experimentation. We believe that as our understanding of vaccinia virus and other poxviruses increases, it will be possible to attenuate them further so that their virulence and ability to spread are minimized. In that regard, the TK$^-$ recombinants described here already exhibit decreased levels of pathogenicity in mice [16].

ACKNOWLEDGMENTS

We thank Robert Lazzarini for recombinant plasmids, Roger Breeze for help and encouragement to T.Y., and Steven Leib and Carol Gallione for technical assistance. This work was supported in part by grants from the United States Department of Agriculture (83-CRSR-2-2189) and (84-CRSR-2-2514) and the Washington State Technology Center. We thank the American Association for the Advancement of Science for permission to use the materials, figures, and tables from our publication Mackett et al., Science Vol. 227, pp. 433-435 (1985).

REFERENCES

1. D. Panicali, E. Paoletti, Proc. Natl. Acad. Sci. USA 79, 4927 (1982).
2. M. Mackett, G.L. Smith, B. Moss, Proc. Natl. Acad. Sci. USA 79, 7415 (1982).
3. M. Mackett, G.L. Smith, B. Moss, J. Virol. 49, 857 (1984).
4. G.L. Smith, M. Mackett, B. Moss, Nature (London) 302, 490 (1983).
5. G.L. Smith, M. Mackett, B. Moss, UCLA Symposia on Molecular and Cellular Biol., New Series 8, 543 (1983).
6. E. Paoletti, B.R. Lipinskas, C. Samsonoff, S. Mercer, D. Panicali, Proc. Natl. Acad. Sci. USA 81, 193 (1984).
7. D. Panicali, S.W. Davis, R.L. Weinberg, E. Paoletti, Proc. Natl. Acad. Sci. USA 80, 5364 (1983).
8. G.L. Smith, B.R. Murphy, B. Moss, Proc. Natl. Acad. Sci. USA 80, 7155 (1983).
9. G.L. Smith, G.N. Godson, V. Nussenzweig, R.S. Nussenzweig, B. Moss, Science 224, 397 (1984).
10. M.P. Kieny, R. Lathe, R. Drillien, D. Spehner, S. Skory, D. Schmitt, T. Wiktor, H. Koprowski, J.P. Lecocq, Nature 312, 163 (1984).
11. M. Mackett, T. Yilma, J.K. Rose, B. Moss, Science 227, 433 (1985).
12. W.C. Patterson, L.O. Mott, E.W. Jenney, J. Am. Vet. Med. Assoc. 133, 57 (1958).
13. D. Ferris, R.P. Hanson, R.J. Dicke, R.H. Roberts, J. Infect. Dis. 96, 184 (1955).

14. R.B. Tesh, B.N. Chaniotis, K.M. Johnson, Science 175, 1477 (1972).
15. T. Yilma, R.G. Breeze, S. Ristow, J.R. Gorham and S.R. Leib, Adv. Exp. Biol. Med. (in press).
16. Manuscript in preparation.
17. J.K. Rose, C.J. Gallione, J. Virol. 39, 519 (1981).
18. C.J. Gallione, J.R. Greene, L.E. Iverson, J.K. Rose, J. Virol. 39, 529 (1981).
19. C.J. Gallione, J.K. Rose, J. Virol. 46, 162 (1983).
20. A.K. Banerjee, D.P. Rhodes, D.S. Gill, Virology 137, 432 (1984).
21. J.K. Rose, J.E. Bergmann, Cell 30, 753 (1982).
22. J. Sprague, J.H. Condra, H. Arnheiter, R.A. Lazzarini, J. Virol. 45, 773 (1983).
23. J.P. Weir, B. Moss, J. Virol. 51, 662 (1984).
24. B. Dietzschold, L.G. Schneider, J.H. Cox, J. Virol. 14, 1 (1974).
25. G.L. Smith, unpublished observations.
26. J.R. Bennink, J.W. Yewdell, G.L. Smith, C. Moller, B. Moss, Nature 311, 578 (1984).
27. G.L. Smith, B. Moss, Gene 25, 21 (1983).
28. G. Bajszar, R. Wittek, J.P. Weir, B. Moss, J. Virol. 45, 62 (1983).
29. J.P. Weir, B. Moss, J. Virol. 46, 530 (1983).

DISCUSSION

Dr. McIntosh: What strain of vaccinia was used to form these recombinants?

Dr. Smith: The chimpanzee experiments were done with a laboratory strain of vaccinia, the WR strain. We have also engineered the same construct into the New York City Board of Health strain. We haven't yet done primate studies with that strain of virus. Mice and rabbits developed similar levels of antibody against the surface antigen with both strains.

Dr. Quinnan: What level of protection in the challenge studies would be sufficient to justify going ahead with field trials, and what type of field trials do you anticipate would be needed, in order that the vaccine could be used in animals?

Dr. Yilma: This particular disease is very important in South America and Mexico. It is endemic in areas of South America. Presently, we are exploring those areas to do the field trials.

Dr. Brown: When you challenged the cattle, did you get any secondary lesions?

Dr. Yilma: No. With foot and mouth disease, you do get secondary lesions. I have made several attempts to reproduce that, but have not obtained secondary lesions on experimental infection. I thought maybe there was a difference between tissue culture-propagated virus and virus isolated from the vesicles. So we passed the virus several times through tongue to attempt to increase its virulence. Even after that, it was never possible to reproduce secondary lesions.

Dr. Brown: International regulations require that foot and mouth vaccines protect against infection with 100,000 ID_{50} administered on the tongue. You do get primary lesions in vaccinated animals on occasion, but protection is great. So 10^2 or 10^3 ID_{50} is a very small challenge dose compared to that used for foot and mouth disease.

Dr. Yilma: That is correct. However, there is some evidence that with very high doses, you may actually observe an interference effect with VSV from interfering particles.

Dr. Boyle: On the revaccination with the vaccinia recombinants, do you get secondary vaccinia lesions or no lesions?

Dr. Yilma: We don't get lesions at all on revaccination.

Dr. Dowdle: Is it possible to do a contact challenge with VSV, as can be done with foot and mouth disease, instead of the tongue challenge?

Dr. Yilma: You cannot do contact challenge with VSV.

Dr. Deinhardt: How does it spread?

Dr. Yilma: The mechanism of natural spread is unknown.

Dr. Deinhardt: Will the vaccinia virus spread among a herd, when you have vaccinated only some of the animals?

Dr. Yilma: We haven't done that study. We have vaccinated about 20 animals and have seen no secondary lesions on them. Probably, it would not spread to other animals either, but that study has not been done.

INFECTIOUS VACCINIA VIRUS RECOMBINANT THAT EXPRESSES THE SURFACE ANTIGEN
OF PORCINE TRANSMISSIBLE GASTROENTERITIS VIRUS (TGEV)

SYVLIA HU,* JOAN BRUSZEWSKI* AND RALPH SMALLING*

*Amgen, 1900 Oak Terrace Lane, Thousand Oaks, California 91320

ABSTRACT

A DNA copy of the surface antigen gene, derived from porcine transmissible gastroenteritis virus (TGEV), has been inserted into the vaccinia virus genome under the control of a vaccinia promoter. Tissue culture cells infected with the recombinant virus synthesize TGEV surface antigen. Mice vaccinated with the TGE-vaccinia recombinant virus produce neutralizing antibodies to TGEV. The potential use of the recombinant virus as live vaccine against TGE is discussed.

INTRODUCTION

TGE is one of the most devastating diseases that can affect newborn pigs. The disease is characterized by vomiting, severe diarrhea and results in high mortality rate in piglets. Although swine of older ages are also susceptible to TGE, the death rate in swine over five weeks of age is usually much lower. In the densely swine-populated areas of the midwestern United States, TGE is recognized as one of the major causes of sickness and death in piglets [1].

TGE is caused by a virus that belongs to the group called coronaviruses. It primarily infects the epithelial cells of the small intestine of swine, resulting in villous atrophy [2]. The small intestine eventually becomes covered with immature enterocytes that cannot function in digestion and absorption.

Shortly after TGE was first recognized in 1946 [3], it became evident that if sows had been infected with TGE virus at least three weeks before farrowing, their suckling pigs were usually well protected against the disease.

Since the character of pigs' placenta does not allow transplacental passage of immunoglobulins, pigs are agammaglobulinemic at birth [4]. Much of the resistance to infection is dependent upon the pigs ingesting colostrum and immediately transferring the colostral antibodies to their own circulation. These transferred colostral antibodies quickly establish a humoral antibody level. Thereafter, the continued ingestion of milk by the pigs, in which secretory IgA is the predominant immunoglobulin class, offers additional protection in the alimentary canal. The milk antibodies are crucial for the survival of neonatal pigs because pigs may not synthesize their own protective levels of antibodies for two or three weeks.

At present, there are five federally licensed TGE vaccines. All contain live, attenuated TGE virus propagated in cell culture and are approved for use in pregnant swine. Available information indicates that they are safe but of limited effectiveness when used to vaccinate previously uninfected pregnant swine.

Intramuscular injection of the sows with the live vaccine in general does not provide satisfactory protection for nursing piglets. The reason could be that this route of inoculation does not result in actual gut infection. Even though the sows do develop circulating serum

IgG antibodies, the amounts of protective antibodies in the milk are usually low and are of the IgG type rather than the IgA type [5]. The IgA type of antibodies provide better protection to the gut cells because they are more resistant to enzymatic breakdown in the gut and are more adherent to mucosal cells.

The oral administration route with the TGE vaccine usually gives better results than the intramuscular injection, but it appears that the attenuated TGE virus fails to adequately infect the gut of pregnant sows and thus fails to initiate the gut-mammary immunologic link which is essential for providing optimal immunity. With this background information in mind, we considered that an effective TGE vaccine when given to pregnant swine must adequately infect or sensitize the gut and stimulate the gut-mammary immunologic system so that protective IgA class antibodies can be made and passed on to the piglets. It is hard to envision that a subunit type of immunogen could fulfill this requirement. Our strategy is then to insert the appropriate surface antigen of TGEV into vaccinia vector and use the recombinant virus as TGE vaccine.

RESULTS AND DISCUSSION

A schematic structure for TGE virion is depicted in Figure 1. The

Schematic of TGEV

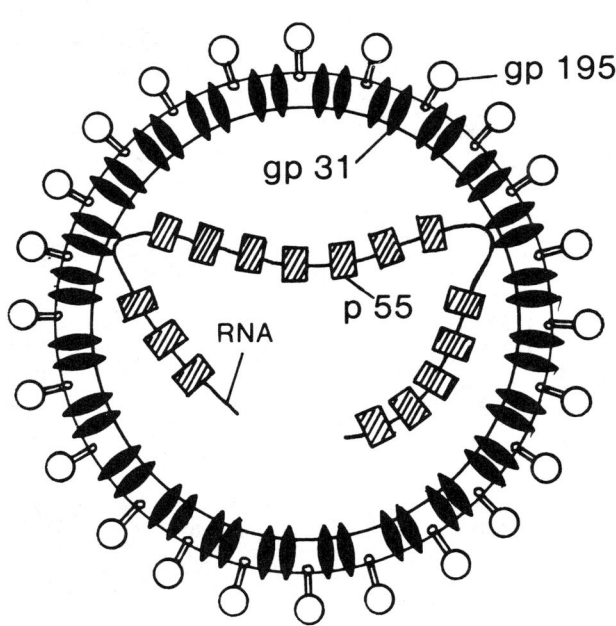

FIG. 1. Schematic model of the location of the three major structural proteins of TGEV: gp195, gp31 and p50, in relation to the viral envelope and genomic RNA.

antigen gp195 that composes the club-like structure on the surface is
of particular interest because it has been shown to induce viral neutralizing response in pigs immunized with this material [6]. This observation
implies the possible use of gp195 as an effective subunit type vaccine.

TGEV is a member of the coronavirus family. It has an 18.5 kilobases
(kb) continuous RNA genome which is of positive (messenger) polarity.
We have previously [7] identified the location of gp195 to be at the 5'
end of a 9.4 kb message as shown in Figure 2. The complete gene for gp195
has subsequently been cloned and expressed in E. coli [8].

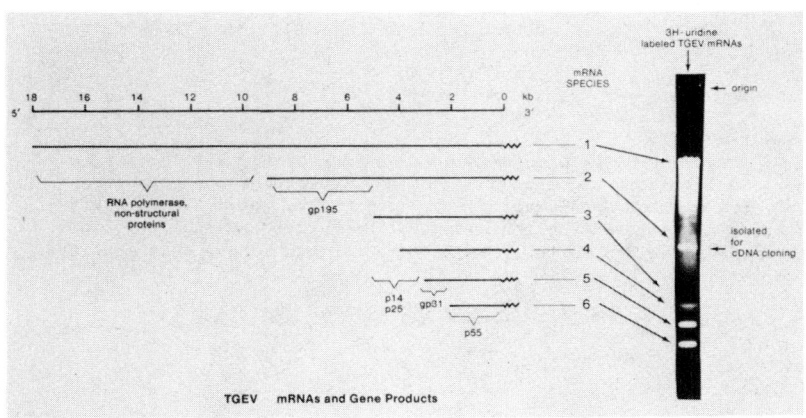

FIG. 2. Transcriptional scheme of TGEV and the six discrete-size TGEV
mRNA's identified by gel electrophoresis. The gene coding for gp195 is
located at the 5' end of the 9.4 kb mRNA.

Figure 3 shows a restriction endonuclease cleavage map of the 9.4 kb
message constructed after a complete cDNA clone. The start and stop
for gp195 gene have been mapped by DNA sequencing, and in between there
is a 3.9 kb long, continuous, translational open reading frame coding
for a protein of 145 kilodaltons, which constitutes the core polypeptide
for gp195.

We have inserted the complete gp195 gene flanked by the second 5'
HpaI and the unique XbaI sites through the BamHI cloning site into one
of Moss's vaccinia expression vector, pGS20 [9]. By following the
selection procedure described by Mackett et al. [10], we obtained
recombinant virus now containing and expressing the gp195 gene of TGEV.
Figure 4 shows a comparison of the gp195 gene product synthesized by
either TGEV or by the TGE-vaccinia recombinant virus, defined by immunoprecipitation using a TGEV specific antiserum. There seems to be a
difference in the extent of glycosylation in these two systems, which
renders the two products to have slightly different electropohoretic
mobilities.

Furthermore, by immunoperoxidase staining, we could detect gp195
on the surface of TGEV infected cells but not on the surface of TGE-
vaccinia recombinant virus infected cells (data not shown). The levels
of expression of gp195 is not great, but can be identified in a pulse-
labeled total cell lysate also shown in Figure 4 (lane 2C).

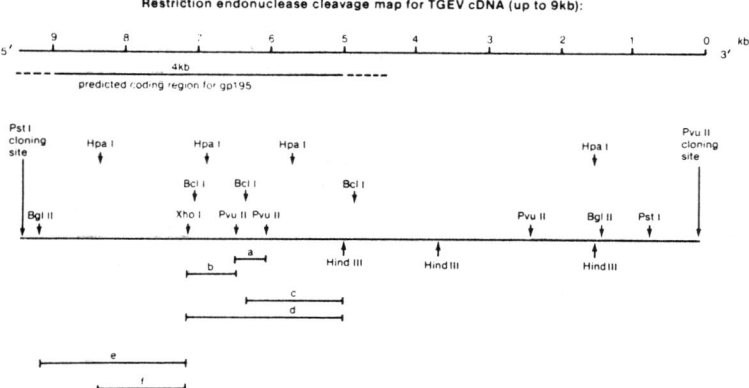

FIG. 3. Restriction endonuclease cleavage map of the 9.4 kb TGEV cDNA clone. Nucleic acid sequence analysis has revealed one continuous, unique, translation open-reading frame coding for gp195, which starts at 8 bases downstream from the second 5' HpaI site and ends at 80 bases upstream from the XbaI site. Fragments a through f have been subcloned for expression in E. coli.

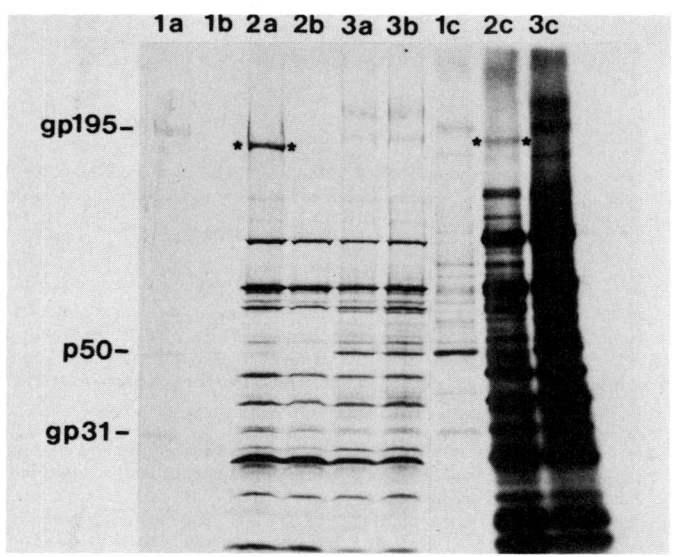

FIG. 4. SDS-polyacrylamide gel analysis of immune-precipitated proteins from (1) ST cells infected with TGEV, (2) CV-1 cells infected with TGE-vaccinia recombinant virus, and (3) CV-1 cells infected with wild type vaccinia virus. "A" lanes were precipitated with TGEV specific antiserum, "b" lanes were precipitated with normal control serum, and "c" lanes were total cytosol extract from corresponding infected cells.

The TCG-vaccinia recombinant virus was purified and used to immunize mice by tail-scarification. Figure 5 shows the results of ELISA tests. Sera from mice inoculated once with the recombinant virus contain antibody binding activities to TGE virion as well as binding activity to vaccinia virion at a level comparable to the control mice that have been inoculated with wild-type vaccine virus.

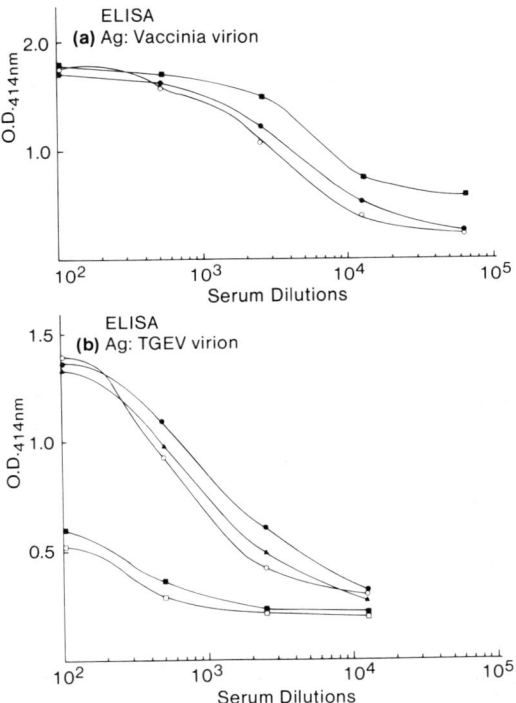

FIG. 5. Antibody titer of mice inoculated with TGE-vaccinia recombinant virus (●, ○, ▲) or a wild type vaccinia virus (■ , □) at six weeks using a standard ELISA test. Only the mice inoculated with the recombinant virus elicit binding activity to TGEV in their sera, whereas the binding titers to vaccinia virus are comparable among all the mice.

More interestingly, sera from all the mice inoculated with the recombinant virus contain viral neutralizing antibodies, not only against vaccinia, but also against TGEV (Table I). The titer against TGEV is only moderate. However, antibody titers of pigs recovered from TGEV infection could also vary from 1:25 to 1:625.

The efficacy of using this TGE-vaccinia recombinant virus as vaccine against TGE is now being tested in isolated gilts. As it has been mentioned before, the presence of IgA type antibody in the colostrum and milk from vaccinated sows will be most indicative of the levels of success for protecting the piglets against TGE.

TABLE I.

Mice No. (Jackson Balb/C)	Neutralizing titer[b]	No. weeks post-inoculation[a]					
		2	4	6	2	4	6
		@ vaccinia			@ TGEV		
1898	vaccinia	40	100	400	<20	<20	<20
1899	vaccinia	60	100	400	<20	<20	<40
1989	vaccinia	70	150	380	<20	<20	<20
1990	TGE/vaccinia recombinant	60	130	345	<20	40	110
1991	TGE/vaccinia recombinant	70	70	75	<20	60	50
1992	TGE/vaccinia recombinant	50	60	350	<20	65	120
1993	TGE/vaccinia recombinant	40	70	370	<20	50	60
1994	TGE/vaccinia recombinant	65	60	250	<20	50	60
1995	TGE/vaccinia recombinant	55	175	400	<20	50	160
1996	TGE/vaccinia recombinant	60	135	350	<20	50	120

[a] Inoculation was done by dabbing a tail scratch with purified viruses with titer of 10^9 pfu/ml.
[b] Neutralizing titer was determined by plaque reduction assay, shown as the reciprocal of serum dilution that reduced 50% of the plaques. Preimmune serum from each mouse was included in each assay as control.

The recent results with the influenza-vaccinia recombinant, in which IgA type antibody could be stimulated by selecting the intranasal route of inoculation demonstrated that a change in the route of administration could result in specific type of immune response (B. Moss, personal communication). Oral delivery of vaccinia virus has been tested in monkeys and shown to induce successful immunization [11]. We feel that this could be the most promising way to stimulate the IgA class of antibody in pigs with the TGE-vaccinia recombinant virus. This approach is currently being tested.

REFERENCES

1. E.H. Bohl in: Diseases of Swine, H.W. Dunne and H.D. Leman, eds. (Iowa State University Press, Ames, Iowa 1975) pp. 195-208.

2. B.E. Hooper and E.O. Haelterman, J. Am. Vet. Med. Assoc. 149, 1580-1586 (1966).
3. L.P. Doyle and L.M. Hutchings, J. Am. Vet. Med. Assoc. 108, 257-259 (1946).
4. Y.B. Kim, S.G. Bradley and D.W. Watson, J. Immunol. 97, 52-63 (1966).
5. E.H. Bohl, P.K.P. Gupta, M.V.F. Olquin and L.J. Saif, Infect. Immun. 6, 289-301 (1972).
6. D.J. Garwes, M.H. Lucas, D.A. Higgins, B.V. Pike and S.F. Cartwright, Vet. Microbiol. 3, 179-190 (1978/1979).
7. S. Hu, J. Bruszewski, T. Boone and L. Souza in: Modern Approaches to Vaccines, R.M. Chanock and R.A. Lerner, eds. (New York: Cold Spring Laboratory 1984) pp. 219-223.
8. S. Hu, J. Bruszewski, R. Smalling and J.K. Browne, International Symp. on Immunobiology of Proteins and Peptides, in press (1984).
9. G.L. Smith, B.R. Murphy and B. Moss, Proc. Nat. Acad. Sci. USA 80, 7155-7159 (1983).
10. M. Mackett, G.L. Smith and B. Moss, Proc. Nat. Acad. Sci. USA 79, 7415-7419 (1982).
11. H.D. Huber, V. Hockstein-Mintzel, P. Rauchenberger and H. Stikl, Zbl. Bakt. Hyg. I. Abt. Orig. B. 157, 102-114 (1973).

DISCUSSION

Dr. Neff: Would you comment on the stability of the biologic properties of these recombinant viruses?

Dr. Hu: In tissue culture, we have done a continuous passage by mass culturing of recombinant virus, and then picked random plaques to recheck. So far, they all seem to be stable. In animals, we haven't done the studies.

Dr. Wallace: To minimize against this disease, it appears that you want to deliver live antigen into the gut. Do you plan to do that with the vaccinia recombinant,, or will you rely on a viremia after giving the virus intradermally?

Dr. Hu: I was hoping that somebody here would have information about the effects of oral administration of pox viruses. There are reports on the use of fowlpox. If you administer fowlpox virus in drinking water, it can establish an infection.

Dr. Welter: One must consider natural point of entry of these infectious agents. We have here a very complex model, one in which the baby pig depends on a continuous source of milk for its lactogenic immunity. Circulating antibody does not protect that pig. We might consider the baby pig, in addition to the sow, as a candidate for immunization. We do know that we can inoculate baby pigs at one day of age with attenuated live viruses, and actively immunize them, even in face of maternal immunity. Many sows, particularly for the first time, may suffer from agalactia, or reduced milk flow.

Dr. Ada: In this particular case, you might consider another possibility, and that is putting the gene into a salmonella vaccine, rather than into the vaccinia.

Dr. D.A. Henderson: Dr. Stickl, from Munich, reported giving vaccinia virus by mouth in the late 1960's or the early 1970's. I am a little dubious, but he did claim good results. He said he got satisfactory takes and neutralizing antibody responses.

<u>Dr. Esposito</u>: At the Centers for Disease Control, vaccinia has been given orally to raccoons, dogs and mongooses. Raccoons and mongooses given vaccinia virus react with HI and neutralizing antibody, but not dogs.

PART IV

OTHER VIRUSES AS VECTORS FOR VACCINE ANTIGENS

Chairpersons: R. Chanock and W. Dowdle

GENETIC ENGINEERING OF HERPES SIMPLEX VIRUS GENOMES FOR ATTENUATION AND EXPRESSION OF FOREIGN GENES

BERNARD ROIZMAN* AND MINAS ARSENAKIS*

*The Marjorie B. Kovler Viral Oncology Laboratories, The University of Chicago, 910 East 58th Street, Chicago, Illinois 60636

THE PROBLEM

Viral Vectors for Live Herpes Simplex Vaccine

Attempts to design vaccines to protect against an infectious disease must take into consideration two factors in addition to safety and efficacy of the product. The first is the human biology of the causative agent. The second is the characteristic of the population susceptible to the disease, particularly as it relates to the opportunities to be vaccinated.

In the case of herpes simplex viruses 1 and 2 (HSV-1 and HSV-2), the usual mode of transmission is through contact of mucous membranes or wounded body surfaces of the recipient with infected body surfaces of the donor. This is the portal of entry into the body and, for most individuals, it is also the target organ. The virus multiplies at the portal of entry, invades sensory nerve endings, ascends to dorsal root ganglia and establishes a latent infection. In the latent state, the virus does not seem to be multiplying, but the precise state of the genome and the mechanism by which it is kept quiescent during latency is not known. During the latent state, the virus appears to be totally shielded from the immune system of the host. The misery and many of the sequelae of herpetic infections stem from the ability of the virus to become activated, as a consequence of physical, emotional or hormonal stress, in the neuron in which it is harbored and to be transmitted preferentially to a site very near the portal of entry but occasionally to distal sites (e.g. central nervous system). Activation of latent virus results frequently, but not always, in the appearance of viral-induced lesions near the portal of entry and, rarely, at distal sites. The virus in the recurrent lesions at the portal of entry comprises the main reservoir for infection of human contacts.

Establishment of latent infection and subsequent recurrences are sequelae of virus multiplication at the portal of entry. To reiterate, the portal of entry is the target organ. In this instance, the objective of vaccination is not merely to stimulate immunity in the expectation that natural exposure to the infectious agent will bolster the immune system before the agent gets to the target organ. To be effective, the virus must not even multiply at the portal of entry! Can an effective vaccine against herpes simplex virus infections be made?

Patient studies suggest that it might be feasible. This conclusion is based on three observations. First, individuals with prior HSV-1 infections have, as a rule, milder first infections with HSV-2 [1]. The two viruses are related and share many antigenic determinants but they are not immunologically identical [2]. Second, although successive infections with the same serotype have been observed in some individuals [3,4], they appear to be rare. The presence of one virus appears to confer partial protection against another serotype and seemingly better protection against superinfection with the same serotype. Lastly, in experimental systems, the presence of latent virus seems to protect against establishment of latent infection by a second virus [5]. This resistance can be overcome [6], but it takes a considerable experimental effort. Given the necessity that the vaccine must protect against multiplication at the portal of entry and that superinfections do occur even in the face of prior infection with the same serotype, expectations that a subunit vaccine will be protective seem rather naive.

The characteristics of the population at risk also argue for a live vaccine. The major stress on the human population is the ever increasing incidence of genital infections. Analyses of the viral DNAs extracted from isolates with restriction endonucleases indicate that the increase in incidence reflects a frenzy of transmission fueled by an epidemic of promiscuity rather than a pestilence caused by a single virus sweeping the land [7,8]. The victim is most often the consenting adult rather than the innocent child. The expectation that the eager adult shall submit voluntarily to vaccination prior to an amorous adventure cannot serve as a basis for public health measures to curtail the incidence of the disease. In the United States, at least, the open and enforceable window for vaccination is the interval of compulsory education, and the vaccine must be effective throughout the sexually active life--a tall order for a live virus vaccine and an impossible one for a subunit vaccine, no matter how attractively presented to the immune system of the host.

These considerations have led us to consider a genetically engineered live virus as a candidate for a vaccine against herpes simplex virus infections. The purpose of this paper is two-fold. First, it is designed to show that techniques have been developed to tailor genomes as large as that of herpes simplex virus to suit the needs of the experimenter, and therefore the technology for constructing viruses with properties suitable for human vaccination is at hand. The second objective is to show that the virus can serve as a vector for expression of foreign genes.

The Properties of the Herpes Simplex Virus Genomes

The genomes of HSV-1 and HSV-2 are very similar in size (150 kbp); both are linear double stranded molecules with similar sequence arrangement and general properties [9]. The two genomes share at least 50% of their sequence with good matching of base pairs [10]. It is convenient to discuss primarily one, since most of the work has been done on HSV-1.

The HSV-1 genome consists of two covalently linked components, L (long) and S (short), each of which consists of unique sequences flanked by inverted repeats [11,12]. The inverted repeats of the L component are each 9 kbp in size and have been designated ab and b'a' whereas the inverted repeats of the S component, each 6.5 kbp in size, have been designated a'c' and ca [12]. Each of the inverted repeats contains at least one gene in its entirety and these genes are therefore diploid. During the viral reproductive cycle, the L and S components invert relative to each other giving rise to 4 equimolar isomers differing solely in the relative orientation of the two components [13,14].

The HSV-1 genome encodes at least 50 genes specifying abundant proteins; the exact genome coding load is not known, but characteristics of the genes encoded in the HSV genome are especially relevant to this report. Unlike the genomes of smaller viruses which encode functions designed to cause the host to replicate their genomes, HSV brings into the infected cell genetic information for a variety of enzymes which both create the necessary deoxynucleotide pools and replicate the genome.

Since cells growing in culture express many of the same enzymes, the viral genetic information specifying the cellular counterparts can be deleted without affecting the ability of the virus to grow in these cells. An example of such an enzyme is the viral nucleoside kinase known better by its misnomer of thymidine kinase (TK). The effect of deleting this enzyme is to reduce the ability of the virus to synthesize its DNA in resting cells with very low pools of deoxy nucleoside triphosphate. The TK has the distinction of being both deletable and specifying a known function. Other genes and domains of the genome are also dispensable in cell culture although their function is less well understood.

Principles of Engineering Insertions and Deletions in HSV-1 Genomes

Because of their size, the construction of altered HSV-1 genomes relies upon selection of specific recombinant genomes generated by spontaneous recombination in infected cells. Efficient generation of desired viral genomic constructs has two requirements. The first is to increase the probability of specific recombinational events by providing "intermediates" or "precursors" to the final construct. In principle, deletions or insertions as a consequence of recombination occur spontaneously. The frequency of a specific deletion or insertion not based on homologous recombination is likely to be very small. To obtain viral recombinants carrying modifications at a specific site, we confront the intact viral DNA with a recombination intermediate--an excess of DNA fragments that provide homologous flanking sequences to introduce the required modification at a specific site. Specifically, we transfect susceptible cells with intact viral DNA and DNA fragments in which the desired modification is inserted between viral DNA sequences homologous to the sequences flanking the site at which the modification is to be introduced into the viral genome.

The second requirement is for a procedure for selection of recombinants. The problem stems from the fact that even homologous recombinations occur at a relatively low rate. Screening of viral progeny for the desirable recombinant can be a slow and tedious job particularly if the recombinant is at a growth disadvantage relative to the wild type virus. The selection procedure we have adopted [15,16] is based on the use of a selectable marker gene--the HSV-1 thymidine kinase. The choice is based on three considerations. First, the enzyme has a broad substrate specificity and phosphorylates a large array of thymidine and other nucleoside analogues. Some of these analogues (e.g. AraT) are phosphorylated preferentially by the viral enzyme and are therefore relatively non-toxic to the uninfected cell. Others, like BUdR, are phosphorylated in uninfected cells uniquely by the host thymidine kinase and therefore are relatively innocuous in cells lacking that enzyme. In each instance, phosphorylation of the analogues by the viral enzyme results in production of non-infectious progeny. These properties of the enzyme and the availability of analogues like AraT and BUdR, render possible rapid selection of viral progeny in which the marker gene, TK, is inactivated or deleted. The second important property of the TK stems from the observation that it is non-essential only in cells capable of maintaining adequate pools of deoxy nucleotides. In TK- cells, the major and only primary pathway for generation of TdRMP is through conversion of UdRMP by thymidilate synthetase. If this pathway in TK- cells is blocked, only cells infected with TK$^+$ HSV-1 are capable of producing infectious progeny and of forming plaques. The availability of drugs (e.g. methotrexate) that block the main pathway for generation of TdRMP permits selection of viral recombinant genomes carrying the TK gene.

Viral constructs utilizing the TK gene for selection of recombinants can be classified into two classes differing primarily in the methods of construction of the vectors. Class 1 vectors carry insertions of the foreign genes within the transcribed domain of the TK gene of the HSV-1 genome. Class 2 vectors carry insertions in all other locations of the genome.

CLASS 1 CONSTRUCTS

General Procedure

This class of constructs consists of viral genomes into which DNA fragments encoding cis or trans- acting functions are inserted into the transcribed domain of the TK gene. One of the key factors that make this type of insertion possible is that the TK gene does not appear to overlap with other genes essential for virus multiplication. The principles of construction of Class 1 recombinant genomes is illustrated in Figure 1. The procedure involves insertion of the desired DNA fragment

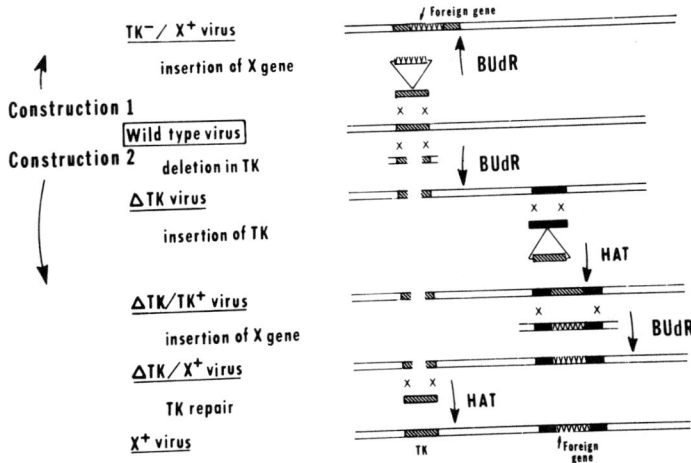

FIG. 1. Flow diagram for the construction of Class 1 and Class 2 recombinant HSV genomes. The HSV DNA is represented as a double line. The phenotype of the recombinant virus is underlined. The symbol delta indicates deletion.

into the transcribed domain of the TK gene cloned in a plasmid, co-transfection of the construct with intact wild type DNA, and selection of TK- recombinants among the viral progeny of the transfection.

This type of constructs has been used to identify the cis-acting sites mediating the inversion of the L and S components, to map the promoter regulatory domains of HSV-1 genes and to express foreign genes.

Identification of the cis-acting sites mediating the inversion of the L and S components of the HSV-1 genome. As noted above, HSV-1 DNA extracted from infected cells and from purified virions consists of four equimolar populations of molecules that differ in the relative orientation of the L and S components [13,14]. To identify the cis-acting sites that mediate inversion, HSV-1 DNA fragments spanning the junction between L and S components were inserted into the transcribed non-translated domain of the HSV-1 TK gene, thus separating the promoter from the structural TK gene [15,17,18]. These constructs were then co-transfected with intact TK+ HSV-1 DNA and the viral progeny of the transfection were plated on cells overlaid with AraT. The drug-resistant progeny consisted predominantly of virus whose TK gene was interrupted by the insertion and only a small fraction of the progeny consisted of spontaneous TK⁻ mutants. Recombinants containing an additional junction fragment in the TK gene formed twelve instead of the usual four isomers, i.e. the insertion of the second junction caused additional inversions. Analyses of these inserts indicated that the cis-acting site that mediates the inversions is located within the 500 bp a sequence. The a sequence has a complex structure consisting of a 20 bp direct repeat No. 1 (DR1), a 64 bp unique sequence (U_b), a 12 bp direct repeat No. 2 (DR2), which is repeated 19 to 22 times, a 37 bp direct repeat No. 4 (DR4), which is repeated 2 to 3 times, a 59 bp unique sequence (U_c) followed by another copy of the 20 bp DR1 [17]. Only DNA fragments flanked by inverted repeats of a sequences inverted [15]. That inversion is mediated by trans-acting viral factors was demonstrated in cells converted to TK+ phenotype with a plasmid containing a viral origin of DNA replication and a TK gene flanked by inverted repeats of a sequences. This plasmid was maintained in head-to-tail concatemers in uninfected cells. Following infection with HSV-1, however, the DNA segment flanked by the two inverted a sequences was both amplified and inverted [19].

The physiological requirements for the inversion of the L and S components relative to each other are not known. The significant finding, that the inversions are mediated by a sequence contained in the internal inverted repeats lead ultimately to the construction of a recombinant lacking the repeats and frozen in one arrangement of the DNA [20]. The construction of this recombinant, described later in the text, indicated that the inversions are not required for virus growth in cell culture.

Regulation of HSV-1 gene expression. Class 1 constructs have been used to identify the promoter and regulatory domains of HSV-1 genes. Although the promoter domain may be deduced from the nucleotide sequence of the gene domain, verification is at times difficult because of technical problems in measuring gene product or vagaries of the expression system. Thus, (a) the amount of protein may not, at all times, reflect the amounts of available mRNA [21]; (b) many HSV proteins are made in small amounts or are insoluble [22-24]; (c) reconstruction of the gene domain frequently presents insurmountable problems because of gene overlaps, and lastly, (d) we have recently shown that identical gene constructs may be regulated differently depending on whether they were introduced into cells in a viral genome by infection or in a DNA fragment by transfection [25]. We [16] solved the problems inherent in the identification of promoter regulatory domains of unknown genes by fusing the putative promoter-regulatory domains to a surrogate gene, the TK, and recombining the chimeric genes into the genome.

The HSV-1 genomes comprise approximately 50 genes that form at
least 3 groups, i.e. alpha, beta and gamma, whose expression is coordinately regulated and sequentially ordered in a cascade fashion [26,27].
Alpha genes do not require prior protein synthesis for their expression.
Alpha gene products induce the expression of two sets of beta genes, $beta_1$
and $beta_2$. $Beta_1$ and $beta_2$ genes differ in the temporal order of their
synthesis but do not require viral DNA synthesis for optimal expression.
Gamma genes may also be subdivided into 2 groups, $gamma_1$ and $gamma_2$.
Maximal expression of both $gamma_1$ and $gamma_2$ genes requires viral DNA
synthesis. $Gamma_1$ genes differ from $gamma_2$ genes in that the expression
of the latter is stringently dependent on viral DNA synthesis.

To identify the promoter and regulatory sequences within the domains
of alpha genes [16] we constructed chimeric genes consisting of portions
of the 5' sequences upstream of the translated domains of alpha genes
fused to the transcribed and translated domain of the HSV-1 TK, a beta
gene. These constructs were then cotransfected with the intact DNA of
a HSV-1 recombinant [HSV-1(F) delta 305] from which 700 bp was deleted
from the TK gene. The progeny of the cotransfection was then plated on
TK⁻ cells and overlaid with medium containing methotrexate. Recombinants
carrying the chimeric alpha-TK gene were shown to regulate the TK gene
as an alpha gene. Similar studies verified the promoter-regulatory
domain of a ($gamma_2$) gene [25].

Studies on chimeric genes have identified the promoters of alpha
genes 4, 0, and 27 [28], and verified the domains of the promoter
regulatory sequences of the genes specifying the HSV-1 glycoproteins gB
and gC deduced from their sequence (Arsenakis and Roizman, work in
progress). Perhaps equally significant, these studies permitted the
dissection of regulatory domains. Thus, in the case of alpha genes, we
were able to separate the promoter and regulatory domains [29] and to
identify within the regulatory domains cis-acting sequences which confer
upon recipients a high constitutive expression level and sequences
which confer the capacity to be induced to a high level of expression
[30] by a structural protein of the virus acting in trans [31]. Detailed
analyses of promoter and regulatory gene domains will ultimately permit
the tailoring of the timing and amount of gene expression to meet the
specific requirement for the gene product.

Expression of foreign genes in Class 1 constructs. HSV-1 characteristically shuts off host macromolecular synthesis in the infected cell
[32-37]. Class 1 constructs were tested for the ability of foreign
genes resident in the HSV-1 genome to be expressed. The foreign genes
include EBNA-1 and EBNA-2 (E. Kieff, M. Arsenakis and B. Roizman,
manuscript in preparation) and hepatitis B virus S gene product [38]. A
requirement for foreign genes in HSV-1 vectors is that they be expressed
from HSV-1 promoter-regulatory domains. To date we have tested alpha
and beta promoter-regulatory sequences and such chimeric genes are
regulated as if they were alpha or beta viral genes, respectively. The
construction of these recombinant viruses follows the same procedure as
described earlier in the text, i.e. cloning of the desired gene under
the control of an HSV promoter, insertion of the chimeric gene into the
domains of the TK gene, recombination with intact TK+ HSV-1 viral DNA
and subsequent selection of TK⁻ recombinants. Figure 2 illustrates the
HSV-1 vector carrying hepatitis B virus S gene linked to alpha and beta
promoter-regulatory domains. The foreign protein is made concurrently
with HSV gene products (Figure 3), but is processed according to
its primary structure. Hepatitis B S protein aggregates to form
typical coreless particles (Dane particles) which are excreted from

cells [38]. In this respect, the gene product made in HSV-infected cells cannot be differentiated from that made in hepatitis B virus infected cells.

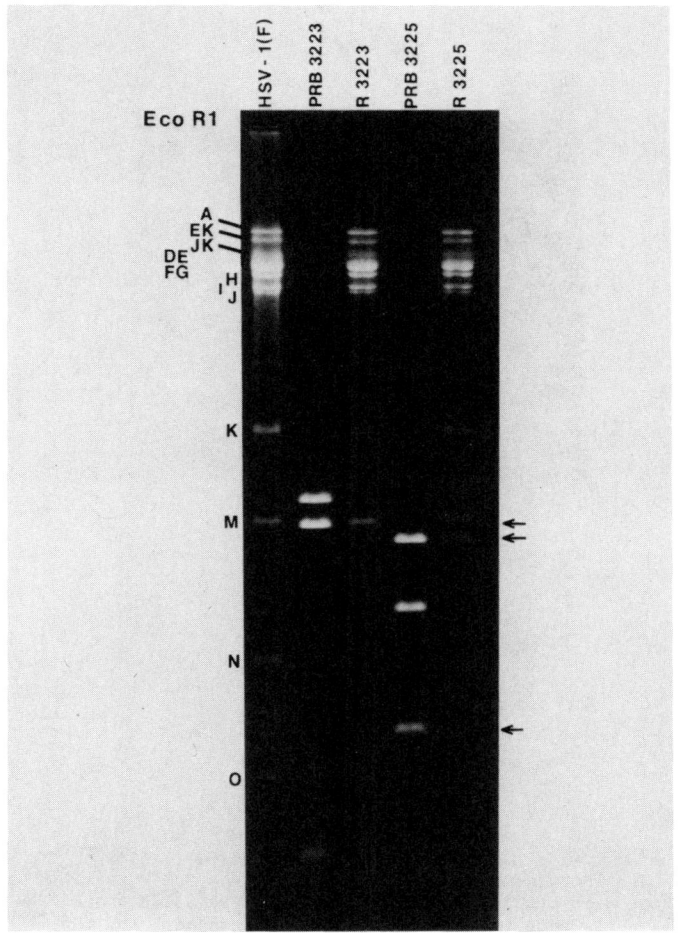

FIG. 2. Photograph of electrophoretically separated EcoRI digests of recombinant plasmids and viruses stained with ethidium bromide. Each DNA was limit digested with EcoRI restriction endonuclease, and electrophoresed on 0.8% agarose gels. HSV-1(F) is the parent virus and R3223 and R3225 are the recombinant viruses carrying the beta- and alpha-regulated HB S gene, respectively. Note that in both the R3223 and R3225 recombinants the EcoRI N fragment is missing and the new fragments carrying the chimeric HBsAg inserts are indicated by the arrows.

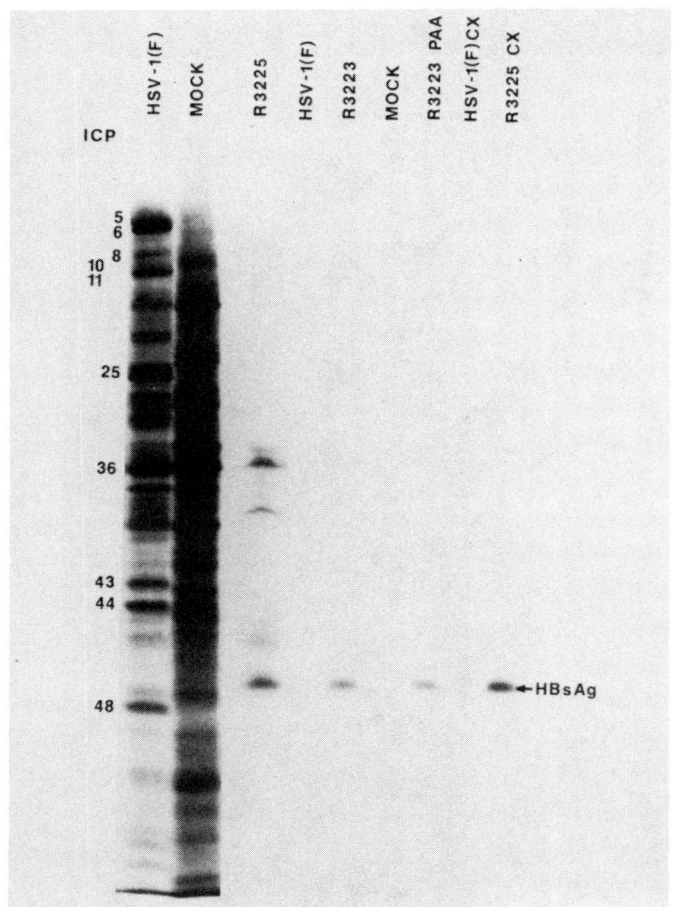

FIG. 3. Photograph of autoradiogram of immune precipitated HB S protein produced by recombinant viruses R3223 and R3225. HEp-2 cells were infected at a moi of 20 pfu/cell and the infected cell proteins (ICP) were labelled with [^{35}S]methionine from 2 to 20 hrs postinfection. In the case of phosphonoacetate (PAA) treatment, the drug was added at the time of virus adsorption and was maintained throughout the infection. In the case of cycloheximide (CX) treated cells, the drug was added 30 min prior to virus adsorption and was maintained for 6 hrs. At that time, it was removed and actinomycin D was added to prevent further viral mRNA synthesis. The proteins synthesized immediately upon removal of cycloheximide were labeled with [^{35}S]methionine until 20 hrs postinfection. The infected cells were solubilized in 1% NP40, 1% DOC, 10^{-5} M TLCK, 10^{-5} M TPCK, and the HBsAg was immune precipitated with a rabbit antiserum to HBsAg. Immune precipitates were adsorbed on protein-A Sepharose, denatured and run on 12.5% SDS-polyacrylamide gels.

CLASS 2 CONSTRUCTS

This type of construction involves the insertion or deletion of genes in locations other than the transcribed domain of the TK gene. In this instance the HSV-1 TK gene is used as the marker for selection of recombinant viruses. As illustrated in Figure 1, the procedure consists of two steps. The first step entails insertion of a copy of the TK gene in the location where the insertion or deletion is to be made. This is accomplished by inserting the TK gene into a cloned copy of a DNA fragment spanning the site of the insertion or deletion. This construct is then cotransfected with intact TK$^-$ [HSV(F)delta 305] DNA and TK$^+$ recombinants are then selected from among the progeny of the transfection. In the case of insertions, the second step entails cloning the gene to be inserted into the same fragment in place of the TK gene. To delete a gene, sequences at the site of the insertion of TK are deleted and the fragment is recloned. These constructs are then cotransfected with the TK$^+$ recombinants obtained in the first step and the desired TK$^-$ recombinants are selected from among the progeny of the transfection.

The Class 2 constructions have been extremely useful in identifying HSV-1 genes that are essential for growth in experimental animals but which are not essential for replication in cell culture. Class 2 constructs are also useful for the expression of foreign genes.

Identification of genes non-essential for virus replication in cell culture.

Although approximately 50 relatively abundant HSV-1 proteins have been identified [39,40], the studies on conditional lethal mutants have yielded approximately 30 complementation groups. The failures to isolate ts lesions in many of the HSV genes may reflects the plasticity of the protein structure in relation to its function or the less likely possibility that any amino acid substitution is lethal. Still another hypothesis is that these genes are not essential for virus replication in cell culture.

An example of the Class 2 constructions designed to test for the latter hypothesis is the engineering of recombinants carrying deletions in the alpha 22 gene by Post and Roizman [41]. This gene is located at the junction between the internal inverted repeats and the unique sequences of the S component. It was constructed as described in Figure 1, i.e. by insertion of the TK gene into the middle of the alpha 22 gene of HSV-1(F) delta 305, a virus carrying a 700 bp deletion in the TK gene, and then replacing the inserted TK gene by recombination with fragments carrying deletions of 100 bp (recombinant R328) and 500 bp (R325) in the domain of the coding sequences of alpha 22 gene.

The construction of the R325 and R328 exemplifies virus attenuation by construction of deletions. In order to test the biologic properties of the R325, it was necessary to restore the TK gene at its natural location by transfecting cells with intact R325 DNA and a DNA fragment carrying the intact TK gene, and to select TK$^+$ recombinants. The R325TK$^+$ recombinant grows as well as the wild type virus in HEp-2 and African Green Monkey (Vero) cells in continuous cultivation [41], but less well in resting human embryonic lung cells. In the latter cells, there appears to be an impairment in the regulation of late gene expression (A. Sears and B. Roizman, manuscript in preparation). The virus is not pathogenic in Balb/C mice (10^7 pfu/LD$_{50}$) as compared to wild type parent ($10^{1.5}$pfu/LD$_{50}$) by intracerebral inoculation, but does establish latency in mouse trigeminal ganglia when inoculated by the eye route (B. Meignier and B. Roizman, manuscript in preparation).

Construction of High Capacity HSV-1 Vector

The use of HSV as a vector required in its initial stages the expansion of the size of HSV-1 DNA. Early studies [42] have shown that the HSV-1 genome can be expanded by at least 7 kbp without affecting the ability of the genome to package into capsids. More recently, F. Jenkins, M. Casadaban, and B. Roizman (manuscript in preparation) were able to insert a 9.7 kbp fragment into HSV-1 DNA. However, the most significant advance was the isolation of recombinant I358 [20]. In this recombinant approximately 15 kbp containing the internal inverted repeats including the L-S junction were replaced by 2 kbp of DNA containing the TK gene. This variant therefore contains space for insertion of approximately 25 kbp of DNA without exceeding the packaging capacity of the virion. An interesting property of this recombinant is that it is arrested in one arrangement (the prototype) and does not invert. Although it does not lack any informational sequences ($\underline{\text{trans}}$-acting genes), the virus is relatively non-pathogenic (10^6pfu/$\overline{\text{LD}}_{50}$) by intracerebral inoculation of Balb/C mice and a reduced capacity to establish latent infections by the eye route. As a vector, I358 expressed the chicken ovalbumin gene under the alpha 4 promoter (M. Arsenakis, K. Poffenberger, and B. Roizman, work in progress) with good results. Notwithstanding the production of viral proteins, approximately 15ug/4 x 10^6 cells/24 hrs was produced and excreted into the extracellular medium.

CONCLUSIONS

The salient features of the studies summarized in this paper are as follows:

(1) Techniques are now available for genetic manipulation of large genomes such as HSV and vaccinia. These techniques are based on the use of the TK gene for selection of recombinant carrying insertions and deletions at specific sites [15,41].

(2) The HSV-1 genome contains sequences that, when deleted by these techniques, generate recombinants (e.g. R325TK$^+$ and I358) capable of growing but which appear to be less pathogenic in experimental systems. The procedures are therefore available for construction of virus recombinants suitable for human vaccination.

(3) HSV-1 genome is capable of serving as a vector for expression of foreign genes notwithstanding the ability of the virus to shut off host macromolecular metabolism relatively early in infection. A strict requirement of the system is that the foreign genes be expressed from viral promoter-regulatory sequences. All of the promoter-regulatory domains of viral genes tested to date have worked; invariably, the expression of the foreign gene is regulated as predicted by the nature of the promoter-regulatory domain to which the foreign gene was fused. Studies to select or construct promoters which confers high level of expression are in progress.

In the Introduction, a case was presented for both vaccination against HSV infections and for the use of a live vaccine. Given this assertion, the question arises as to what advantages accrue with the use of HSV rather than that of another virus as a vector for foreign genes. If cost were irrelevant and the opportunities for vaccination were infinite, the vaccine for each infectious agent could be dealt with on its own merits in accordance with the biologic properties of the agent and requirements for protection against disease. This is not the case, and the use of vectors is clearly "cost and opportunity" effective, if in fact, the vaccine administered in this fashion prevents disease. The distinction between HSV and other vectors like vaccinia is that vaccination with an HSV vector could protect against both HSV and an infectious agent whose informational sequences are expressed by the vector, whereas in the case of vaccinia the requirement is solely for the informational sequences of another infectious agent. Why then immunize against 200 vaccinia proteins to elicit an immune response against one antigen?

ACKNOWLEDGEMENTS

The studies described in this paper were aided by grants from the United States Public Health Service (CA 08494 and CA 19264) from the National Cancer Institute, by grant MV-2T from the American Cancer Society. M.A. is a postdoctoral fellow of the Damon Runyon-Walter Winchell Cancer Fund.

REFERENCES

1. L. Corey in Herpesviruses, Volume 5, B. Roizman and C. Lopez, eds. (Plenum Press 1985) pp. 1-26.
2. P.G. Spear and B. Roizman in The Molecular Biology of Tumor Viruses, (Cold Sring Harbor, Laboratory, 1980) 2nd Edition, Part 2, pp. 615-746.
3. T.G. Buchman, B. Roizman and A.J. Nahmias, J. Infect. Dis 140, 295-304 (1979).
4. R. Whitley, A.D. Lakeman, A. Nahmias and B. Roizman, New Engl. J. Med. 307, 1060-1062 (1982).
5. Y.M. Centifanto-Fitzgerald, E.D. Varnell and H.E. Kaufman, Infection and Immunity 35m 1125-1132 (1982).
6. B. Meignier, B. Norrild and B. Roizman, Infection and Immunity 41, 702-708 (1983).
7. T.G. Buchman, T. Simpson, C. Nosal, B. Roizman and A.J. Nahmias, Ann. N.Y. Acad. Sci. 354, 279-290 (1980).
8. B. Roizman and M. Tognon, Current Topics Microbiol. & Immunol. 104, 275-286 (1983).
9. E.D. Kieff, S.L. Bachenheimer and B. Roizman, J. Virol. 8, 125-132 (1971).
10. E.D. Kieff, B. Hoyer, S.L. Bachenheimer and B. Roizman, J. Virol. 9, 738-745 (1972).
11. B. Sheldrick and N. Berthelot, Cold Spring Harbor Symp. Quant. Biol. 39, 667-668 (1975).
12. S. Wadsworth, R.J. Jacob and B. Roizman, J. Virol. 15, 1487-1497 (1975).
13. G.S. Hayward, R.J. Jacob, S.C. Wadsworth and B. Roizman, Proc. Nat. Acad. Sci. USA 72, 4243-4247 (1975).
14. H. Delius and J.B. Clements, J. Gen. Virol. 33, 125-134 (1976).
15. E.S. Mocarski, L.E. Post and B. Roizman, Cell 22, 243-255 (1980).
16. L.E. Post, S. Mackem and B. Roizman, Cell 24, 555-565 (1981).
17. E.S. Mocarski and B. Roizman, Proc. Nat. Acad. Sci. USA 78, 7047-7051 (1981).
18. E.S. Mocarski and B. Roizman, Cell 31, 89-97 (1982).
19. E.S. Mocarski and B. Roizman, Proc. Nat. Acad. Sci. USA 79, 5626-5630 (1982).
20. K.L. Poffenberger, E. Tabares and B. Roizman, Proc. Nat. Acad. Sci. USA 80, 1690-2694 (1983).
21. D.C. Johnson and P.G. Spear, J. Virol. 51, 389-394 (1984).

22. K. Wilcox, E.I. Sklyanskaya, A. Kohn and B. Roizman, J. Virol. 33, 167-182 (1980).
23. D.K. Braun, B. Roizman and L. Pereira, J. Virol. 49, 142-153 (1984).
24. M. Ackermann, D.K. Braun, L. Pereira and B. Roizman, J. Virol. 52, 108-118 (1984).
25. S. Silver and B. Roizman, Mol. and Cell Biol., in press, March 1985.
26. R.W. Honess and B. Roizman, J. Virol. 14, 8-19 (1974).
27. R.W. Honess and B. Roizman, Proc. Nat. Acad. Sci. USA 72, 1276-1280 (1975).
28. S. Mackem and B. Roizman, J. Virol. 44, 939-949 (1982a).
29. S. Mackem and B. Roizman, Proc. Nat. Acad. Sci. USA 79, 4917-4921 (1982b).
30. T.M. Kristie and B. Roizman, Proc. Nat. Acad. Sci. USA 81, 4065-4069 (1984).
31. W. Batterson and B. Roizman, J. Virol. 46, 371-377 (1983).
32. B. Roizman, G.S. Borman and M. Kamali-Rousta, Nature (London) 206, 1374-1375 (1965).
33. R.J. Sydiskis and B. Roizman, Science 153, 76-78 (1966).
34. R.J. Sydiskis and B. Roizman, Virology 34, 562-565 (1968).
35. E.K. Wagner and B. Roizman, J. Virol. 4, 36-46 (1969).
36. M.L. Fenwick and M.J. Walker, J. Gen. Virol. 41, 37-51 (1978).
37. G.S. Read and N. Frenkel, J. Virol. 46, 498-512 (1983).
38. M.-F Shih, M. Arsenakis, P. Tiollais and B. Roizman, Proc. Nat. Acad. Sci. USA 81, 5867-5870 (1984).
39. R.W. Honess and B. Roizman, J. Virol. 12, 1346-1365 (1973).
40. L.S. Morse,, L. Pereira, B. Roizman and P.A. Schaffer, J. Virol. 26, 389-410 (1978).
41. L.E. Post and B. Roizman, Cell 25, 227-232 (1981).
42. D.M. Knipe, W.T. Ruyechan, B. Roizman and I.W. Halliburton, Proc. Nat. Acad. Sci. 75, 3896-3900 (1978).

DISCUSSION

Dr. Small: You can engineer many of the adverse qualities out of the virus, to use it as a vector, but what about things like temperature stability?

Dr. Roizman: Generally, the virus in lyophilized form is quite stable. We have maintained virus in lyophilized form for a long time. We have a box of lyophilized viruses that we keep at room temperature, and ship to people who ask for it.

Dr. Ellis: When you delete the internal repeat, how many base pairs of repeat sequence can you leave behind and still have a non-invertible genome?

Dr. Roizman: I cannot answer the question, because we deleted all of it. I can speculate. About 500 base pairs is all that is required for inversion. One of the reasons for doing all of this engineering is to find out what is required for inversion, and the answer is 500 base pairs. If we take the terminal 500 base-pair sequence, and put it anywhere in the genome, we now get three components instead of two that invert. Instead of getting four isomers, we get 12. So, if you only delete 500 base pairs, you probably will make it a non-inverting virus.

Dr. Ada: One would expect that at least some of those 200 proteins would be very important for carrier effects, particularly with revaccination with vaccinia.

__Dr. Roizman:__ Yes, and I hope that for herpes simplex, this same thing holds true.

PART V

CONSIDERATIONS OF THE SAFETY, EFFICACY AND POTENTIAL
APPLICATIONS OF RECOMBINANT VACCINIA VIRUSES

Chairperson: G. Noble

POTENTIAL APPLICATIONS OF VACCINIA VIRUS VECTORS FOR IMMUNOPROPHYLAXIS

FRED BROWN*

*Wellcome Biotechnology Ltd, Beckenham, Kent, United Kingdom

The impact of recombinant DNA technology in the field of immunoprophylaxis has so far been rather muted. Although the expression of protective antigens in bacterial and eukaryotic cells has been achieved for several different diseases, sometimes in quite remarkable yields, the biological activity of the products has been disappointing. With virus antigens, for example, only the gene coding for the surface antigen of hepatitis B virus has given a product possessing an acceptable level of biological activity. The highly promising result with hepatitis B surface antigen expressed in yeast cells is almost certainly the consequence of the expressed protein assembling into the highly antigenic 22nm particle found in the blood of carrier patients. The results with antigens such as the haemagglutinin of influenza virus and the protective protein VP1 of foot and mouth disease virus have been very disappointing despite the high levels of expression that were achieved.

The work of Moss and Paoletti and their colleagues on the use of vaccinia virus as a carrier for the expression of genes coding for protective antigens is thus both timely and of great potential value in the control of disease. Already its potential value for immunization against hepatitis B has been demonstrated in animals and it seems likely that the basic molecular biology of the system will be applicable to any gene, i.e. that any gene, suitably inserted into the vaccinia virus genome, will express its product.

It is important to recognise, however, the commercial aspects of the work. Vaccination against virus diseases has been one of the greatest achievements in both human and veterinary medicine and many of them have been brought under control. Indeed smallpox has been eradicated by the rigorous application of vaccination with vaccinia virus. Since cheap and effective vaccines are available for most virus diseases, any new vaccine must be superior to those currently available, either in effectiveness or in reduced cost, but preferably in both. For these reasons it is highly likely that the first application of the recombinant vaccinia viruses will be in those diseases where an effective vaccine is not available or where its cost is so high that it is essentially not available to a large proportion of the world's population.

Any list of diseases affecting the human population for which effective vaccines are not available, whether for reasons of cost or lack of potency or occasionally the present inability to produce the protective antigen in adequate amounts, would include hepatitis A and B, influenza and other respiratory diseases, Dengue fever, rabies and diarrhoea caused by rotaviruses. The genes coding for the protective antigens of hepatitis B, influenza, rabies and rotaviruses have been identified and the first three have been expressed following inoculation with recombinant vaccinia viruses into which they have been integrated. All three of these diseases are of such enormous importance that if the recombinant vaccines prove to be effective in man the investment of scientific skill in vaccinia virus vaccines will have been fully justified. However, the potential of the recombinant vaccinia virus approach is so great that there seems to be no valid reason why the technology should not be applied to all virus diseases.

A crucial step in this work which is well recognised is the identification of the gene(s) coding for the protective antigen(s) for each virus disease. It is possible, however, that we may have been taking an over simplified view of the application of vaccinia virus as a carrier for important protective genes. It is becoming increasingly apparent, that there are huge gaps in our knowledge of the immunology of infectious diseases. The type of immunity required for protecting the body against influenza virus, which infects the respiratory tract, is clearly different from that required to protect against a virus such as rotavirus which infects the gastrointestinal tract. Whether recombinant vaccinia viruses will provide the universal panacea is doubtful so it is essential as a first step that the target diseases we select should be amenable to control by the immunity elicited by antigens which are expressed when the recombinant vaccinia virus grows in the skin. It seems unlikely that the response to rotavirus antigens expressed in this way would afford protection against infection.

The low cost of many of the currently available vaccines makes it unlikely that they will be replaced by recombinant vaccinia virus vaccines unless there is a significant advantage in terms of effectiveness and price. There is, however, another factor which may be brought into the equation. Vaccinia virus in its freeze-dried form is extremely stable, even at tropical temperatures. Provided the recombinant viruses have a similar stability, vaccines based on vaccinia virus would not require the cold chain which is so necessary for the retention of potency of many traditional vaccines. This is an important factor to consider in determining our future vaccine requirements.

Any discussion about the possible targets for the application of the recombinant vaccinia virus technology must include reference to acquired immune deficiency syndrome (AIDS). Our knowledge of the causative agent of the disease is rather small at present but if the increasing evidence that it is a retrovirus is confirmed, by using the information emerging from work on feline leukemia virus, for which a potentially effective vaccine has been produced by expression of the appropriate gene, there seems no reason why AIDS should not become a target for the vaccinia virus approach.

Antibiotics have solved so many of our disease problems with bacteria that the list of targets for bacterial vaccines is much shorter. However, it is clear that an effective and safe vaccine for whooping cough would be of great value. Similarly successful vaccination against malaria would have a major impact on the quality of life and life expectancy of many millions of people in the underdeveloped countries. The successful application of the recombinant vaccinia virus approach to these two diseases would have a major social impact throughout the world.

DISCUSSION

Dr. Warren: I would like to suggest that there ought to be some sense of what the priorities are for vaccine development based on what the most important diseases are on a global level in terms of prevalence, morbidity, mortality, and feasibility of control. Also, there are certain diseases that are not the most important but for which there are no adequate treatments. Two examples of such untreatable diseases, although one may be changing now, are onchocerciasis, river blindness, and Chagas' disease.

The three most important disease complexes or diseases in the world are diarrheal diseases, respiratory diseases, and malaria. We know which diarrheal diseases ought to be targeted in that area. We have no adequate strategies at all for dealing with respiratory diseases in the developing world. The impact of different disease complexes on a global basis has been studied extensively and priorities established for 24 of them.

Dr. Jordan: The National Institute of Allergy and Infectious Diseases has a program named Accelerated Development of New Vaccines, to exploit the kind of technology you have been hearing about. Our staff worked together with a group of experts convened by the Institute of Medicine to identify priorities for development of vaccines for both domestic use and international use. The draft report on domestic vaccines has been submitted. It very thoroughly documents, not only the state of the art, but the disease burden and variables that you might use to decide what your priorities would be. They are now working on international vaccines. They have 24 candidate diseases that they will establish priorities for.

CONSIDERATIONS OF SAFETY, EFFICACY AND POTENTIAL APPLICATIONS OF VACCINIA VECTORS FOR IMMUNOPROPHYLAXIS: AN ALTERNATIVE APPROACH FOR CONTROL OF HUMAN DISEASES FOR WHICH VACCINES ARE AVAILABLE

DAVID T. KARZON*

*Professor and Chairman, Department of Pediatrics, Vanderbilt University, School of Medicine, Nashville, Tennessee 37232

INTRODUCTION

The prospects which are offered by recombinant vaccinia vaccines require translation into public health practice. The availability of alternative vaccines imposes the burden of documentation of comparative performance and the development of a data base for each new recombinant vaccine candidate eventually matching our knowledge of contemporary vaccines. Further, considerations of assessment of risk versus benefit of such vaccines should be in terms of specific and local ecological settings rather than designations such as industrialized or developing countries.

REQUISITES FOR VACCINIA RECOMBINANT VACCINE CANDIDATES

We may begin with some requisites necessary for the development of a desired vaccine candidate. Molecular genetic information must be available, including: (a) identification of specific protective antigen(s), (b) availability of gene clones to be incorporated into the vaccinia genome, (c) production of an adequate mass of authentic gene product during dermal recombinant vaccinia replication, and (d) successful immunization, resulting in immune response and wild type challenge protection in animal models and then man. In addition to the successful production of a protective recombinant, a central concern is the documentation of a satisfactory level of safety of the altered vaccinia virus. The as yet incompletely defined performance of vaccinia recombinants poses significant questions to be answered prior to public health acceptance. What are the important undefined areas of concern?

SAFETY

The general use of vaccinia as a recombinant vector brings up the first issue, namely the severe but infrequent adverse reactions known to be associated with wild type vaccinia [1]. An unmodified primary take of wild type virus itself carries greater morbidity than is desirable. Studies are necessary to determine whether the recombinant vaccinia carries the same risk. Thus, the relative or absolute contraindications identified for wild type vaccinia, i.e. patients or their contacts with skin lesions, altered immune state (e.g. severe malnutrition) and pregnancy will need evaluation [2]. The danger of secondary virus transfer from the dermal site in man, especially to individuals where vaccination may be inappropriate or dangerous, must be reckoned with.

Good genotypic and phenotypic laboratory markers are necessary which are reliably predictive of stable attenuation on primary immunization of individuals of different ages. It cannot be assumed that suppressed local replication in an animal model, or even man, predicts reduced risk of invasive disease in an individual with altered immune state or risk of post-vaccinal encephalitis in a susceptible individual. The species specificity of attenuation challenges our ingenuity [3]. The latter suggests specificity of cell receptors, a problem which theoretically can be approached genetically [4]. The molecular and immunological mechanisms of vaccinia encephalitis are not understood. Can introduction of one or more novel surface peptides change the recognition and attachment properties of the recombinant vaccinia and thereby alter tissue trophism or affect the induction of an untoward "hypersensitivity" state?

If further attenuation of the vaccinia vector is attained, it would broaden consideration of its use for more antigens in more population groups. Experience so far indicates that substitutions or deletions in the TK region of the vaccinia genome are accompanied by attenuation [3,5]. However, in final analysis, laboratory markers of attenuation must be correlated with experience in man gained through field trials. Insofar as recombinant vaccinia carries any "intrinsic risk" for severe adverse reactions, this should be known and quantitated. In situations where contemporary vaccines are acceptably safe and effective, the need for persuasively favorable risk/benefit ratios is sharpened. In settings where the benefit heavily outweighs even a significant risk, new recombinant vaccines may be desirable as an early priority.

It has been suggested [6,7] that a further attenuated vaccinia mutant, LC16m8, might be a safer candidate. The mutant was derived from the Lister strain and has been shown to have reduced capacity to grow in the CNS of the monkey and rabbit. Although the strain was used for smallpox prophylaxis in Japan for several years, there is inadequate documented experience in man to justify discarding the vast knowledge obtained with the N.Y.C. Board of Health (Wyeth) strain. Similarly, there is inadequate experience with the Rivers derived CV-1-78 strain [8].

MULTIPLE ANTIGENS

This brings us to the second issue which will affect immunization strategy. It is possible to engineer vaccinia recombinants which contain multiple antigens [9]. This should allow economy of administration, perhaps of a constellation of antigens selected for a given population, e.g. one or more childhood diseases plus HBV, or plus malaria [10]; or for other populations, HBV plus HSV [11]. An alternative to polyvalent antigens is the development of monospecific recombinants administered dermally as mixtures, or in multiple sites. The effect of simultaneous administration of recombinant antigens with classical non-replicating or live immunizations must be examined. Careful planning is required to account for anti-vaccinial immunity in a total lifelong immunization program for any population. Hopefully the system designed will permit a level of flexibility which will allow for individual variances in scheduling, changes in public health priorities, or technical advances in vaccine development.

EFFICACY

Third is the issue of efficacy. The initial animal serological and challenge studies are promising [12-15,5]. In addition, conceptually, the immunizing antigen, at least as studied in influenza, is presented in a manner resembling live replicating virus which should be immunologically advantageous [14]. However, the dermal site of replication may have drawbacks in the failure to produce an immune response in the respiratory secretory compartment [16]. Studies in animals and in man are necessary to determine protective efficacy against wild type challenge in human volunteers or under field conditions when compared to available vaccines. Initial studies indicate that the recombinant retains the thermal stability characterizing the wild type parent. In addition, as a practical matter of great significance, it would be useful to retain standards permitting production of recombinant in calf lymph rather than the technically more difficult and costly culture methods.

REVACCINATION

The fourth issue, and one affecting efficacy, can be defined broadly as the dependency of antigenic mass of the targeted immunogen upon replication of the unrelated vaccinia virus with its own set of immunologic controls. In the usual situation with which we have experience, one administers inert antigen or a replicating agent where the immune response is modulated by controls which are homologous. Thus, individuals who are immunologically naive or with minimal immune dampening are most frequently successfully immunoconverted or boosted. In the vaccinia vector system, the effectiveness of the desired priming or booster doses in developing an effective antigenic mass involves the anti-vaccinial immune status and its modulation of replication of the attenuated recombinant. Universal or selective smallpox immunization was discontinued in the 1970's as the disease smallpox was eliminated. This provides a favorable time "window" of waning immunity in adults as well as a population of children who are vaccinia-naive. Also, infants who may be endowed with variable transplacental immunity will be a target population for several antigens, such as HBV. This complex epidemiological setting will be the backdrop for assessing options for use of recombinant vaccines. To overcome immune-modulated recombinant vaccinia replication, the gene expression may be maximized using optimal promoters [17].

COMMENTS REGARDING SPECIFIC VACCINES

Common Childhood Diseases

Currently available vaccines against common childhood diseases have a very good public health record with the possible exceptions of pertussis with less than optimal safety and efficacy, and OPV with a low frequency of invasive disease and a questioned efficacy in highly endemic areas. Measles vaccine is effectively blocked by maternal transplacental antibody, and BCG is a less than optimal vaccine. It is notable that none of the agents causing the common childhood illnesses has as yet been derived as a vaccinia recombinant. Measles is theoretically approachable, rubella as well, although the molecular genetics are inadequately defined. With poliovirus, further information about stability of protective peptides remains under study [18]. Bacterial vaccines may be feasible where toxins are single gene products (e.g. diphtheria, tetanus). Pertussis, which would be of special interest, requires clarification of protective antigens(s). Expression of bacterial polysaccharide or lipopolysaccharides, probably requiring multigenic control, will be difficult. Instances where immunizing antigens have required multiple, relatively closely spaced doses to attain adequate immune response, will pose special problems when they are presented as vaccinia components.

Influenza A Hemagglutin Vaccinia Recombinant

The influenza A hemagglutinin recombinant looks encouraging in animal models, producing circulating antibody, cytotoxic lymphocyte (CTL) responses, and reducing virus titers in the lung [12,14]. Incorporation of more than one hemagglutin could broaden the coverage. There is a suggestion that inclusion of the NP gene may induce subtype-cross-reacting CTL responses [19]. Evaluation of influenza vaccinia recombinant must consider not only currently available inactivated and subunit vaccines but also live attenuated gene reassortant vaccines currently under test.

Intradermal influenza HA recombinant failed to induce secretory antibody or dampen nasal influenza replication but interestingly, intranasal immunization did produce local antibody and protection in addition to serum antibody and lung protection [16]. The information derived from influenza-vaccinia recombinant studies can be extended to other agents. When secretory and alimentary antibody are important in protection, such as with respiratory or enteric viruses, such dermally administered recombinant vaccines may be handicapped. Systemic virus infections with a mandatory viremia predictably will be more amenable to dampening by stimulation of persistent circulating antibody and possibly CTL [5].

HBV Vaccinia Recombinant Vaccine

The HBV recombinant is a logical candidate for early use [15]. It would seem to provide an economical and feasible approach to a compelling medical problem in a large segment of the world's population. At present, the cost of plasma derived HBV vaccine effectively makes it unavailable in most areas with high endemicity. A low cost, easily administered vaccine would allow consideration of immunizing whole populations in order to halt the high rate of spread in infancy and early life. Initial trials would logically be done in endemic areas with a high rate of antigenemia and hepatitis and its chronic consequences. The design should encompass efforts to intervene in vertical as well as horizontal transmission. The persistence of antibody, protection after primary immunization, and need for repeated stimulation remains to be demonstrated. The desirability of obtaining protection with a single administration of HBV recombinant vaccine should be stressed [5]. High risk populations in areas of low endemicity provide different types of opportunities for study in varied epidemiological settings and age groups. Comparisons with plasma and yeast [20] derived vaccines would be instructive.

Rabies Vaccinia Recombinant Vaccine

In man, the target group for rabies vaccine is narrow, namely postanimal bite exposure in endemic areas and pre-exposure prophylaxis in selected individuals at high risk. The cost and significant adverse reactions associated with the current rabies vaccines suggests that a rabies recombinant vaccine is a logical candidate for veterinary and possibly human use. Many questions remain, including the potential danger of transfer of rabies recombinant virus from vaccinated animals to man and the delicate prospect of relying upon rabies recombinant virus for post-bite exposure prophylaxis. On the other hand, one could visualize the prospect of using a tailored rabies surface glycoprotein recombinant to delete the CNS reactions which have been present to some extent in all rabies vaccines [4].

Other Vaccinia Recombinants

Theoretically other viruses such as the Flaviviruses, yellow fever and Japanese B encephalitis are potential candidates for recombinant vaccine. Cholera and enterotoxigenic E. coli toxins would be interesting candidates, although secretory antibody may be limiting. Choice of vectors other than vaccinia may be appropriate, such as a benign recombinant Salmonella or E. coli administered orally.

FIELD TRIALS

Many questions must ultimately be answered in human field trials. The trials must be designed to address issues specific to the epidemiology and pathogenesis of the agent in targeted population groups. The following principles may act as guides to field trial design:

1) A population should be selected which is at significant risk for the disease to be prevented. The vaccine should have a substantial prospect for benefiting the recipients.

2) The incidence and severity of anticipated adverse reactions should provide a wide margin of safety compared to the expected risk of disease to be prevented and its complications.

3) The population should normally have no access to current vaccine or there should be substantive evidence that the vaccinia recombinant is as good as, or better than current vaccines in its expected ratio of efficacy/safety. Trials in settings with a relatively successful control program for a given disease may have to await such assurance.

4) Inclusion of double-blind, randomized controls is the desired design. Controls may be unvaccinated and/or at least in a subset, immunized with current vaccine.

5) The number of individuals to be studied is based upon the usual calculations of expected cases and adverse reactions in control (or current vaccine) and recombinant vaccinia groups. The design must provide for attaining significant numbers of vaccine-related reactions as well as rates for similar events in controls.

6) Efficacy may be estimated by surrogate markers such as quantity, quality and half-life of circulating plus secretory antibody and measures of CMI where useful. Use of multiple antigens and need for revaccination impose special design requirements.

7) Special surveillance for illness and other disease markers is necessary. Longitudinal followup is required to determine persistence of challenge immunity and remote complications of vaccine and disease.

8) Finally, in principle, each field trial should be designed to learn as much as possible within the limits of feasibility, in order to contribute to a universal data pool.

CONCLUSION

The remarkable capacity to design vaccinia vaccines which include relevant foreign antigens or epitopes and which hopefully can be recognized as live virus and also permit structuring of defined levels of vaccinia attenuation or trophism will continue to unfold. The next set of hurdles involves understanding the immune perturbation of the host and the specific effects of intervention on human pathogenesis and ecology of the agent. The biological and sociological strictures which apply to other immune intervention systems will continue to operate with recombinant vaccines as a class and must be understood in order to develop definitive guidelines for dose, target groups, and integration into a total schedule of immunoprophylaxis.

REFERENCES

1. J.M. Lane and J.D. Millar, Amer. J. Epid. 93, 238-240 (1971).
2. Recommendation of the Public Health Service Advisory Committee on Immunization Practices. MMWR 27, 156-158 and 163-164 (1978).
3. M. Buller. Workshop on Vaccinia Viruses as Vectors for Vaccine Antigens, Nov. 13-14, 1984.
4. B. Dietzschold, W.H. Wunner, T.J. Wiktor, A.D. Lopes, M. Lafon, C.L. Smith and H. Koprowski, PNAS 80, 70-74 (1983).
5. B. Moss, G.L. Smith, J.L. Gerin and R.H. Purcell, Nature 311, 67-69 (1984).
6. M. Morita, Y. Aoyama, M. Arits, H. Amano, H. Yoshizawa, S. Hashizume, T. Komatsu and I. Tagayo, Arch. Virol. 53, 197-208 (1977).
7. S. Hashizume, H. Yoshizawa, M. Morita and K. Suzuki. "Properties of Attenuated Mutant of Vaccinia Virus, LC16m8, Derived from Lister Strain." Unpublished data (1984).
8. K. McIntosh, Workshop on Vaccinia Viruses as Vectors for Vaccine Antigens, Nov. 13-14, 1984.
9. G.L. Smith and B. Moss, Gene 25, 21-28 (1983).
10. G.L. Smith, G.N. Godson, V. Nussenzweig, R.S. Nussenzweig, J. Barnwell and B. Moss, Science 224, 397-399 (1984).
11. E. Paoletti, B.R. Lipinskas, C. Samsonoff, S. Mercer and D. Panicali, PNAS 81, 193-197 (1984).
12. G.L. Smith, B.R. Murphy and B. Moss, PNAS 23, 7155-7159 (1983).
13. D. Panicali, S.W. Davis, R.L. Weinberg and E. Paoletti, PNAS 80, 5364-5368 (1983).
14. J.R. Bennink, J.W. Yewdell, G.L. Smith, C. Moller and B. Moss, Nature 311, 578-579 (1984).
15. G.L. Smith, M. Mackett and B. Moss, Nature 302, 490-495 (1983).
16. P.A. Small, Jr., G.L. Smith and B. Moss, Workshop on Vaccinia Viruses as Vectors for Vaccine Antigens, Nov. 13-14, 1984.
17. M. Mackett, G.L. Smith and B. Moss, J. Virol. 49, 857-864 (1984).
18. B.E. Enger-Valk, J. Jore, P.H. Pouwels, P. van der Marel and T.L. van Wezel in: Modern Approaches to Vaccines, R.M. Chanock and R.A. Lerner, eds. (New York, Cold Spring Harbor Laboratory 1984).
19. J.W. Yewdell, J.R. Bennink, G.L. Smith and B. Moss, "Influenza A Virus Nucleoprotein is a Major Target Antigen for Cross-Reactive Anti-Influenza A Virus Cytotoxic T Lymphocytes." Unpublished data (1984).
20. W.J. McAleer, E.B. Buynak, R.Z. Maigetter, D.E. Wampler, W.J. Miller and M.R. Hilleman, Nature 307, 178-180 (1984).

DISCUSSION

Dr. Koprowski: Considering the high susceptibility of different species of animals to vaccinia, perhaps one should consider performing initial vaccine trials in susceptible animals. They could then be investigated for intraspecies and interspecies transmission. Animals in close contact with man would be of particular interest.

Dr. Karzon: There is a great opportunity to learn from veterinary vaccines if they are studied appropriately. Animals are valuable not only as laboratory models, but also for field studies. There is one thing that bothers me about your proposal, though. That is, unless these animals are sequestered, we will be exposing humans to an agent before we have tested it in humans in any other way. I don't like this backdoor method of learning what happens when the agent might be put into a human.

CONSIDERATIONS OF SAFETY, EFFICACY, AND POTENTIAL APPLICATION OF VACCINIA VECTORED VACCINES FOR IMMUNOPROPHYLAXIS AGAINST ANIMAL DISEASES

FREDERICK A. MURPHY*

*Division of Viral Diseases, Centers for Disease Control, Atlanta, Georgia 30333

From the first days of the genetic engineering revolution it was felt that bioengineered vaccines for animal diseases would be a seminal success --veterinary vaccines were seen as the proving ground for human vaccines because licensing is simpler and markets are much larger. But, in the past year there has been a partial collapse of this premise and more and more biotechnology companies are shying away from the veterinary vaccine market. The disillusionment which led to this situation should be examined in regard to the new potential for vaccinia vectored vaccines in the animal vaccine marketplace. Perhaps a new optimism is called for, perhaps a new catalog of veterinary vaccines will emerge from the concept of viruses as vectors for heterologous genes coding for protective antigens.

Certainly there are many livestock diseases for which much better vaccines are needed. It is not appropriate to include here a prioritized list of the important diseases of each species of livestock in the U.S. --such lists are produced by the USDA and other agencies for general and specific purposes. These lists are impressive because infectious diseases are the most important health-related constraint to profitable livestock production. The quality of presently available, conventionally derived, livestock vaccines is arguable--certainly there is much room for improvemet in efficacy, if judgements are made from the perspective of the overall quality of human virus disease vaccines. In several livestock industries, the use of vaccines is considered crucial--in the poultry industry this is certain, in the swine industry likewise, but in other industries, such as the beef industry, vaccines are used with skepticism and with constant question of cost/benefit. In livestock agriculture, there is no equivalent of the kind of ethical risk/benefit consideration which must dominate thinking in human vaccine development. Cost/benefit considerations dominate in the business decisions of the livestock industries and cost containment is practiced to an extreme. All production costs, including health costs (prevention and treatment), are built into economic equations. Endemic disease losses are regularly figured into the cost of production. For example, in the beef feedlot industry there is about a 2% loss to disease which is passed on to us in the cost of the meat we buy. Introduction of a new health product, like a vaccinia vectored vaccine for an endemic disease, must in this context be perceived as being valuable enough to influence the cost/benefit equation--it must do this in competition with the use of nothing--the minimum cost production systems in which very little use of biologics is made.

The initial enthusiasm which faced the new biotechnology companies when they looked at the livestock vaccine market was the extraordinarily large numbers of doses of vaccines produced in this country annually. The USDA publishes an annual list: in 1982, the total number of doses of all vaccine formulations produced was over 21 billion doses--for example, there were 52 million doses of IBR (infectious bovine rhinotracheitis) vaccine produced in various combinations with other immunogens and there were 2.8 billion doses of Marek's disease vaccine produced for the poultry industry. The initial enthusiasm wanes in the realization that these very large numbers of doses of vaccine only support a biologics industry with sales of about $300 million/year. The question facing

Published 1985 by Elsevier Science Publishing Co., Inc.
VACCINIA VIRUSES AS VECTORS FOR VACCINE ANTIGENS, Quinnan, Editor

biotechnology companies has been how to make a profit by expanding this market, not just be redividing it. Perhaps the very low cost of vaccinia vectored vaccines will require a reevaluation of this bleak market reality. The perception by the livestock producer of a better product will be influential in building larger vaccine markets.

There are two exceptions to the above view of the potential market for livestock vaccines produced by vaccinia vectoring, both of which involve public responsibilities for animal disease prevention and control:

a) exotic diseases--those foreign diseases which upon introduction would cause epidemics and great impact on the supply and cost of food and fiber. Vaccines for foot-and-mouth disease, rinderpest, African swine fever, exotic Newcastle disease, African horsesickness, Rift Valley fever, and other similar diseases must be developed and stockpiled in anticipation of introduction into the U.S.

b) wildlife diseases-- those diseases which upon introduction into new wildlife habitats would cause irreparable damage or zoonotic foci for human disease. The single practical example at this time is rabies; the concept of wildlife immunization for the control and eradication of wildlife rabies is well-developed and vaccinia vectored vaccine adds an exciting new element in terms of safety and low cost to the concept.

Of course, one overriding issue in considering vaccinia vectored vaccines in livestock and companion animals is the great diversity which must be considered--diversity in species, breed (and inbreeding), age at time of immunization, immunological maturity at birth, placental transfer of immunity, colostral transfer of immunity, etc.

a) We would have to know more about the particular strain of vaccinia in each species to be vaccinated than we do today.

b) We would want to consider the use of other poxviruses, avian pox viruses, parapox viruses, etc., in each virus + host combination. There will be advantages and disadvantages in each pair, but these are yet to be determined; for example, a vector which in a given host exhibits long-term expression might be excellent for allowing continuous expression of viral and non-viral antigens. Could such vectors be used to express growth hormone or reproductive hormones?

c) We would want to consider the possibility of achieving the practical termination of infections which are already established. The important herpesvirus diseases of animals might require such a tactic because of logistical problems of vaccine delivery to young animals before infection.

d) We would want to offer protection on day of birth--there are many important diseases of the newborn of livestock species for which we must be prepared to deliver vaccine at birth. We must also consider vaccinia vector vaccination of pregnant dams so as to provide passive immunity to the newborn.

The five attributes of vaccinia described by Dr. D.A. Henderson which would make human vaccinia vectored vaccines most useful in developing countries would also make them useful in the animal agriculture of developing countries. Vaccinia vector vaccines for use in developing countries would have the following advantages:

a) Ease of administration. This is crucial--it is very expensive to round up animals for multiple course vaccine regimens. In subsistence agriculture this is nearly impossible.

b) Ease of manufacture. This is crucial--the infrastructure for animal vaccine production in developing countries is far more primitive than that for human vaccine production.

c) Vaccine stability. This would be as important as it is in human vaccine programs.

d) Duration of immunity. This is a relative matter--long or lifetime immunity is not important because livestock do not usually live very long, but a practical duration of immunity is very important. For example, some foot-and-mouth disease vaccine protocols call for 3 vaccinations per year; the cost savings from even an annual cycle would be very large.

e) Acceptability by local people--for veterinary vaccines, livestock farmers everywhere in the world would wish that vaccines did what they are supposed to do--acceptability is measured by the saying, "the proof is in the pudding."

Some international agencies have stated that conventional vaccine production infrastructure can be leapfrogged and biotechnology-based vaccine production started from scratch in developing countries. Not everyone agrees. One major problem is that there is no agency to set standards in this environment--no international agency like WHO, no national agency like FDA, which would determine safety on an ongoing basis. Who would constantly monitor vaccine efficacy (for exammple to exclude the practice of using as seed stock serially passaged virus)? Who would provide QA? There are many international agencies trying to build vaccine factories in developing countries by bilateral agreement but there is no central oversight agency. The question is whether FAO will play the necessary role. USDA's and EPA's new role in the same kind of necessary oversight on the domestic level needs to be developed.

In addition to the need for international oversight in the animal disease research and vaccine development sector, there is a need for funding--one key to raising and directing public and private sector funding is to develop priority exercises so as to influence funding agencies.

One such exercise was conducted at a 1982 workshop on "Priorities in Biotechnology Research for International Development," sponsored by the National Academy of Sciences, National Research Council, the Agency for International Development, the World Bank, and the Rockefeller Foundation. A high priority was given to vaccine development relative to all other areas of biotechnological research and development. The following animal diseases were identified as having highest priority internationally:

a) Neonatal diarrheas of all species--including rotavirus diseases.
b) Bovine respiratory disease complex--Pasteurella pneumonia is central to this disease complex.
c) Foot-and-mouth disease of cattle.
d) African swine fever.
e) Hemotropic protozoa--African trypanosomiasis, theileriosis, babesiosis and anaplasmosis.
f) Animal tuberculosis.

g) Rabies.
h) Rift Valley fever of ruminants.
i) Newcastle disease of fowl.
j) Rinderpest of cattle.
k) Bluetongue of sheep.
l) Hog cholera.
m) African horsesickness.
n) Equine encephalitis.
o) Pulmonary adenomatosis and other retrovirus diseases of sheep.
p) Pseudorabies of swine.
q) Vesicular stomatitis of cattle and horses.

In this workshop, a bleak picture was painted in regard to the possibilities for technology transfer to developing countries. DNA-recombinant technology requires very sophisticated expertise and facilities. Vaccinia vectored vaccines, on the other hand, in final form for production, may represent the first truly transferable technology--they certainly must be tried.

DISCUSSION

Dr. Ada: You did not mention the companion animal area and, of course, there are obviously potential public health problems there. Would you care to comment on that? It seems like that could be a very large market, too.

Dr. Murphy: There is a very large market. I am not sure any public support is needed in this regard because, at least in this country, the dog, cat, and equine markets can, and probably should be self-sustaining commercially.

Dr. Millar: In view of the fact that veterinary vaccines offer a tremendous market (a possibly transferable technology that might be developed in this country and then shipped overseas for implementation), somebody needs to worry about the safety of workers making these products. I would make a plea that if this technology will be shipped somewhere else to be implemented we must assume some responsibility, since there are no agencies like the Occupational Safety and Health Administration in most countries.

Dr. Murphy: I think that point is relevant to both the research laboratory and the production facility.

PANEL DISCUSSION OF BASIC AND CLINICAL RESEARCH NEEDS, ETHICAL AND
SAFETY CONCERNS PERTINENT TO RECOMBINANT VACCINIA VIRUS VACCINES.

BASIC RESEARCH NEEDS

FRIEDRICH DEINHARDT, M.D.

Max V. Pettenkofer Institute, Pettenkoferstrasse 9a, D8000, Munich, Germany

I will try to be somewhat provocative by focusing on a few concerns that have not really been addressed. First of all, I think it is clear that those who are engineering vaccinia viruses can integrate virtually whatever gene they want wherever they want to put it. It can be done not only with vaccinia but also with other viruses. One possibility I see is that other vectors, such as herpes simplex virus, or other methods of forming vaccinia virus recombinants may result in better expression of the gene products we are interested in and provide stronger stimuli to the immune system with longer lasting immunity. Additional studies of gene expression in other types of vaccinia virus recombinants and in other types of vectors will be of great interest.

Another concern is how genetically stable these recombinant viruses really are, not only stable in that they will continue, passage after passage, to express the genes, but also in the stability of their other biological characteristics, such as virulence and neurovirulence.

There is the question of where these genes are expressed in the virus, and how is the behavior of the virus changed by the presence of these genes? In particular, if they are on the surface of the virus particle, does this alter their host range and thereby increase their virulence? I would be particularly interested in a situation like vaccinia virus carrying genes of Epstein-Barr virus, if such a virus could suddenly infect and multiply in human B cells. What would then happen? Would we have a B-AIDS? I am not trying to be funny about this. One has to consider the same question about hepatitis B virus surface antigen in vaccinia. Can expression of the surface antigen on the surface of vaccinia virus make it hepatotropic?

Direct experiments pertaining to this question are difficult to do. We did hear that the vaccinia virus which was used to immunize chimpanzees did not cause hepatitis and, obviously, did not multiply in and destroy the livers of those chimpanzees. Of course, there were only a few animals. In general, I think more information on this subject is badly needed.

The last question I wish to raise pertains to vaccine cost. Some current vaccines, such as hepatitis B and others, are much too expensive. You can't use them in developing countries. Vaccinia vaccines appear incredibly inexpensive. But we have heard many reasons why the factors responsible for the low cost of smallpox vaccines may not result in equally low-cost recombinant vaccinia vaccines. Now, if that is the case, other types of expression systems for vaccine production such as transfection of mammalian cells, or the use of yeast and other microorganisms, might be competitive on a cost basis. We should continue to study these methods.

I will end with these few examples. There are really a great many basic research needs that should be addressed.

CLINICAL RESEARCH NEEDS

KENNETH WARREN, M.D.

Rockefeller Foundation, New York, NY 10036

There are many clinical issues that will need to be addressed regarding recombinant vaccinia virus vaccines. First of all, the diseases for which these vaccines can be applied depend on their cost. Many of the vaccines that are being developed are for sexually transmitted diseases, such as genital herpes, hepatitis B and AIDS. For the developing world, if any safe and effective vaccines can be made from recombinant vaccinia viruses against diseases unique to those parts of the world, they will be important, not only because of the cost of the vaccine itself, but also the cost of administration.

To give all of the usual childhood vaccines in the developing world, the vaccines cost about 69 cents. To administer them, to build the infrastructure to administer them, costs between $5 and $10. So the cost of the labor and the gasoline for the automobiles and everything else involved is far more important than the cost of the vaccine itself. Despite the significance of delivery costs, the availability of low-cost production methods is still essential. Because production of vaccines in tissue culture is likely to have many advantages over production in calves, it is important with respect to application of vaccines in developing countries that vaccine produced in tissue culture cost less than it did in calves.

Other clinical issues that are important include the duration of immunity induced and the effect of booster doses. The booster effect was described for veterinary vaccines, indicating that there were no local lesions after revaccination but that there was a good antibody response. Those results were very encouraging.

The route of administration is also an important issue. I would be very hesitant to begin giving vaccinia virus by atypical routes, such as intranasally, orally or intravenously.

We must also give some special attention to the choice of diseases for which vaccines will be developed. First of all, we can sit back as scientists and try to identify what the priority diseases are. But there are additional requirements. There must be researchers interested in the diseases, if they are going to do good work. Another requirement is, is there enough basic information known to approach prevention of the disease? Obviously, you have to know which antigens to look for. Much progress has been made in virology in this respect, and even greater progress has been made in protozoan and helminthic diseases.

You also need information on pathogenesis. For example, if you choose certain antigens in certain infections, immunization may actually make the disease worse.

Finally, there is a need to study what the best vectors might be under given circumstances. In the case of diseases involving mucosal surfaces, like gastrointestinal diseases or pulmonary diseases, vaccinia virus might not be the best vector. In intestinal diseases bacterial vectors might be preferred.

Published 1985 by Elsevier Science Publishing Co., Inc.
VACCINIA VIRUSES AS VECTORS FOR VACCINE ANTIGENS, Quinnan, Editor

ETHICAL CONCERNS

WILLIAM JORDAN, M.D.

National Institute of Allergy and Infectious Diseases, NIH, Bethesda, MD 20205

It is easiest for me to begin by recounting my own travels with this ethical problem. I am not sure if I have had a conversion, but my viewpoint has changed. For some years it was my pleasure to serve as a member of the Advisory Committee on Immunization Practices. They were, of course, concerned with the prevention of smallpox, and were very delighted when the world was declared free. The disease was eradicated and the vaccine no longer had to be used. There was a struggle for several years to persuade the manufacturers not to keep selling it, since it became clear that it was creating more complications than any possible good.

Another group that I participate with is the Armed Forces Epidemiology Board. They are concerned with the continuing use of smallpox vaccine in their personnel. The Board has advised the Department of Defense that smallpox is no longer a military problem, that there are no health indications for the use of this vaccine. The military has seen complications in its dependents as military personnel went home with primary takes. In fact, one could characterize a primary take now as an adverse reaction to vaccinia because it leaves one with a sore, it lasts for a while, and it is dangerous because it may spread to contacts. The nature of primary takes induced by recombinant vaccinia virus vaccines, for that reason, should be given special attention.

In my capacity at the National Institutes of Health I have to write annual reports. The year that the use of vaccinia virus to make recombinant viruses as potential vaccines was described, I characterized it as a "hollow victory," in writing, because of my past experiences. I thought, "they've done it, but they've done it with the wrong virus. Just at the time the world is rid of this disease, who in the world is going to bring it back? Are the pediatricians in the United States willing to see vaccinia re-introduced for whatever reasons?"

Since that time, I have continued to consider this issue. For example, I have heard Frank Fenner, who knows a little bit about this, review the pros and cons of the use of vaccinia recombinants. He has made a very strong case for the advantages outweighing the disadvantages. So that is probably where my conversion began.

The World Health Organization has raised the ethical issues. Here is high technology in the developed world. Are we going to impose this technology on the developing world without using it ourselves? There can be no double standard. We could stop now and not pursue this any further, assuming no one would ever use this type of vaccine. That, to me, doesn't make much sense.

It seems to me that the conventional approach to vaccine development will work. We are a long way from having a human candidate, but we will have one one day. The conventional approach is to do step-wise trials to determine safety, efficacy, and indications for use. There are certain diseases in the developing world or in the tropics that don't occur in the United States. There is no way we could fully assess the efficacy of a malaria vaccine, for example, in the United States. Other diseases like hepatitis, are highly endemic in certain parts of the world. If newborns could be protected over a period of time, a great benefit would be achieved. There is a vaccine against hepatitis B, but it is very expensive, multiple doses are required and, in infancy, immune globulin may be required as well. An inexpensive hepatitis B vaccine that was easily administered and effective in a single dose could be a major advance for people of all countries. However, it should be tested in developing countries to determine if local factors, such as nutrition, relate to efficacy. Those participating in clinical trials may benefit before the vaccine is available otherwise. Even if there was a complication rate of ten per million, the probable benefits of a hepatitis B vaccine shown first to be effective in chimpanzees should far outweigh even that complication rate, justifying clinical trials.

Having viewed vaccinia virus from many perspectives over the years, my current attitude is that it would be unethical not to proceed.

SPECIAL SAFETY CONCERNS

GERALD V. QUINNAN, JR., M.D.

Director, Division of Virology, Center for Drugs and Biologics, FDA, Bethesda, MD 20205

The evidence for safety of smallpox vacine and the possibility of improving this significantly by genetic engineering have been reviewed here by others. Rather than summarize those data once again, I will discuss a few safety topics that are relevant here, and perhaps to all vaccines.

The first is the concern that when you change a virus you don't always make it better. We can't assume that vaccinia is going to behave as vaccinia just because it is mostly vaccinia. The great likelihood is that it is going to remain the same, or be better, but we have to be aware of the possibility that it may develop new properties. Studies should be done on individual recombinant viruses as they are developed, to address this concern.

The second concern regards methods of vaccine manufacture. I would strongly encourage movement towards production of vaccines in tissue culture. I do not mean to categorically reject in vivo methods of manufacture. However, I think the feasibility of producing vaccines in tissue culture, where there is better control over sterility and other aspects of consistency, should be considered seriously before assuming that in vivo production in developing countries is something that is desirable again. Production in tissue culture will probably allow for better control of genetic stability of recombinant viruses and consequent greater assurance of safety.

The third issue involves clinical studies and what it takes to demonstrate adequate safety. There is a paradox in that we are focused on vaccinia because it has been so extensively used. The complication rate is well-known, better known than with most other viruses and, in particular, other viruses that are currently on the horizon as alternate vectors, like herpes simplex, adenoviruses, even retroviruses. There may be a tendency to use as the yardstick for acceptable safety a demonstration that vaccines are as good as smallpox vaccine was. I am not sure that is a realistic yardstick. Clinical trials to demonstrate that level of safety and obtain accurate estimates of serious complication rates would require hundreds of thousands of vaccinees. That is where the paradox lies. Despite the fact that so much is known about the safety of vaccinia virus, the safety of these new recombinants cannot be fully known in advance. The real measure of safety in the case of these new vaccines is likely to be from clinical trials that demonstrate that the adverse effects actually observed are acceptable in terms of the benefits achieved.

The last point I would focus on has also been mentioned before. That is the need to understand the biology of the infections we are trying to prevent and to recognize that immunization may have adverse effects because of the way it affects the course of subsequent infection. The two examples with which most people are familiar are measles and respiratory syncytial viruses. Inactivated measles virus vaccine induced neutralizing antibodies but didn't protect against later disease and actually predisposed to serious atypical disease on exposure to natural measles. To the extent that we don't understand the immunology of any given infection, concerns regarding possible similar problems become progressively greater. As genetic engineering moves rapidly ahead, we must be careful to continue to emphasize research on pathogenesis and immunology of diseases we are trying to prevent.

DISCUSSION

Dr. D.A. Henderson: I would like to make three points and follow up on what Dr. Jordan was saying. I see some real difficulties in standard setting in a paternalistic sense. The developing countries themselves need to have a say in this and the choice of producing it in vivo or in vitro, and having it or not having it.

Secondly, we may be overstating just how severe vaccinia virus infection is. The data with the New York Board of Health strain that Dr. Neff reviewed indicate that the death rate per million primary vaccinations was approximately one. Admittedly, there were other complications, but they were usually not permanently incapacitating. The rate for oral polio vaccine is four paralytic cases of polio per million children vaccinated. Vaccinia virus does cause complications but it is not that far away, perhaps, from the oral polio virus vaccine.

Thirdly, I wonder whether there will be a commercial interest anxious to produce a vaccine using vaccinia virus. I hope we have a sense of urgency to get out and look at the issues with this vaccine to make decisions at some reasonable point in time, perhaps before all possible answers are in.

Dr. Koprowski: I would like to emphasize that one of the most urgent needs in the United States for rabies prevention is vaccination of wildlife and the only possible vaccination is by oral bait. Therefore I think that the question of using the vaccinia recombinant with rabies and the possibility to vaccinate by the oral route represents for us a very real problem. A small trial in the United States would seem justified in a captured population of raccoons. Since we know that oral vaccination has been successful in Germany and in Switzerland by bait with live attenuated rabies virus.

Dr. Deinhardt: I have a question for Dr. Koprowski. Assuming that a recombinant rabies antigen-vaccinia virus vaccine could be used for immunization orally, would you assume that would be more effective than the feeding of the live attenuated rabies virus?

Dr. Koprowski: It may be a question of cost, and that will have to be evaluated. An attenuated virus may have been highly concentrated and recombinant vaccinia virus may be less costly. Please do not misunderstand me. I do not mean that tomorrow we should capture 100 raccoons, vaccinate them and set them loose in the United States. I think, however, that a study in a contained population in the United States seems eminently justified.

Dr. Maynard: I would like to comment on the ethical issue raised by Dr. Jordan. Considerations pertinent to hepatitis B vaccine may be relevant to the general issue of ethics. The unacceptable situation is that of a two-tiered system, a vaccine that would be utilizable only in the developing world because of either cost benefit or risk benefit considerations. In the United States hepatitis B is not hyperendemic, but it is endemic in certain high risk populations. In fact, at the present time the Indian Health Service is trying to mount an effort to vaccinate all Eskimo infants. We are, in addition, trying to screen all pregnant women and vaccinate all babies of mothers who are chronic carriers. There are high risk groups for which mass vaccination is being proposed. Similarly, in the case of many recombinant vaccinia virus vaccines it would be possible to do the initial safety and immunogenicity studies in the country where the vaccine was developed. Would we be able to justify the use of a recombinant vaccinia vaccine in a high risk group in a developing country and not use it for mass vaccination in a high risk group in the United States because of adverse reaction considerations?

I feel, personally, that it is necessary to do at least the initial studies in man in the country of origin. One might then proceed to the large-scale efficacy trials in the developing countries where the vaccines would be most used.

Dr. Jordan: I am in agreement with what you said. Another high risk target group in the United States, both for hepatitis B and for a candidate AIDS vaccine is male homosexuals. In the case of the Alaskan Eskimo there is money already being provided and there already are programs ongoing in Alaska to immunize those children. The low cost of recombinant vaccinia virus vaccines may be a consideration in selecting additional target groups for initial studies.

Dr. Yilma: It should be recognized that these ethical questions also pertain to veterinary vaccines in Third World countries. I was involved in what was probably one of the largest attempts at eradication of disease in east and west Africa, eradication of rindepest disease. You can develop all the vaccines you want for human usage, and use these vaccines to eradicate malarias, hepatitis and the like, but you must also address at the same time what those nomadic populations are going to have for food. For nomadic people in east Africa the main source of food is milk. If you eradicate human diseases and have larger populations that you cannot feed, you have, in a sense, aggravated the situation. So I think that approaches to eradication of human and animal diseases should be developed in parallel. People are dependent on the animals for their livelihood.

Dr. Warren: I would just like to say that I agree with you. Fortunately, I work for an organization that has both a health sciences program and an agricultural sciences program. It played a major role in the green revolution and is also involved in ILRAD, the International Laboratory for Research in Animal Diseases, in Kenya, that is trying to deal with some of these problems. We also have a population sciences division which we consider equally important. It should be understood by everybody that we have to try to deal with all three of these issues. But that doesn't mean that if you have some major breakthroughs in the health areas that you can actually say that we shouldn't use them because we are going to have other problems. That poses quite an ethical issue.

Dr. Schild: Many here have mentioned high priorities for use of potential vaccines in developing countries. I think we should recognize that hitherto the standardization of potency, safety, etc., of vaccines has been based almost completely on biological tests. But for this new generation of vaccines, these are going to be clearly inadequate. We will need to have detailed molecular characterization both of the virus and its product to ensure that it is going to do what it is intended to do. And, of course, these techniques are only available in about two or three control laboratories in the world. So it is not adequate just to give the organism and say, get on with it. We have to transfer detailed technology for the standardization of the product.

Dr. Quinnan: I think that point is a very important one. To date, we have dealt successfully with the seed lot system, for viral vaccines, demonstrating consistency of the product based on a consistent method of manufacture. For most viruses presently in vaccines we don't know the genome structure and we don't know that it never changes from lot to lot. I can envision the possibility that genetic consistency of recombinant vaccinia viruses might be dmonstrated by intensive study during development and initial usage, so that simplified methods for product characterization might eventually be established. Until and unless simplified release criteria can be established, it will be necessary to plan for transfer of technology for vaccine control. Even for use in developed countries, criteria for vaccine release need to be established.

Dr. Dumbell: I have an answer to suggest for the problem of sophisticated laboratory control of vaccines made in the Third World countries. There is a precedent in the smallpox program where the World Health Organization did exactly that for all batches of smallpox vaccine for the last 20 years.

Dr. Boyle: Certainly recombinant vaccinia viruses will be used as veterinary vaccines. However, I see a danger there in risk of spread to man by infected animals and from animal products. Also, there is the possibility that recombinant vaccinia viruses may circulate in animal populations, such as raccoons, and cause major ecological problems or disease problems in domestic animal populations. I think those are two risks which haven't been addressed.

Dr. Neff: There is a concern about vaccinia spreading from person to person, but that risk can be blown out of proportion. There were many, many years when there were literally millions of people who were vaccinated and the incidence of transmission from vaccines to others was relatively low, and only occurred when there was very close body contact. So even though it may happen and is a concern, the incidence is likely to be low and acceptable.

There is a comment on a different issue that I want to make. With regard to revaccination, vaccinia has been shown to confer good protection against itself. On revaccination there is a very limited amount of virus replicating at the site. Although the animal experiments indicate a good booster effect, I think it is still a question whether in humans the primary vaccination will provide enough immunity to limit local replication after a second vaccination. You may not get the kind of booster effect that was seen in animals.

Dr. D.A. Henderson: Part of the concern regarding transmission of vaccinia virus from animals to man may be based on incorrect impressions of transmission of cowpox viruses to man. Dr. Baxby has studied the history of cowpox virus and has searched for human cases in the United Kingdom, finding very few. The only significant outbreaks that have occurred have involved five or ten individuals working in dairy herds milking cows. Another case occurred in a veterinarian who did an autopsy on an elephant that had died of cowpox. There aren't too many people exposed that way. Beyond that there have been very few cases of cowpox in humans, and very few cases of cowpox in animals even though this is a circulating virus.

Dr. Deinhardt: Monkeypox virus can spread to man, but usually there is no second or third generation spread from man to man. There are a few tertiary cases in the literature, but the number is very, very limited. The danger may not be so terrible, but I think we are all aware of how carefully we have to proceed, anyway.

I would like to stress another issue which has been raised several times during this meeting. Obtaining more detailed information on the immune responses which follow vaccination with recombinant vaccinia viruses may simplify decisions regarding which risks are acceptable in clinical trials and considerations of ethics of using the vaccines in various populations. In particular, in those cases where alternative vaccines already exist, this information may be important. For example, in the case of hepatitis B, is the response to antigen in replicating vaccinia virus different than the immune response to a dead antigen? Are there differences in cellular immune responses, or IgA, IgM, IgG responses? Is the persistence of antibodies possibly longer? If differences were found, risks of serious illness at rates of one in a million may become much less important. If the immunology suggests these vaccines are better than the others, then they should be tried. If that is not the case, however, and the motivation is only a question of finances, then we are always open to the attack. If it is not good for your own children, then it is not good enough for the children in Africa only because you or society are not willing to come up with the money. If there was evidence that an antigen presented in a replicating virus might be a much better immunogen, we could move forward in the near future.

Dr. Ada: This is essentially the point I brought up yesterday, that we could do a lot of work very simply, very soon, on the local immune response to these antigens incorporated into the vaccinia virus. It wouldn't take a large effort. We could look at the primary response quite readily. In three or four weeks' time you could look at the secondary response by in vitro stimulation and in vivo. To me, it is one of the things that should be done fairly soon.

Dr. McIntosh: With regard to safety and ethical issues, it is important to remember, I think, that thse vaccines will probably be capable of immunizing against multiple diseases. The risks will probably depend on the vaccinia virus itself and not the number of antigens. So once you have taken those into account, the more antigens you put in, the greater the benefit-risk ratio. You could add multiple antigens with presumably very little, or no, additional risk.

Dr. Noble: I wonder whether the vaccinia strain described by Dr. Kato should be considered by the laboratories working on this issue. Is anyone currently planning to add that to their strains?

Dr. Paoletti: I think it has characteristics which obviously are very nice to look at, and I think it is a strain that we should obtain.

Dr. Widdus: Much of the talk has been about multicomponent vaccines, but I haven't heard a great deal about how many different antigens can be responded to in a protective fashion, if delivered in this way. If someone has a comment, I would be interested.

Another piece of information I would like to transmit regards two reports from the National Academy of Sciences which have been mentioned during the course of the discussions, one from the Institute of Medicine on setting vaccine priorities for diseases within the United States, and that will be available shortly. The study on international diseases will probably be available in February. The other report from the Board of Science and Technology for international development is available.

Dr. Noble: Would anyone like to respond to the question of how many antigens the body can respond to at once?

Dr. Moss: The serum from a rabbit that has been vaccinated with vaccinia virus will immunoprecipitate over 100 proteins.

Dr. Noble: Before we disperse, I would like to make a comment about the use of smallpox vaccine in laboratory workers. I think it is an important issue for those new laboratories beginning work with vaccinia. It is well to remind them of the need for smallpox vaccination.

Dr. Quinnan: I want to express a word of thanks to everyone on behalf of the other Public Health Service agencies, the World Health Organization and the National Institute for Biologic Standards and Control for what I think has been a tremendously successful meeting. The data and discussion presented here should provide the needed basis for additional progress in this exciting area of research.

INDEX

Actinomycin D, 218
Acquired Immunodeficiency Syndrome, 228
Adenovirus, 23
Advisory Committee on Immunization Practices, 77, 243
African horse sickness, 238, 240
African swine fever virus, 238-239
African trypanasomiasis, 245
Agency for International Development, 102, 239
Animal and Plant Health Inspection Service, 187
Antibodies, hemagglutination inhibiting, 74, 77-83, 88, 96
    Neutralizing, 70, 72, 77-83, 88, 96, 98, 104, 107, 154, 203-204
    Passive, 107
Aphasia, postvaccinal, 52
Armed Forces Epidemiology Board, 243
Avian leukosis virus, 113
Avian poxviruses, 238

Babesiosis, 239
Bacillus Calamette Guerin vaccine, 232
Bacteria, anaerobic, 110
Bifurcated needle, 62, 105, 122
Bluetongue of sheep, 240
Board of Science and Technology for International Development, 249
Bovine respiratory disease complex, 239
Brain edema, postvaccinal, 52-54
BS-C-1 cells, 39
Buffalo, vaccinia virus infection in, 9, 38
Burkitt's lymphoma, 179

Calf lymph, 70, 74, 80, 87, 109
Calves, in smallpox vaccine production, 109-110, 117
Camel pox, 3, 9, 12, 15
Camels, vaccinia virus infection in, 37
Carona virus, 201-203
Cat, vaccinia in, 10
Cattle, 117
Cell mediated immunity, 107
Centers for Disease Control, 75, 101-104
Center for Disease Control Smallpox Eradication Program, 101
Cerebrum, 91
Chagas disease, 228
Chicken embryo cells, 39, 70, 72, 89
Chorioallantoic membrane, 16, 37, 39, 64, 70, 80, 87, 89, 110, 113, 117
Choroid plexus, 98-99
Circumsporozoite antigen, 129-131
Cold chain, 63, 117, 228
Coliforms, 110
Complement, 107
Connaught Laboratories, Ltd., 109, 119
Convulsions, postvaccinal, 52
Cortisone, 93-96
Cotton top tamarin, 188
Cowpox, 307, 9-13, 15-22, 37-38, 69, 109, 248
CV-1 cells, 203
Cyclohexamide, 218

Cynomologous monkeys, 74, 90
Cytosine arabinoside, 50
Cytotoxic T cells, 106-107, 169-174

Dane particles, 216
Delayed type hypersensitivity, 103-107
Demyelinization, postvaccinal, 52-54, 99
Dengue virus, 227
Diarrheal disease, 229
Dog, vaccinia in, 208
Duvenhage virus, 165

Ectromelia virus, 3, 9, 12-13, 15, 22, 38-39, 43, 106-107
Eczema, 72
Electron microscopy, 4
Encephalitis, postvaccinal, 12, 37, 52-57, 65, 69-74, 85, 87, 98, 231
Encephalopathy, postvaccinal, 12, 52-57, 87, 98
Enveloped vaccinia virus, 106
Environmental Protection Agency, 124, 239
Epidermal hyperplasia, 5
Epstein-Barr virus, 179-186
    membrane antigen, 179-186
    nuclear antigen, 216
    transformed cell lines, 180-183
Equine encephalitis, 240
Erythema multiforme, postvaccinal, 55

Feline leukemia virus, 228
Flaviviruses, 233
Food and Drug Administration, 110, 239
Foot and mouth disease, 107, 198, 227, 238-239
Fowlpox virus, 207
Franklin, Benjamin, 58

Glial proliferation, 92
Green Revolution, 247
Growth hormone, 238

Hela cells, 38
Hemiplegia, postvaccinal, 52
Hemolytic protozoa, 239
Hepatitis, 106
Hepatitis A virus 227
Hepatitis B virus, 49, 58, 129-135, 146-149
    surface antigen, 33, 131-136, 137-149, 154, 195, 216, 227-228
Hepatocellular carcinoma, 131
Herpes simplex virus, 33, 41, 137, 140, 146, 153-162, 211-219, 241
    Class I and II constructs, 214
    genes, 216
    latency, 211
    neutralizing antibodies, 143
Herpesviruses, 22, 107, 238
Hog cholera, 240
Horsepox, 3-4, 69
Human amnion cells, 70
Human embryonic lung cells, 70-72

Immune complexes, 107
Immunity, colostral transfer, 201-207, 238
    persistence, 61, 107-108

placental transfer, 238
Immunodeficient children, vaccinia in, 107
Immune response genes, 169
Indian Health Service, 246
Infectious bovine rhinotracheitis virus, 237
Infectious mononucleosis, 175
Influenza virus, 33, 146-149, 169-177, 227
International Laboratory for Research in Animal Diseases (Kenya), 247

Japanese B encephalitis virus, 233
Jenner, Edward, 78, 137
Jet injector, 61, 102-104

Lagos bat virus, 165
Leptomeningitis, 91
Lister Institute, 63
Livestock, 237
London School of Hygiene and Tropical Medicine, 104

Major histocompatability complex, 169
Makola virus, 165
Malaria, 34, 49, 58, 129-131, 137, 228
Mammilitis, 6
Marek's disease, 237
Marmoset herpesvirus, 41
Mass vaccination, 102
Measles, 4, 52, 60, 106
Merozoite antigens, 131-136
Methotrexate, 213, 216
Metisazone, 50, 53
Ministry of Health (United Kingdom), 56
Mongoose, vaccinia in, 208
Monkeypox, 3, 9, 12-13, 15, 22, 37-38, 248
Moscow Institute of Virus Preparation, 69
Mousepox, 38
Mucous membranes, 211

Nasopharyngeal carcinoma, 179, 183
National Academuy of Sciences, 239, 249
National Institute of Allergy and Infectious Diseases, 77, 229
National Institute of Public Health (Utrech), 118-119
National Institutes of Health, 243
National Research Council, 239
Neonatal diarrhea, 239
Neurovirulence, 85, 87-99
Newcastle Disease virus, 238, 240
Nuecleoside kinase, 212

Onchocerciasis, 228
Orthopox viruses, 3-6, 9-13
Ovalbumin, 219

Parapox viruses, 238
Pasturella, 239
Phenol, 110
Phosphonoacetate, 218
Pig kidney cells, 37
Pigs, vaccinia virus infection in, 37
Pk-15 cells, 38
Plasmodium falciparum, 129-131

knowlesi, 129-131
Pock-forming units, 71, 78
Poliovirus, 4
Primary rabbit cells, 72
Pseudorabies virus, 240
Pulmonary adenomatosis, 240

Rabbit cornea cells, 37
Rabbit kidney cells, 87-88, 113, 153
Rabbitpox virus, 4, 15, 22, 27, 37, 38, 41
Rabbit scarification test, 124
Rabbit testes, 70, 124
Rabies virus, 34, 137, 163-167, 227, 235, 240
Raccoonpox, 3, 9
RCT marker test, 88, 90
Red Book Committee, 77
Reproductive hormones, 238
Retroviruses of sheep, 240
Rhabdoviruses, 188
Rifampicin, 50
Rift Valley Fever virus, 238, 240
Rinderpest virus, 238-239, 247
Rockefeller Foundation, 239
Rotaviruses, 227, 239
Rubella virus, 107
Rubeola virus, 107

Saint Louis Record Center, 75
Salmonella, 207
Seed lot system, 124
Shakespeare, William, 101
Sheep, 117
Smallpox Global Eradication Program, 49, 61, 69, 103, 117-123
Smallpox vaccine complications,
    accidental infection, 50-60
    eczema vaccinatum, 50-60, 65, 72-73
    fatal infection, 52
    generalized vaccinia, 50-60
    lymphadenopathy, 107
    major reactions, 64, 70, 83, 97, 104
    parainfectious encephalopathy, 60
    vaccinia necrosum, 74
    viremia, 93
Smallpox vaccine,
    in pregnancy, 52
    primary takes, 64-66, 79-83
    pulp, 109-110
    quality control, 120
    stability, 118
Smallpox Vaccine Research Committee (Japan), 96
Spongy degeneration, 92
Staphylococcus, coagulase positive, 110
Streptococcus, hemolytic, 110
Surveillance containment operations 105

T cell immunity, 75
Tatera pox, 3, 9
Tissue culture, 70, 109, 113-115, 117-122
Thielerosis, 239
Thymidine kinase, 27-35, 41, 180-181, 188, 212

Thymidyllate synthetase, 213
Transmissible gastroenteritis virus, 201-208
Tuberculosis, 109

Uasin Gishu, 7, 9
UNICEF, 61, 126
United States Army, 102
United States Army Research and Development Laboratory, Fort Totten, NY, 102
United States Department of Agriculture, 187, 237, 239

Vaccinia immune globulin, 50, 52-53, 58, 70-71, 99
Vaccinia virus,
    comet formation, 39, 44
    early cell surface antigen, 85
    host range, 5, 39
    inverted terminal repeats, 22-24
    outbreaks in farm workers, 6
    strains:
        Ankara strain, 98
        Bern strain, 56, 69
        CV-I strain, 43, 70-72, 77-83, 87-99, 232
        CV-II strain, 70-71, 81, 98
        Copenhagen strain, 37, 39, 69, 71
        Copenhagen-hr strain, 38
        DIs strain, 43, 89, 98
        Em-63 strain, 69-74
        Ecuador strain, 69
        Elstree strain, 69-75, 77, 113
        G9 strain, 49
        LC16m8 strain, 49, 85, 87-99, 232
        Lister strain, 37, 43, 55-58, 74, 77-83, 85, 87-99, 232
        MVA strain, 72, 98
        Massachusetts strain, 69-70
        New York Board of Health strain, 41, 55-58, 69-75, 77-83, 198, 232, 246
        TK$^-$16 strain, 181
        Temple of Heaven strain, 121
        WI-38 strain, 72
        WR strain, 22, 39, 41, 181, 198
        WR-6/2 strain, 38
        Yugoslavian strain, 72
    ts mutants, 39
    ulcerated pock variants, 37
    white pock variants, 12, 22-24, 37
Varicella virus, 50
Variola virus, 3, 9, 12-13, 15, 22, 64, 69, 106-108
Vero cells, 88
Vesicular stomatitis virus, 107, 187-199, 240
    glycoprotein G, 187-197
    neutralizing antibodies, 195
    serotypes, 33, 187-197
Veterinary vaccines, 237-240

Water buffalo, 117
West and Central African Smallpox Eradication and Measles Control Program, 101-105
Whooping cough, 228
Wildlife,
    diseases, 238

immunization, 237
World Bank, 239
World Health Assembly, 104, 124
World Health Organization, 49, 62, 65, 69, 110, 113, 117-124, 137, 243-248
    Collaborating Center for Orthopox Virus Research, 119
    Collaborating Center for Smallpox Vaccine, 120
    International Commission for the Certification of Smallpox
        Eradication in South America and Somalia, 101
    Smallpox Eradication Unit, 101
    Special Account for Smallpox Eradication, 122
World War II, 74, 102
Wyeth Laboratories, 61

Yellow fever virus, 233